Topics in Environmental Epidemiology

Topics in

Environmental

Epidemiology

Edited by

KYLE STEENLAND, Ph.D.
National Institute of Occupational Safety and Health

DAVID A. SAVITZ, Ph.D.
Department of Epidemiology
University of North Carolina, Chapel Hill

New York   Oxford
OXFORD UNIVERSITY PRESS
1997

Oxford University Press

Oxford   New York
Athens   Auckland   Bangkok   Bogota   Bombay   Buenos Aires
Calcutta   Cape Town   Dar es Salaam   Delhi   Florence   Hong Kong
Istanbul   Karachi   Kuala Lumpur   Madras   Madrid   Melbourne
Mexico City   Nairobi   Paris   Singapore   Taipei   Tokyo   Toronto

and associated companies in
Berlin   Ibadan

Copyright © 1997 by Oxford University Press

Published by Oxford University Press, Inc.
198 Madison Avenue, New York, New York 10016

Library of Congress Cataloging-in-Publication Data
Topics in environmental epidemiology / edited by
Kyle Steenland, David Savitz.
p.   cm.   Includes bibliographical references and index.
ISBN 0–19–509564–2
1. Environmentally induced diseases—Epidemiology.
I. Steenland, Kyle, 1946–   . II. Savitz, David A.
[DNLM: 1. Environmental exposure—adverse effects.
2. Epidemiologic Factors.
3.   Epidemiologic Methods.
4. Environmental Pollutants—adverse effects.
WA 670 T674 1997]
RA566.T67   1997
614.4'2—dc20
DNLM/DLC
for Library of Congress   96–29398

9 8 7 6 5 4 3 2 1

Printed in the United States of America
on acid-free paper

Preface

THIS book provides an overview of environmental epidemiology, integrating a review of existing knowledge with a discussion of methodologic issues for the major environmental exposures. An introductory chapter defines the field and supplies a context for what follows. The second chapter focuses on common issues in the design and analysis of environmental studies, including clusters, ecologic biases, and measurement error. The third chapter considers risk assessment and meta-analysis, generic topics for all epidemiology but particularly relevant for environmental epidemiology. Environmental epidemiologic studies are often grouped for meta-analysis and are often subject to risk assessment for regulatory purposes.

Subsequent chapters are arranged by exposure. Our focus is on involuntary exposures of the general public, which are suspected of playing a role in endemic disease, although epidemic outbreaks due to contamination of diet and water are also covered. Chapter 4 considers diet, describing outbreaks of disease since WWII due to consumption of food contaminated with chemicals, in which the specific responsible toxin is often unknown. This chapter also includes a short discussion of diet and cancer. Chapter 5 addresses water contamination, both chemical contaminants resulting from water treatment and by infectious agents present because of inadequate treatment.

Chapters 6–8 deal with air pollution. Chapter 6 covers particulates in the air and their short-term effects on both mortality and morbidity. This issue has become particularly urgent in recent years as there is increasing evidence that the current, relatively low, levels of particulates in the air are linked to cardiovascular and respiratory disease, although it has been difficult to disentangle the role of particulates from that of other air pollutants. Chapter 7 considers nitrogen dioxide, of concern particularly in indoor environments, where it is produced by gas appliances. Chapter 8 discusses the health effects of tropospheric ozone; there is evidence that ozone exacerbates asthma, affects short-term pulmonary function, and may be linked to overall mortality.

Chapters 9–11 are concerned with environmental tobacco smoke (ETS). Chapter 9 focuses on childhood exposure and respiratory disease, presenting the large body of evidence linking the two. Methods of measuring exposure, including biomarkers and environmental measurement, are also discussed in this chapter. Chapter 10 covers ETS and lung cancer; it reviews the accumulated evidence as well as the continuing controversy, including the problem of measuring dose by "cigarette-equivalents" as determined by different biomarkers. Chapter 11 focuses on ETS and heart disease, about which there is an increasing body of epidemiologic and toxicologic evidence that indicates an effect, although the potential for confounding is still unresolved.

Ionizing radiation is a confirmed lung carcinogen at high levels encountered occupationally, but it is not clear whether low-level radon in homes increases lung cancer risk. Chapter 12 reviews the literature to date on this subject. Chapter 13 considers one form of nonionizing radiation, the electric and magnetic fields produced by electric currents in residential settings. The potential cancer risk of these fields remains highly controversial, and here as in many areas exposure assessment is the fundamental challenge.

Chapter 14 covers lead, both its neurologic effects in children and its effect on blood pressure in adults. The former are by now relatively well documented, although issues of confounding by socio-economic status are still relevant. The latter is not as universally recognized, but there is again a body of epidemiologic and toxicologic evidence that suggests a real but small effect.

The last chapter takes a brief, crystal-ball look at the future of environmental epidemiology, with special attention to stratospheric ozone depletion and global warming.

All the chapters based on specific exposures provide summaries of the literature and discuss the issue of exposure assessment that can be so difficult in environmental epidemiology, a field which is concerned with low-level but common exposures. Each chapter also makes explicit the key methodologic issues that must be resolved to move the field forward.

The exposures covered in the book all entail some degree of controversy as to whether they cause disease at low levels when high-level exposures are known to be harmful—or whether they cause disease at all. In virtually all cases the diseases in question are caused by a number of different environmental agents in combination with genetic factors and voluntarily chosen exposures such as smoking. The environmental exposures are important because, although they are low-level, they are ubiquitous. If exposure–disease relationships are in fact confirmed, each exposure discussed here would be responsible for a significant fraction of diseases that affect large numbers of people. Finally, virtually all these exposures are potentially subject to remedial action, i.e., intervention to reduce or eliminate them.

This book should be useful to a wide variety of readers, including public-health practitioners, epidemiologists, and those specifically interested in environmental health. It can be used as a text in introductory or in more advanced courses on environmental epidemiology, along with supplementary readings from the current literature.

Contents

1. Introduction, 3
   Kyle Steenland and David A. Savitz

2. Design and Analysis of Studies in Environmental Epidemiology, 9
   Kyle Steenland and James A. Deddens

3. Meta-analysis and Risk Assessment, 28
   Catherine Wright, Peggy Lopipero, and Allan Smith

4. Diet and Food Contaminants, 64
   Manuel Posada de la Paz

5. Water: Chlorinated Hydrocarbons and Infectious Agents, 89
   David A. Savitz and Christine L. Moe

6. Outdoor Air I: Particulates, 119
   Douglas W. Dockery and C. Arden Pope III

7. Outdoor Air II: Nitrogen Dioxide, 167
   Jordi Sunyer

8. Outdoor Air III: Ozone, 184
   Victor Hugo Borja-Aburto and Dana Loomis

9. Environmental Tobacco Smoke I: Childhood Diseases, 200
   Ruth A. Etzel

10. Environmental Tobacco Smoke II: Lung Cancer, 227
    Anna H. Wu

11. Environmental Tobacco Smoke III: Heart Disease, 256
    Kyle Steenland

12. Radiation I: Radon, 269
    Ross C. Brownson and Michael C.R. Alavanja

13. Radiation II: Electromagnetic Fields, 295
    David A. Savitz

14. Effects of Lead in Children and Adults, 314
    David Bellinger and Joel Schwartz

15. Future Trends in Environmental Epidemiology, 350
    Kyle Steenland and David A. Savitz

    Index, 359

Contributors

Michael Alavanja
Division of Cancer Etiology
National Cancer Institute
Rockville, Maryland 20892

David Bellinger
Neuroepidemiology Department
Children's Hospital
300 Longwood Ave.
Boston, MA 02115

Victor Borja-Aburto
Instituto Nacional de Sulud Publica
Cuernavaca, Morelos, Mexico

Ross C. Brownson
St. Louis University Health Sciences
   Center
School of Public Health
3663 Lindell Blvd.
St. Louis, MO 63108–3342

James A. Deddens
National Institute of Occupational
   Safety and Health R13
4676 Columbia Parkway
Cincinnati, OH 45256–1998

Douglas W. Dockery
Department of Environmental Health
Harvard School of Public Health
665 Huntington Ave.
Boston, MA 02115

Ruth A. Etzel
NCEH F39
Centers for Disease Control and
   Prevention
4770 Buford Highway NE
Atlanta, GA 30341–3724

Dana Loomis
Department of Epidemiology
University of North Carolina
CB# 7400
Chapel Hill, NC 27599–7400

Peggy Lopipero
School of Public Health
Earl Warren Hall
University of California, Berkeley
Berkeley, CA 94720

Christine L. Moe
Department of Epidemiology
University of North Carolina
CB# 7400
Chapel Hill, NC 27599–7400

C. Arden Pope III
Department of Economics
Brigham Young University
142 FOB
Provo, UT 84602

Manuel Posada de la Paz
Ministeria de Sanidad y Consumo
Sinesio Delgado 6
28029 Madrid, Spain

David A. Savitz Ph.D.
Department of Epidemiology
University of North Carolina
CB# 7400
Chapel Hill, NC 27599–7400

Joel Schwartz
Department of Environmental Health
Harvard School of Public Health
665 Huntington Ave.
Boston, MA 02115

Allan Smith
School of Public Health
Earl Warren Hall
University of California, Berkeley
Berkeley, CA 94720

Kyle Steenland, Ph.D.
National Institute of Occupational
    Safety and Health, R13
4676 Columbia Parkway
Cincinnati, OH 45226–1998

Jordi Sunyer
Institut Municipal d'Investigacio
    Medica (IMIM)
Doctor Aiguader 80
E–08003 Barcelona, Spain

Catherine Wright
School of Public Health
Earl Warren Hall
University of California, Berkeley
Berkeley, CA 94720

Anna H. Wu
USC/Norris Comprehensive Cancer
    Center
Department of Preventive Medicine
1441 Eastlake Ave., MS #44
PO Box 33800
Los Angeles, CA 90033–0800

Topics in Environmental Epidemiology

Introduction   1

KYLE STEENLAND

DAVID A. SAVITZ

NVIROMENTAL epidemiology may be defined as the epidemiologic study of the health consequences of exposures that are involuntary and that occur in the general environment. Such exposures may occur in the air, water, diet, or soil. Examples in these generic categories are respirable particulates in the air, chlorinated hydrocarbons in treated water, toxic contaminants in cooking oil, and lead in the soil. The involuntary nature of these exposures separates environmental epidemiology from other realms of epidemiology. For example, passive smoking falls within the scope of environmental epidemiology because it is involuntary and a public exposure, whereas active smoking is not. Community exposure to lead coming from a local plant is an issue of environmental epidemiology, whereas worker exposure to lead in the plant itself is a problem of occupational epidemiology; study design and methods typically would be quite different for these two populations. Much of infectious disease epidemiology is also excluded when transmission of the infectious agent is person-to-person. However, infectious agents encountered in the general environment (e.g., in water supplies) are within the scope of environmental epidemiology.

Environmental epidemiology may be divided into the study of epidemics and endemics. *Epidemics* are characterized by acute outbreaks of disease in a limited population shortly after the introduction of an unusual exposure, which may or may not be known. The disease is often specific to the exposure in question, and may or may not be previously known. The poisonings at Bhopal involved a known exposure with predictable effects. In contrast, the epidemic of deaths from toxic oil syndrome in Madrid involved an unknown agent and a previously unknown disease.

Endemics are characterized by either acute or chronic disease occurring at "usual" frequency in a large general population, caused in part by some common and often unsuspected exposure. Examples include diarrhea caused by microbes commonly found in drinking water, or bladder cancer caused by chlorination by-products in drinking water. A great challenge to epidemiologists is to identify these endemic relationships between exposure and disease. Typically the diseases of interest have multiple causes, some of which are known and some of which are not. Environmental exposures are usually suspected of causing some fraction (often small) of the cases of the disease.

Endemics are a more common issue in the environmental epidemiologic literature than epidemics. Epidemics with unknown causes are relatively rare, especially in industrialized developed countries where environmental epidemiology is most commonly practiced. The most important issues in less developed countries often involve control of known hazards, such as cholera from contaminated water. In more developed countries, known hazards are usually well controlled, and epidemiologists have the luxury of investigating possible environmental contributors to baseline disease occurrence.

This book emphasizes epidemiology as it is used to determine disease etiology, rather than descriptive epidemiology. Thus, it is primarily concerned with the suspected causes of endemic disease, although the chapters on diet and on water do discuss specific epidemics as well, including several for which the causes are still not well understood.

Environmental epidemiology often involves low-level exposures to the general public, which are difficult to measure and difficult to link to disease. Low-level exposure may be difficult to measure for many reasons. In some cases we may lack the technical ability to measure the environment or biological samples with enough sensitivity to detect low levels. Only recently for example, have we been able to measure low levels of dioxin in the serum. The development of this technology has had important consequences, for example permitting us to know that Vietnam veterans did not have elevated levels of dioxin in the blood compared with veterans who served at the same time but did not go to Vietnam. In other instances we may not even know exactly what exposure to measure. In the case of electric and magnetic fields, observations regarding leukemia in association with configurations of electrical wiring led to hypotheses about low-level magnetic fields produced by common electrical frequencies (60 Hertz). But it is not clear, if electric and magnetic fields do cause leukemia or other cancers, exactly what type of fields are implicated (electrical or magnetic, peak or average exposures).

In many studies we seek historical estimates of exposure to predict future disease. Direct historical measures often are impossible to obtain for common low-level exposure to agents that are only now thought to be potentially dangerous. Hence we are often forced to rely on current measurements, the recall of subjects, or attempts at historical reconstruction of exposure. In some cases we are fortunate, and current measurements are likely to reflect past exposures to some degree, such as radon measurements in homes. More frequently, current measurements (e.g., cotinine in urine to measure environmental tobacco smoke) reflect only current exposures, and we must rely either on the study subject's memory to assess past exposure, or on educated guesses about how exposures may have changed over time. Remembering one's personal exposure to agents that are ubiquitous and that occur at low levels may prove especially difficult; for example, remembering the frequency of eating certain foods or drinking tap water. Historical reconstruction of exposure by investigators has become a field of its own ("retrospective exposure assessment") and can range from little more than intuition and common sense to elaborate use of historical data correlated with the exposure of interest, or even actual physical reconstruction of past exposure scenarios.

Measuring relatively small effects of low-level common exposures on common diseases with multifactorial etiologies is sometimes beyond the capacity of epidemiology. We are dependent on identifying natural "experiments" that, unlike controlled experiments, are subject to bias due to confounding by other risk factors, many of which may be unknown. Nevertheless, even when detection of effects is at the margins of epidemiology's capabilities, there can be important potential impacts on public health from the exposures of concern. Small effects in large populations can have large attributable risks if the diseases are common. Consider environmental tobacco smoke and heart disease. Findings to date suggest that there may be a small relative risk associated with exposure, on the order of 1.2–1.3. If this is true, the estimated annual toll attributable to this exposure is large, on the order of 40,000 deaths per year in the United States.

Our goal in this book is both to provide an overview of some of the main topics in environmental epidemiology organized by exposures, and at the same time to elucidate some of the methodological issues in the field. Toward this end, the literature reviews in each chapter devoted to specific exposures are succinct rather than comprehensive. Exposure assessment, typically the Achilles heel of environmental epidemiology, is a theme in each of the exposure-specific chapters.

We begin with two chapters on study design and meta-analysis/risk assessment. Although not specific to environmental epidemiology, these topics are discussed with special reference to their applications in this field. The chapter on study design covers three issues: clusters, ecologic studies, and measurement error. Clusters of disease in the general population are often the motivation for environmental studies; they may announce the beginning of an epidemic or be nothing more than an expression of random variation in disease occurrence. Ecologic studies are typically conducted in environmental epidemiology because there may be little variation of exposure within specific populations of interest, motivating ecologic studies across different populations (e.g., countries) that do have different exposure levels. Little variation in common but low-level exposures within a population also contributes to exposure measurement error, which plagues all of epidemiology but is perhaps even more troublesome in environmental studies. Exposure measurement error (or exposure misclassification) tends to distort relative risk estimates, and the old dictum that nondifferential errors or misclassification lead to bias toward the null is not always true.

The chapter on meta-analysis and risk assessment covers two types of analysis which are typical of environmental epidemiology. Meta-analysis combines studies to calculate a common estimate of exposure effect. It is often used in cases in which there appears to be a small exposure effect though single studies are not definitive, and some studies may be inconsistent. A quantitative estimate across all studies is then desired, as opposed to qualitative summaries typical of literature reviews. Risk assessment is usually understood as the attempt to calculate individual excess lifetime risk of disease or death due to exposure at a given level to a specific agent. Regulatory agencies use risk assessment to set a level of exposure in which individual lifetime risk is below a certain threshold, e.g., one in a million for some environmental carcinogens. Risk assessment may be based on either animal or human epidemiologic data.

Subsequent chapters are organized by exposure. The chapter on diet is concerned largely with past epidemics of known etiology, but it also includes a brief section on diet and cancer. The chapter on water covers both infectious agents in water, which may cause epidemic outbreaks, and chlorination by-products that have been associated with cancer.

A set of three chapters on air covers particulates, nitrogen dioxide (NO_2), and tropospheric ozone. Small particulate matter has increasingly been linked to short-term increases in cardiorespiratory mortality and morbidity, even though current levels are far below those that caused the well-known epidemic of deaths due to the London "fog" in 1955. NO_2 is commonly a concern in indoor air, although outdoor levels have also been studied. Indoor contamination has been linked to respiratory health in some studies. Ozone, typically a product of automobile emissions and sunlight, has been linked both to mortality and to increased asthma in some studies, but the data are inconsistent.

Another set of three chapters reviews environmental tobacco smoke (ETS). The link between ETS and childhood respiratory illness is perhaps the best established of all health effects, but the subject remains controversial and better exposure measurement is leading to better studies. The ETS/lung cancer association among never-smokers is somewhat more controversial. Most studies have found a small but measurable increase in lung cancer risk due to spousal exposure, but there are still questions about the effects of exposure during childhood or in the workplace, and the relevance of particular biomarkers of exposure in estimating risk. The link between ETS and heart disease is perhaps the most controversial. The effects observed to date are small, and heart disease is caused by many factors that are difficult to fully adjust for in most studies.

Two chapters on radiation cover both ionizing radiation at low levels and non-ionizing radiation of low frequencies. Radon is a gas that at high levels, is known to cause lung cancer in miners, but whether radon in homes at much lower levels causes lung cancer remains unclear. In some studies electromagnetic fields in homes have been linked to brain cancer and leukemia, but the strength of association has been small, the studies are inconsistent, and biological mechanisms are unknown, making this subject one of the most controversial in epidemiology.

A single chapter on lead covers both the neurologic effects on children and the effect on blood pressure in adults. Childhood neurologic effects are reasonably well established, but there are questions about effects at lower levels. Effects on adult blood pressure are more uncertain; however, meta-analyses suggest that there are significant effects. A final chapter covers likely future directions in environmental epidemiology.

This text is concerned largely with exposures for which the evidence of health effects is not conclusive but rather suggestive. Some of these exposures may prove to be innocuous; some will certainly be confirmed as toxic. Epidemiology will have a critical role in making this assessment. Two points deserve mention regarding the scope of exposures that have been included here. First, there is a broader definition of environmental epidemiology, which we have not adopted. For example, socioeconomic status can be considered an etiologic agent (probably acting as a surrogate for more specific but unknown risk factors, such as access to health care). Although socioeconomic "exposures" may have a larger public health impact than the narrow range of exposures to environmental agents covered here, a thorough discussion of them draws extensively on sociology, economics, and behavioral research, and is beyond the scope of this text.

Second, there are several exposures of increasing importance for which we have no applicable epidemiologic data yet, so that they are also omitted here. Increased ultraviolet radiation due to depletion of stratospheric ozone is one example, and global warming due to increased man-made production of carbon dioxide (CO_2) is another. These exposures are considered briefly, however, in the concluding chapter.

Environmental epidemiology is an exciting research area, with growing prominence in the scientific community in public consciousness. It is a challenging field because the questions are of such broad importance but the answers so fraught with uncertainty. To meet these challenges, environmental epidemiologic studies have become increasingly sophisticated and sensitive, and increasingly linked to other environmental sciences such as toxicology, molecular biology, and industrial hygiene. Due to these past improvements and anticipated future methodological advances, we can expect that in most cases we will eventually be able to determine whether suspected environmental agents are in fact associated with disease—or at least to narrow the bounds of uncertainty.

Design and Analysis of Studies in Environmental Epidemiology

2

KYLE STEENLAND

JAMES A. DEDDENS

BASIC study designs and analytic methods are covered in all textbooks of epidemiology, and we will not trod through this familiar terrain again. Rather this chapter focuses on three areas of study design and analysis that are uniquely important in environmental epidemiology: ecologic studies, cluster analysis, and errors in measuring (or classifying) exposure.

In ecologic studies the unit of observation is a group rather than an individual. Such studies are often done because low-level common exposures may not vary much within a given population, making a study of exposure and disease based on individuals within that population difficult. Ecologic studies will be informative when exposure is homogeneous within groups and heterogeneous across groups (although this ideal is rarely attained in practice). For example, arsenic levels within public water supplies may vary little in the United States, being in general rather low. This may make it difficult to detect a possible effect of arsenic in drinking water on cancer rates within the United States. However, other countries may have much higher natural levels of arsenic in their water, and the association between arsenic and cancer might be studied by determining if there is a positive correlation across countries of arsenic levels and cancer rates. Although such studies can be very informative, they may suffer from "ecologic bias": i.e., their results are not the same as when individuals are studied. Often this occurs because of ecologic confounding, in which a confounding variable at the group level causes a spurious correlation (such as the apparent negative correlation between radon in homes and county lung cancer rates, resulting from high radon levels in the western U.S. where smoking rates are relatively low). This chapter provides an overview of ecologic studies and ecologic bias, and cites some empirical evidence on the likely magnitude of ecologic bias.

Clusters are unusual temporal and spatial aggregations of disease that are often identified by the public and then brought to the attention of pubic health authorities. An environmental agent is frequently suspected of causing the disease, based on the assumption that such exposures have varied over time or space. As a first step one must confirm that a statistically unusual event has occurred—that is, that the cluster really exists. Such clusters can provide a rich source of etiologic information to detect previously new associations between exposure and disease. Unfortunately, epidemiologic investigations of environmental clusters almost never lead to discovering an etiologic agent, for reasons discussed later.

Aside from the cluster investigations prompted by public recognition, this chapter also discusses the systematic search for clusters. While such systematic surveillance will indeed detect clusters, little valuable etiologic information is usually gained from such detection. On the other hand, surveillance systems set up to monitor disease rates in small geographic areas can be useful for rapidly assessing putative clusters that attract public attention and placing those clusters in a broader context.

The final section of this chapter covers errors in exposure measurement or exposure classification. Such errors plague all of epidemiology but affect environmental epidemiology perhaps even more seriously because of the difficulty of measuring low-level common exposures, which often must be done retrospectively in situations where no historical measurements exist. It is commonly assumed that exposure measurement error (or exposure misclassification for categorical variables), which is nondifferential (unrelated to disease status), will bias exposure–disease associations toward the null. This chapter provides an overview of recent evidence that in certain situations this assumption does not always hold, and that estimates may be either unbiased or even biased away from the null. However, it is of some comfort to know that bias away from the null usually arises only in certain very specific situations that are not likely to occur in most analyses in environmental epidemiology. Nonetheless, the ability to predict direction of bias is a poor substitute for avoiding bias through refinements in exposure assessment. A theme common to all the chapters in the book is the need for improvements in this area because imperfect measurement of exposure is usually the key limitation in environmental epidemiologic studies.

Observational epidemiology that seeks to ascertain cause-and-effect relationships (i.e., etiologic epidemiology) is usually based on studies of individuals for whom exposure, potentially confounding variables, and disease outcome are measured. The data analysis then seeks to evaluate the exposure–disease relationship while controlling for other variables (confounders) that might otherwise distort (bias) this relationship. In addition, the investigator seeks to determine if the exposure–disease relationship may vary according to the level of other variables (effect modifiers). Ecologic studies represent one variant of this general model.

Ecologic Studies

Ecologic studies are based on groups as the units of observation, rather than individuals. The disease rate and the average level of exposure are known for each group or unit, and sometimes the average level of potential confounders or effect modifiers. Typically a regression analysis then seeks to determine whether the disease variable (often a disease rate) varies in relation to the exposure, taking into account confounding and/ or effect modification. Often the units of observation are different geographical units or time periods. For example, one might measure the percent of homes using chlorinated surface water in a county as the exposure variable and the outcome variable might be the county rate of bladder cancer. Another example would be the mean radon level in a county and its lung cancer rates. Similarly, one could seek to determine if the rates of childhood leukemia were increasing over time in a given geographical area as the quantity of electric power used (and presumed electromagnetic field [EMF] exposure) increased.

There are a number of different types of ecologic studies; a general description can be found in Morganstern and Duncan (1993). Some ecologic studies are purely descriptive, in which only data on disease are considered (e.g., cancer rates between countries). Here we will focus on ecologic studies in which the investigator seeks to link exposure to disease (etiologic studies).

One variant of ecologic studies worthy of special mention is a *time series study*, in which disease occurrence over time in a specific population (one time series) is correlated with the occurrence of some exposure variable over time in the same population (a second time series). For example, one might correlate the occurrence of daily deaths in London with daily air pollution levels. Time series are characterized by a large number of observations, units of time that are typically short (e.g., days or months), and an assumption that the effect of exposure is acute. Time series are attractive because they are less subject to confounding than many study designs—many variables do not change over time for the same population—but only a limited range of outcomes and exposures can be studied via time series.

Some studies have a seemingly mixed design, with data on exposure being for entire groups but data on disease occurrence and confounders available on an individual level. For example, Pope et al. (1995) studied air pollution and mortality across many cities in a cohort study in which data on individuals were available from the American Cancer Society. A single air pollution level was assigned to all individuals in a given city. This design is perhaps best thought of as an individual-level study in which exposures to individuals are measured with error because they have been assigned (see later discussion of measurement error). Some variables such as altitude are inherently "ecological" and group levels can accurately be assigned to individuals (Susser, 1994). Air pollution and temperature are somewhat like this, but an individual may stay inside and be less affected by these variables than another individual who spends more time outside.

Perhaps the most common motivation for ecologic studies using groups instead of individuals is that data permitting such analyses are often routinely collected for other reasons and are therefore readily available. Another motivation, again common to environmental epidemiology, may be that analysis across geographical regions permits study of many different exposure levels, which might be impossible in a single geographical region (e.g., the percentage of fat in the diet may vary little within a country but greatly between countries).

Ecologic data on disease, exposure, and potential confounders are often collected separately, and may be of varying quality. Exposure data may often be a mean taken from a limited survey that did not cover the entire population of the unit of observation, such as the mean indoor radon level in a survey of a subset of homes in a county. Data on confounders may also not reflect a mean of measurements on all individuals in the group—for example, smoking levels in a county may be assessed by overall cigarette sales. Disease data, however, often do accurately represent data aggregated across all individuals in the group, such as county lung cancer rates.

Ecologic studies are often viewed as subject to more biases than studies based on individuals, and their results generally are held in less regard than comparable results for individuals (Greenland and Robins, 1994). Ecologic studies are often recommended only for hypothesis generation rather than hypothesis testing (although there are some situations in which an ecologic design will be inherently superior to an individual-level design; see below).

One problem in ecologic studies lies in determining the temporal sequence of exposure and disease in ecologic studies. Most ecologic studies are cross-sectional; both exposure and disease are measured at the same point in time. For example, in our example above, the percentage of homes with treated water may be ascertained at the same time as bladder cancer rates in different counties. However, it is likely that the relevant exposure period would be some years before the development of bladder cancer (if indeed there is a true exposure–disease relationship). Hence, it might be preferable to determine treated water use some years before as the exposure variable. The same problem will occur in individual-level studies, but in ecologic studies there is the additional problem of migration: the target exposed population may have left the area by the time disease is measured, or others may have moved in, and various selection biases can result. Often it is simply assumed that the current exposure variable reflects the relevant exposure in the past.

Aside from temporal sequence, however, there are other intrinsic difficulties in ecologic studies. They are often summarized by the term ecologic fallacy, or ecologic bias, which refers to the incorrect assumption that the same results that were obtained in an ecologic study would have been obtained in a study based on individuals (implicit here is the assumption that individual-level studies are the gold standard). The term ecologic fallacy or ecologic bias actually covers several distinct biases, which can affect ecologic studies more than studies of individuals.

Much bias in ecologic studies is due to confounding (Greenland and Robins, 1994). Ecologic confounding refers to confounding at the ecologic or group level by variables that are not of intrinsic interest but which are correlated both with aggregate measures of disease and exposure. Ecologic and individual-level confounding may be independent. There can be individual-level confounding within ecologic groups by variables that are not confounders on an ecologic level, or vice versa. For example, within a county, older people might live in homes with more indoor radon, making age a confounder that needs to be controlled. However, the mean age across counties may be the same, so that age is not an ecologic confounder.

Ecologic studies are often subject to ecologic confounding by unmeasured covariates because they rely on data that are routinely collected for purposes other than epidemiologic studies. For example, smoking data by county may not be available for a study of indoor radon and lung cancer rates. Ecologic studies of this issue have suffered from precisely the lack of such data—indoor radon levels are higher in Western states where smoking is less prevalent, creating an apparent negative dose-response relationship due to confounding by smoking.

Even when data are available on an ecologic confounder, those data may not be adequate to control for the confounder. One example (see Greenland and Robins, 1994) would be the use of percent smokers by county in an ecologic study without knowledge of the level of smoking. If counties with more smokers had smokers who smoked less, then the percent smokers would inadequately control for smoking. Poor control over confounders of course will affect individual-level studies as well, but can lead to even more bias in ecologic studies due to model misspecification.

The issue of model misspecification is a bit more complicated, and involves the general question of when ecologic study results would be expected to be the same as a study based on individuals. One would hope that the quantitative exposure–disease relationship estimated from an ecological study could be assumed to apply for an individual-level study also. However, quantitative results for ecologic studies and individual-level studies can be expected to be the same only when exposure-disease relationships can be well described by a limited group of linear additive models without multiplicative terms.

Suppose we have a model in which the predicted response (Y) is a function of an exposure variable (X) and a confounder (C) (Piantadosi, 1994), and all variables are continuous. Suppose a suitable model is a linear additive one such that

$$Y_{ij} = \beta_o + \beta_1 X_{ij} + \beta_2 C_{ij} + \varepsilon_{ij} \tag{1}$$

where the subscript "i" indexes the individual, "j" indexes the ecologic unit (e.g., county), and ε represents a random error. If we sum over all observations in each ecologic unit and divide by the number of subjects in each group (n_j), we have

$$\overline{Y}_j = \beta_o + \beta_1 \overline{X}_j + \beta_2 \overline{C}_j + \overline{\varepsilon}_j \tag{2}$$

as the model for each group "j". Note that this equation is what would be used in an ecologic analysis using mean values across ecologic units. Assuming that the exposure effect does not vary by group, then β_1, the coefficient of interest, would have the same value in the ecologic analysis as in the individual analysis, which is what is desired (although its variance would be different). However, suppose instead that the appropriate model is log linear, and the individual-level model is

$$\log Y_{ij} = \beta_o + \beta_1 X_{ij} + \beta_2 C_{ij} + \varepsilon_{ij} \tag{3}$$

Now if we sum over the n_j subjects in each group and take means, we no longer have the mean of Y in our equation, but the mean of the log Y_{ij}'s, which is not available for an ecologic analysis. The corresponding log-linear model for an ecologic analysis is

$$\log \overline{Y}_j = \beta^*_o + \beta^*_1 \overline{X}_j + \beta^*_2 \overline{C}_j + \varepsilon_j \tag{4}$$

Here the resulting exposure coefficient β_1^* will differ from the β_1 from the individual-level analysis, so that results of ecologic and individual-level analyses are no longer equivalent.

Similarly, if there is an interaction (multiplicative) term in the linear model such that

$$Y_{ij} = \beta_o + \beta_1 X_{ij} + \beta_2 C_i + \beta_3 X_{ij} C_{ij} + \varepsilon_{ij}, \tag{5}$$

then averaging over the individual values in each jth group yields

$$\overline{Y}_j = \beta_o + \beta_1 \overline{X}_j + \beta_2 \overline{C}_j + \frac{\beta_3}{n_j} \sum_{i=1}^{n_j} X_{ij} C_{ij} \tag{6}$$

in which the multiplicative term contains individual-level variables, which are not available in ecologic studies. The comparable model with interaction in an ecologic study would be

$$\overline{Y}_j = \beta^*_o + \beta^*_1 \overline{X}_j + \beta^*_2 \overline{C}_j + \beta^*_3 \overline{X}_j \overline{C}_j + \overline{\varepsilon}_j \tag{7}$$

in which the multiplicative term contains means. The β_1^* coefficient for exposure in Equation 7 is again not the same as the corresponding coefficient in Equation 6.

Aside from ecologic confounding and model misspecification, there is another problem that may occur in ecologic studies. A oft-cited example of the ecologic fallacy is the study by Durkheim of the rate of suicide in Prussia, which he found to be positively correlated with the percentage of Protestants in the provinces he studied (Durkheim, 1951). One might conclude that Protestants are *more* likely to commit suicide (assuming that the ecologic results apply to individuals). However, it is possible that within the province those committing suicide were Catholics, possibly due to the stress of being a minority group within a mostly Protestant province. If this were true then on an individual level being Protestant meant you were *less* likely to commit suicide. The potential ecologic fallacy here results from group membership acting as an effect modifier of individual risk, e.g., in a study of individuals, the relative risk of committing suicide for Protestants versus Catholics would vary by province, according to the percentage of Protestants in the province. Another example of group membership acting as an effect modifier might be differing genetic susceptibility across populations; for example, the ability to metabolize (detoxify) a carcinogen might differ between populations. Some authors (Greenland and Robins, 1994) have called this particular ecologic bias a "cross-level" bias. In some cases, such as the Durkheim study described above, this effect modification can be eliminated if the exposure variable were homogeneous within ecologic groups; for example, if the provinces studied were all Catholic or all Protestant. Homogeneity of exposure within groups is in general desirable in ecologic studies, as is heterogeneity of exposure between groups, because these conditions make it easier to detect effects of exposure.

Another issue in ecologic studies that can lead to different biases than in individual-level studies is misclassification of exposure. In general, nondifferential exposure misclassification (equal misclassification for diseased and nondiseased) will lead to biases toward the null hypothesis in individual-level studies (see the discussion later in this chapter), but for certain types of ecologic studies the bias will be away from the null. This occurs in ecologic studies in which the exposure variable is the proportion of individuals exposed in the group (Brenner et al., 1992). Nondifferential misclassification of exposure for individuals within groups results in proportions exposed for groups that tend to be more similar to each other than the true proportions. For a given true effect of exposure on disease (groups with higher proportions exposed have more disease), the estimated effect using misclassified data is judged to be greater than it actually is.

Taken together, the above caveats about ecologic studies raise concern, but the practical question concerns the degree to which ecologic studies actually lead to different (often biased) results than individual-level studies. The degree of ecologic bias in empirical data has been estimated by Piantadosi et al. (1988). These authors conducted individual-level and ecologic analyses of the nutrition data from the Second National Health and Nutrition Examination Study (NHANESII) for 13 variable pairs (univariate regression), and found no consistent pattern to results—that is, the estimated regression coefficients for the ecologic regressions are sometimes higher and sometimes lower than the individual-level regressions. Although in no case do the coefficients actually reverse sign, in several cases one estimated coefficient was two to four times bigger than the other, and the confidence bounds for one coefficient excluded the point estimate of the other. Greenland and Robins (1994) and Stidley and Samet (1994) have used simulated data to provide examples of ecologic studies of indoor radon and lung cancer in which some combination of poor or no control over ecologic confounding, measurement error, and model misspecification lead to an observed negative relationship between radon and lung cancer, while an individual level analysis yields a positive relationship. Stidley and Samet (1993) reviewed existing ecologic studies of indoor radon and lung cancer and concluded that the shortcomings of ecologic studies are so severe as to make these studies useless.

The discussion above should make clear that ecologic studies must be interpreted with caution. For refined hypotheses focusing on subtle effects or for quantitative dose-response evaluation, ecological studies may be of little value. On the other hand, there are situations in which they are particularly apt (Susser, 1994). They are likely to have value for broad hypotheses related to strong associations, which are unlikely to be the product of confounding. In addition, some exposure variables are inherently ecologic (Susser, 1994). A ecologic study of melanoma and latitude, for example, fulfills the above conditions. Another scenario where ecologic studies may be particularly useful would be studies of public health interventions in which the intervention is applied to all individuals in a group, such as study of infectious disease rates before and after a vaccination program, or study of dental caries before and after fluoridation.

Clusters

Clusters are aggregations of disease, typically aggregations defined by space or time. Such aggregations imply an unusually high occurrence of disease rates in specific populations. In the general sense, clusters of disease are the basic subject of epidemiology, which studies variation in disease rates across populations with the goal of uncovering the causes of such variation. Beyond this general sense, however, clusters are usually thought of as something more specific. Clusters often refer to a relatively small number of cases of disease occurring in a particular place and time, which appear unusual, come to public attention, and which often require some response from public health authorities. This response is directed toward determining whether the cases really represent an unusually high disease rate in a given population. If so, an investigation into the causes of such high rates may be warranted. Clusters may be distinguished from outbreaks or epidemics, in which such large numbers of cases occur that it is apparent without further investigation that disease rates are excessive and authorities must immediately investigate.

The first problem is determining whether the cluster really represents a high occurrence of disease. Typically, one first must verify the cases. Assuming the cases are real (have been diagnosed properly), one must verify that disease incidence within the cluster area or time period is in fact elevated beyond random variation. Typically one might calculate an incidence rate for the defined geographical area (and/or time period) where the cluster was discovered and then compare this rate to the rate for some referent populations. A cancer cluster in a neighborhood might lead to the calculation of an incidence rate for the census tract where the neighborhood is located, and comparison of this rate (with appropriate adjustment for known demographic variables such as age, race, and sex) with the incidence rate for adjoining census tracts, or perhaps for an entire region such as a county or state. Alternatively, one might compare the disease rate in the cluster area with the rate in the same area 5 years previously. Comparison of the observed "cluster" rate with comparison rates can confirm or refute the apparent cluster, in the sense of determining if it is unusual statistically.

One problem that arises initially is defining the boundaries of the area or time frame for the cluster to be used in calculating rates. If one defines the boundaries around the cluster sufficiently narrowly, a higher observed than expected rate will normally be found. This has been referred to as the Texas sharpshooter's method: the marksman fires at the side of the barn, and subsequently draws a circular target around the bullet hole, so that his shot is always accurate (Grufferman, 1982). Often the definition of boundaries is somewhat arbitrary.

Assuming the cluster has been confirmed, in the sense that a true excess disease rate is evident, there is then the issue of whether the cluster results from a specific common cause or from many different causes. Rothman (1990) has provided a succinct discussion of this problem. If the cases in the cluster have occurred due to different causes, then epidemiologic investigation into a common specific hypothesized cause will be negative. Most clusters of diseases with multi-factorial etiologies that are identified and investigated by public health authorities are in fact of this type—no common cause can be found. Caldwell (1990) summarized 108 cancer clusters investigated by the Centers for Disease Control and concluded that no clear single cause was found for any of them. Similarly, Shulte et al. (1987) summarized 61 investigations of occupational cancer clusters and found that only 16 were confirmed, and in none was a specific cause discovered.

Rothman (1990) has pointed out that the more fruitful clusters will be those of rare diseases or of diseases in which the increased incidence is extremely marked. Such clusters are more likely to involve a single specific cause. For example, an occupational cluster of angiosarcomas of the liver, an extremely rare disease, was found to be associated with vinyl chloride exposure (Creech and Johnson, 1974). Similarly, an occupational cluster of men who were impotent led to the discovery that DBCP (dibromochloropropane) causes infertility (Whorton et al., 1977). Fleming et al. (1991) have pointed out that occupational clusters, rather than environmental ones, are more likely to yield etiologic discoveries because (1) they often have well-defined geographical boundaries (avoiding the Texas sharpshooter problem), (2) they often have shared and easily defined exposures, and (3) there are other workplaces with similar exposures that can be studied to confirm an association.

Rothman has pointed out five reasons why most cluster investigations are unlikely to lead to discovery of environmental causes: (1) clusters are often too small to be well studied epidemiologically, with proper control of confounding, (2) the diseases may be too heterogeneous to be caused by a single agent (e.g., a cancer cluster composed of different types of cancer), (3) the boundary problem in verifying a cluster, (4) poor characterization of exposures, and (5) publicity surrounding the cluster may make an epidemiologic study difficult.

Despite all these caveats and the data documenting how few reported clusters yield new scientific information, it is worth remembering that many exposure–disease associations have been discovered as a result of identification of clusters. Infectious disease clusters often lead to discovery of the infectious agent (e.g., Legionnaires' disease at an American Legion Convention). Fleming et al. (1991) have listed the large number of occupational associations found after investigation of clusters. Successful investigations of environmental clusters have also occurred, such as the investigation of an apparent cluster of asthma cases in Barcelona, which led to the identification of soybean dust as the etiologic agent (Anto et al., 1989), or the association between the pesticide trichlorfon and congenital abnormalities (see Czeizel et al., 1993)

In recent years there has been some increased interest in the routine surveillance of disease data to detect clusters, partly as a result of the discovery of a cluster of leukemias near the Sellafield nuclear plant in England. This cluster sparked a spirited debate, as well as numerous epidemiologic studies to test the hypothesis advanced by Gardner that paternal exposure to radiation prior to conception resulted in childhood leukemia (Inskip, 1993). A study by Gardner et al. (1990) did find such an association in the Sellafield area, but other investigations of leukemia clusters near other nuclear facilities did not.

Subsequent to this controversy, there has been an attempt to detect leukemia clusters in England, and then to investigate whether the detected clusters can be associated with environmental exposures. This generalized seeking of clusters is different from the occurrence of clusters discussed above, in which single clusters come to attention via local discovery and publicity. Generalized cluster identification can be conducted as long as a complete list of cases across space and time is available. Investigators then may calculate a large number of incidence rates based on small geographical areas (e.g., cancer rates for all counties in the United States). Alternatively, other techniques may be used based only on the cases to determine whether geographical and temporal "closeness" between cases is occurring more than would be expected by chance alone. For example, the investigator may form all possible pairs of cases and calculate distance in space and time between them, and then determine if the distribution of these distances differs from what would be expected by chance. Refinements are possible to allow for different densities of population within different areas, migration of populations over time such that the population at risk is changing, and possible latency periods between putative exposures and disease.

For example, Knox and Gilman (1992) have conducted an investigation of leukemia cases in England, and determined that there was a statistically significant excess of cases occurring jointly within 0.5 kilometers and 60 days of each other. The motivation for such studies is the presumption that identification of such clustering can yield useful etiologic hypotheses about the causes of such clustering, but this is often not the case. In many cases, detection of clustering may lead to no testable hypotheses at all. Hypotheses regarding possible environmental causes of clustering can be investigated by seeking common environmental exposures for the detected clusters, but these kinds of ecologic analyses may yield little useful information. For example, Knox (1994) has studied both leukemia cases and leukemia clusters in England; he purportedly showed that compared to controls, both occurred most commonly around railroads, with possible exposures to fossil fuels (railways being near oil refineries or oil storage facilities). However, Bithell and Draper (1995) have subsequently shown that failure to appropriately account for population density in control selection may have biased the Knox analysis sufficiently to explain the observed association; they also pointed out that the Knox analysis failed to account for issues of temporal sequence and possible migration. Furthermore, even if the association of leukemia cases and railroads could be upheld, this "exposure" is probably too nonspecific to be of much use.

Hypothesized causes of clusters that occur in one area can be tested if they occur in other areas. The Sellafield controversy also sparked the routine collection of denominator and numerator data for small geographical units, which can be useful for rapidly determining the occurrence of suspected clusters, and in turn determining whether similar clusters have occurred at other sites sharing some environmental exposure. Elliot et al. (1992) have described a system in which postal codes are used to identify the residence of cases, and the postal codes are linked to denominator data that are available down to the level of census enumeration districts averaging only 400 people. These data enable investigators to compare disease rates in concentric circles around a suspected point source, or to compare disease rates around one point source with disease rates around other such point sources to determine if a pattern of elevated disease is occurring. These authors illustrate the use of their data by confirming a cluster of mesothelioma and asbestos in residences near a naval dockyard where asbestos was used.

The evaluation of clusters is an important public health problem because of public demand, even though thorough epidemiologic investigation of the cluster is extremely unlikely to find any etiologic association. Public health authorities must adopt a triage method to determine where to invest scarce resources. Rapid use of good databases to confirm a cluster statistically and to test hypotheses about point sources of exposure can help with a rapid response to public demand. Useful scientific data on environmental risks, on the other hand, is more likely to be found by designing good studies to investigate specific etiologic hypotheses, in populations in which no cluster has been noted.

Errors in Measuring Exposure

In many epidemiologic studies, it is very difficult or even impossible to measure the true exposure exactly. Hence the observed exposure is measured with error (for continuous variables) or misclassified (for categorical variables). It is usually assumed that the error or misclassification is nondifferential and unbiased. This means that the error is independent of the disease status and that the expected value of the observed exposure is the true exposure.

In general, epidemiologists have assumed the nondifferential exposure measurement error or misclassification biases effect estimates to the null. Effect estimates might be regression coefficients for exposure in a regression model relating exposure to disease, or odds ratios or relative risks for categorical data arranged in 2×k tables. This assumption of bias toward the null has been made as a generalization of the special case of exposure misclassification in 2×2 tables for categorical data, or of the special case of usual linear regression for continuous exposure and outcome variables, using a "classic error" model (see below). Recent work has considered the case of multiple levels of exposure for categorical data, the case of nonlinear regression for continuous data, and the case of regression in which the classic error model may not hold. It has been shown that for some of these situations, exposure measurement error or misclassification can lead either to no bias in the estimated exposure effect, or to bias away from the null, rather than bias toward the null. We will describe and attempt to summarize some of this work here.

Exposure-disease models and error models

In order to understand the measurement error problem, one needs to understand the relevant models. First, one has a model for the exposure/disease relationship. Suppose Y is the response variable of interest. Y can be continuous (linear regression), dichotomous (logistic regression), or discrete (e.g., Poisson regression). Suppose Z denotes the true exposure and that X denotes the observed surrogate exposure. The true relationship between disease and exposure models $Y|Z$ as a function of Z. For example, in ordinary linear model $E(Y|Z) = \alpha + \beta Z$, while in logistic regression $P(Y=1|Z) = 1/(1+\exp(-\alpha-\beta Z))$.

A second model, the error model, relates Z and X. The classic measurement error model is given by $X = Z + \varepsilon$, where the error term ε is independent of Z. If the error term ε has expected value 0, then the measurement error is unbiased, which means that on the average the value of the measured X equals the true exposure Z. An example of the classic error model in an environmental study might be the case when Z is the true indoor radon exposure of an individual, while X is the estimated personal indoor radon exposure for the individual based on dosimeters placed in the home. In this case it is natural to assume that the error is independent of the true level, in the sense that the errors in measuring high levels are no greater than the errors in measuring low levels.

However, there are many instances in environmental epidemiology in which a single measured exposure level is assigned to a large number of people who are all in some category; for example an air pollution index may be assigned to everyone in a city, or the average radon level in a small survey of homes is assigned to all homes in the county. This leads to a different type of error model, called the Berkson model. In this case it is natural to assume that the true exposure for all individuals in the same area vary randomly about the assigned value. Hence the error is independent of the observed value. The Berkson error may be written as $Z = X + \varepsilon$, where ε is independent of the observed covariate X. Z and ε are not independent but positively correlated (Thomas et al., 1993).

In both the classical and Berkson models, one also usually assumes a specific distribution for the error term in the model, for example a normal distribution with mean 0 and variance σ_e^2 (Thomas et al., 1993).

In general, if the observed exposure is an individual measurement, then the classic error model applies, but if the observed exposure is assigned on a group basis, then the Berkson model will apply.

Errors in measurement of continuous variables in a regression context

It is well known that in ordinary linear regression with the classic error model and normal error distribution, the estimate obtained by using the observed X values in regression is always biased toward the null value (Cochran, 1968). Hence using the observed values X will result in a "conservative" estimate of the true effect of Z. Furthermore, this same bias toward the null will generally hold for log linear regression (e.g., logistic regression) as long as the classic error model holds (Armstrong et al., 1994).

Wacholder (1995) has studied the situation for ordinary regression when the assumptions of the classic error model are violated because the measurement error is correlated with the true value (i.e., $X = Z + \varepsilon$, where Z and ε are correlated). In general in this case the error model leads to bias, so that the errors do not have mean 0. One example in which this kind of error model might hold would be if those who eat smaller amounts of nutrients tend to overreport, whereas those who eat larger amounts tend to underreport. In this case the measurement error is negatively correlated with the true value. Another example would be when people systematically underreport their weight, but the underreporting errors are greater at higher weights. Then the measurement error is positively correlated with the true value. When the correlation between the true exposure Z and the error ε is positive, the resulting bias in the effect measure (e.g., the exposure regression coefficient in a model relating exposure to disease) is always toward the null. When the correlation is negative, the resulting effect bias can be either toward the null, away from the null, or even in the opposite direction. Wacholder advises using caution in interpreting epidemiologic results in the presence of measurement error.

Although epidemiologists generally recognize that measurement error with the classic error model leads to bias toward the null, it is less well appreciated that if the Berkson model holds, then the estimate of exposure effect (the coefficient for X) obtained by ordinary linear regression obtained by using the observed X values is in fact unbiased (Berkson, 1950). However the standard error is increased, resulting in less power or precision.

On the other hand, in log linear regression (e.g., logistic, Cox, Poisson regression) when the Berkson error model holds, measurement error can lead to bias away from the null value, but only if the variance of the errors is not constant. For example, this would occur if the errors were greater for larger values of the observed variable X; this situation would not be uncommon in environmental studies. For example, this might occur for radon in homes when the average level for an area based on a sample is assigned to each home in the study (Berkson error). The variance of the true values, and hence the measurement errors, might be greater within areas of higher radon levels, and hence the error variance would not be constant.

One of the first examples using the Berkson model was given by Prentice (1982). Deddens and Hornung (1995) have expanded on the earlier work of Prentice. They have shown that unbiased nondifferential measurement errors can bias the risk estimate away from the null value in log linear regression when the measurement error variance is not constant. However the exposure effect estimate (exposure regression coefficient) is unbiased when the error variance is constant.

Exposure misclassification in categorical data

When the exposure variable is discrete or categorical, then errors in measurement are often called misclassification. As in measurement errors, misclassification can be nondifferential or differential. Instead of error distributions, one describes the misclassification probabilities, for example $P(i|j)$, the probability of classifying the exposure as i when in fact it is j.

Dosemeci et al. (1990) described the case of $2 \times k$ tables, in which $k-1$ odds ratios or relative risks are typically calculated, each in reference to the first (often lowest) exposure level. For example, in the 2×3 case one might compare high exposure to low, and medium exposure to low. These authors showed that, in theory, in the case of $2 \times k$ tables, nondifferential misclassification can result in biasing the true exposure effects either toward the null value or away from the null value. However, the examples in which bias away from the null occurs are rather extreme—in some cases their observed exposures are actually negatively correlated with the true exposure, meaning that the incorrectly classified data is classified worse than if it had been classified by chance alone.

As a follow-up to Dosemeci et al., Correa-Villasenor et al. (1995) have considered numerous scenarios of misclassification in 2×3 tables. These authors show that in general the bias is toward the null, whether one is considering the odds ratio of the middle level versus the lowest, or the highest level versus the lowest. Exceptions occur only for extreme cases of misclassification or small sample sizes.

Flegal et al. (1991) have considered the special case in which continuous data suffering from nondifferential measurement error are categorized for analysis. Investigators typically categorize continuous data to check for monotonic trends and to provide effect estimates that are less model-dependent, while accepting some resulting loss of precision. Such categorization typically leads to misclassification of exposure level subjects around the cutpoint(s). This misclassification will be differential (affecting diseased and nondiseased differently) when there is a true exposure–response relationship, e.g., more exposure increases disease rates. This occurs because cases and noncases are not distributed randomly around the cutpoint. Flegal et al. conducted simulations in which the bias in the effect measure was always toward the null, as with nondifferential misclassification, although the authors point out that this will not always be the case.

Summary, measurement errors

There is little known empirically regarding bias caused by measurement error, because we generally lack a gold standard of correctly measured data with which to compare results based on mismeasured data. Hence most of the work done on measurement error has been theoretical or based on simulated data, and work in this area is still evolving.

Recent work has made it clear that nondifferential measurement error in measuring the exposure variable, or misclassification of exposure in the categorical case, can lead not only to effect estimates biased toward the null, but also to no bias or bias away from the null. The direction and/ or existence of the bias depends on the true error model, the type of data, the type of analysis, and the true exposure–response relationship. This is tantamount to saying it depends on everything, so that no generalizations can be made. However, it is somewhat comforting to find that in most cases, bias is generally absent (many Berkson error cases) or again usually conservative (toward the null). With the exception of some cases of nonlinear regression with Berkson errors and nonconstant error variance, bias *away* from the null (perhaps of most concern to epidemiologists) seems to occur only in rather extreme and unusual cases.

References

Anto J, Sunyer J, Rodriguez-Roisin R, et al. 1989. Community outbreaks of asthma with inhalation of soybean dust. N Engl J Med 320:1097–1102.

Armstrong B, White E, Saracci R. 1994. Principles of Exposure measurement in Epidemiology. Monographs in Epidemiology and Biostatistics, Vol 21. Oxford University Press, New York.

Berkson J. 1950. Are there two regressions? J Am Stat Assoc 45: 164–180.

Bithell J, Draper G. 1995. Apparent association between benzene and childhood leukemia: methodological doubts concerning a report by Know. J Epidemiol Community Health 49:437–439.

Brenner H, Savitz D, Jockel K, et. al. 1992. Effects of nondifferential exposure misclassification in ecologic studies. Am J Epidemiol 135:85–95

Caldwell G. 1990. Twenty-two years of cancer cluster investigations at the Centers for Disease Control. Am J Epidemiol 132, suppl 1:S43–S62.

Cochran W. 1968. Errors of measurement in statistics. Technometrics 10:637–666.

Correa-Villasenor A, Stewart W, Franco-Marina F, Hui S. 1995. Bias from nondifferential misclassification in case-control studies with three exposure levels. Epidemiology 6:276–281.

Creech J, Johnson M. 1974. Angiosarcoma of the liver in the manufacture of polyvinyl chloride. J Occup Environ Med 16:150–151.

Czeizel A, Elek C, Gundy S, et al. 1993. Environmental trichlorfon and cluster of congenital abnormalities. Lancet 341:539–542.

Deddens J, Hornung R. 1995. Quantitative examples of continuous exposure measurement errors that bias risk estimates away from the null. In: Smith C, Christiani D, Kelsey K, eds. Chemical Risk Assessment and Occupational Health. Auburn House, Westport, CT

Dosemeci M, Wacholder S, Lubin J. 1990. Does nondifferential misclassification of exposure always bias a true effect toward the null value? Am J Epidemiol 132:746–748.

Durkheim E. 1951. Suicide: a Study in Sociology. The Free Press, New York.

Elliot P, Westlake A, Hills M, et al. 1992. The Small Area Health Statistics Unit: a national facility for investigating health around point sources of environmental pollution in the United Kingdom. J Epidemiol Community Health 46:345–349.

Flegal K, Keyl P, Nieto F. 1991. Differential misclassification arising from nondifferential errors in exposure measurement. Am J Epidemiol 134:1233–1244.

Fleming L, Ducatman A, Shalat S. 1991. Disease clusters: a cental and ongoing role in occupational health. J Occup Environ Med 33:818–825.

Gardner M, Snee M, Hall A, et al. 1990. Results of case-control study of leukemia and lymphoma among young people near Sellafield nuclear plant in West Cumbria. Brit Med J 300:423–429

Greenland S, Robins J. 1994. Invited commentary: ecologic studies—biases, misconceptions, and counterexamples. Am J Epidemiol 139:747–771.

Grufferman S. 1982. Hodgkin's disease. In: Schottenfeld D, Fraumeni J, eds. Cancer Epidemiology and Prevention. Saunders, Philadelphia.

Inskip H. 1993. The Gardner hypothesis. BMJ 307:1155–1156.

Knox E. 1994. Leukemia clusters in childhood: geographical analysis in Britain. J Epidemiol Community Health 48:369–376.

Knox E, Gilman E. 1992. Leukemia clusters in Great Britain 1. Space-time interactions. J Epidemiol Community Health 46:566–572.

Gardner M, Snee M, Hall A, et al. 1990. Results of case-control study of leukemia and lymphoma among young people near Sellafield nuclear plant in west Cumbria. BMJ 300:423–429.

Morganstern H, Thomas D. 1993. Principles of study design in environmental epidemiology. Environ Health Perspect 101, suppl 4:23–38.

Piantadosi S. 1994. Invited commentary: ecologic biases. Am J Epidemiol 139:761–771.

Piantadosi S, Byar D, Green S. 1988. The ecological fallacy. Am J Epidemiol 127:893–904.

Pope C, Thun M, Mohan M, et al. 1995. Particulate air pollution as a predictor of mortality in a prospective study of US adults. Am J Respir Crit Care Med 151:669–674.

Prentice RL. 1982. Covariate measurement errors and parameter estimation in a failure time regression model. Biometrika 69:331–342.

Rothman K. 1990. A sobering start for the cluster busters' conference. Am J Epidemiol 132, suppl 1:S6–S13.

Schulte P, Ehrenberg R, Singal M. 1987. Investigation of occupational cancer clusters: theory and practice. Am J Public Health 77:52–56.

Stidley C, Samet J. 1993. A review of ecologic studies of lung cancer and indoor radon. Health Physics 65:234–251.

Stidley C, Samet J. 1994. Assessment of ecologic regression in the study of lung cancer and indoor radon. Am J Epidemiol 139:312–322.

Susser M. 1994. The logic in ecological: the logic of design. Am J Public Health 84:830–835.

Thomas D, Stram D, Dwyer J. 1993. Exposure measurement error: influence on exposure-disease relationships and methods of correction. Annu Rev Public Health 14:69–93.

Wacholder S. 1995. When measurement errors correlate with truth: surprising effects of nondifferential misclassification. Epidemiology 6:157–161.

Whorton D, Krauss R, Marshall S, et al. 1977. Infertility in male pesticide workers. Lancet 2:1259–1261.

Meta-analysis and Risk Assessment

3

CATHERINE WRIGHT

PEGGY LOPIPERO

ALLAN SMITH

THE most important questions about the relationship between environmental agents and human disease are often the most difficult to answer. Does the weight of the evidence indicate that exposure causes disease? If so, what is the quantitative dose-response relationship? What does that relationship imply for regulation? Risk assessment is usually defined as the process by which these questions are answered. Within the terminology of risk assessment, the first question is often called hazard identification, the second concerns dose-response assessment, and the third question combines estimates of the prevalence of exposure with risk quantification. Risk assessment can be done with animal or human data.

Meta-analysis is a tool often used in risk assessment to combine results across studies, usually human studies, with the goal of estimating measures of association with improved precision. It is commonly used at the hazard identification stage to combine a number of studies of exposed versus nonexposed populations and provide a quantitative summary of results. It is sometimes also used to assess dose-response relationships when there are several studies with dose-response results and one wishes to combine them.

Meta-analysis is increasingly replacing the traditional review of the literature because of its ability to provide a quantitative estimate with corresponding confidence intervals. It is done by calculating a weighted average of results across studies, with the weights usually being the inverse of the variance of the result for each study (i.e., larger studies with more precise results are given greater weight).

A problem with meta-analysis is its tendency to combine apples and oranges; well-designed studies may be combined with poorly designed ones. One way to confront this problem is to conduct analyses of subsets of studies that are deemed to be better designed versus those less well designed. Results may help decide whether an exposure truly causes disease. For example, if better-designed studies with good control over confounding show no exposure effect but less well designed studies do show such an effect, one might conclude that confounding was responsible for biased results in the latter studies and that exposure did not cause disease.

A second problem in meta-analysis is publication bias, meaning that "negative" studies tend not to be published and thus are unavailable for the meta-analysis. This produces results that may be biased toward finding an effect. There is no ideal solution to this problem beyond searching diligently for all studies on a given topic, including if possible any that are lying on some investigator's back shelf.

Once a hazard has been identified, typically by a meta-analysis, risk assessment has the more ambitious goal of quantifying potential health risks in relation to exposure. Typically this involves determining a dose-response relationship, and then using the resulting excess risk associated with each unit of exposure to estimate an acceptable level of exposure over a lifetime.

By definition, the process of risk assessment is a speculative exercise, laden with assumptions. The underlying question of the quantitative impact of exposure on disease is truly the bottom line for all environmental health research. Instead of hedging with vague terms of "small risk" or "likely to be substantial," risk assessment seeks the best possible quantitative estimate of the risk. Debate over risk assessment is predictable, given the direct application to regulatory policy and untidiness inherent in the generation of quantitative results. Informal or implicit risk assessment is part of everyday life at the individual and societal level. The unique feature of formal risk assessment is its explicitness in delineating each step in the process and the assumptions involved for each step.

One of the important products of risk assessment, in addition to the quantitative results, is the identification of critical gaps in our knowledge that prevent the assessment from being more definitive. Among the lists of assumptions and data sources, there are often just a few key issues that are the dominant sources of uncertainty. Most commonly, in risk assessments based on animal data, the limitation is in extrapolation across species and from high to low doses. In risk assessments based on epidemiologic data, estimates of the level of exposure for study subjects— key to dose-response analyses—are often subject to substantial uncertainty. Data on confounders may also be minimal. It is not always appreciated that the proper comparison is not between the clarity of toxicologic studies compared to epidemiologic studies, which must favor the toxicologic research because of tight experimental control. The real question is the information value for human risk assessment, and perfect toxicology may be roughly equivalent to adequate epidemiology, with high-quality epidemiology superior to all other approaches.

The methods of risk assessment have evolved principally to address cancer, and extrapolation from animals to humans is most advanced for addressing this set of health end points. The combination of extensive experimental results, a substantial body of epidemiologic findings, and some general ideas of mechanisms makes risk assessment for cancer relatively advanced, at least compared to the kind of assessment that is possible for such outcomes as reproductive health or neurological disease. There may be some circular reasoning, in that regulation is most often based on carcinogenicity, and the tools for risk assessment, which serves as the basis for regulation, are most fully developed to address carcinogenicity. However, the general principles of risk assessment are applicable to all health outcomes, and creative approaches are needed to apply those principles to a more comprehensive array of health considerations.

Environmental risk assessment is the quantification of potential adverse health effects of human exposure to environmental hazards. To estimate health risks at low environmental exposure levels often requires extrapolating from studies with high exposures to chemical or physical agents. High-exposure studies include epidemiologic studies of occupationally exposed cohorts, epidemiologic studies involving high environmental exposures in the community, and experimental animal studies. Results of risk assessments are used by risk managers to set regulatory policies regarding acceptable levels of chemical contaminants in the environment.

Risk assessments contain some or all of the following four steps: hazard identification, dose-response assessment, exposure assessment, and risk quantification (EPA, 1989). Hazard identification involves determining whether an agent can cause an adverse health outcome, such as cancer or other disease. Dose-response assessment involves determining the relationship between the magnitude of exposure and the probability of occurrence of the health effects in question. Exposure assessment is the evaluation of the extent of public exposure to the chemical or physical agent; it may include environmental or occupational exposure measurement, emission or effluent quantification, modeling of environmental transport and fate, identification of exposure routes, identification of exposed populations, and estimation of short-term and long-term exposure levels. Risk quantification requires calculation of the magnitude of human risk at various exposure levels, and often includes an analysis of uncertainty inherent in the risk estimates.

Risk assessments may be based on experimental animal data or epidemiologic data. Although epidemiologic data are considered the most convincing evidence of human risk in the regulatory setting, risk assessments are often performed with animal data because adequate human data are often lacking. There are a number of advantages and disadvantages in conducting risk assessment based on either type of data.

The advantages of using long-term studies in animals for risk assessment are that exposure levels and conditions are known, and the toxicity and carcinogenicity of individual chemicals can be clearly identified. However, animal experiments are conducted at exposure levels far in excess of those anticipated for humans, and they are often conducted using a route of exposure that may not be relevant to human exposure scenarios. Animal experiments also do not reflect human exposure circumstances, because animal tests are typically conducted with single chemicals whereas humans experience multiple exposures during their entire lives (Huff and Hoel, 1992). The relevance of animal experiments to humans is also questionable because of biological differences between humans and laboratory animals.

Little is known about the true correlation between carcinogenic effects in animals and those in humans. Allen et al. (1988) argue that there is a relatively good correlation between known human carcinogens and animal carcinogenicity. This conclusion is based on a limited number of chemicals, however. Some work has been done looking at interspecies correlations between rats and mice (Piegorsch et al., 1992; Haseman and Lockhart, 1993). If mice and rats are similar in regard to carcinogenesis, this provides some evidence in favor of interspecies extrapolations. Haseman and Lockhart (1993) examined a database of 379 long-term carcinogenicity studies in rats and mice to evaluate sex and species correlations in site-specific carcinogenesis response. Within a species, target sites showed only 65% agreement between males and females. The overall concordance in carcinogenic response between rats and mice was 74% when all target sites were considered collectively. However, the correlation between rats and mice in site-specific carcinogenic response was only 37%. In fact, no significant interspecies correlations were observed for lung tumors, which are a common concern in environmental epidemiology and health risk assessment.

A number of articles have also been published on the correlations between carcinogenic potencies in rats and mice. Crouch and Wilson (1979) demonstrated a strong correlation between carcinogenic potencies in rats and mice, supporting the extrapolation from mouse to humans.

However, others have suggested that this observed correlation is mainly a statistical artifact of bioassay design (Bernstein et al., 1985a,b; Freedman et al., 1993).

As stated above, there is only a small (37%) correlation between rats and mice in site-specific cancer causation. Extrapolating causation even between rodent species is difficult, so it is expected that extrapolating actual cancer risks from rodents to humans would involve large degrees of uncertainty.

Because of the uncertainties in using animal data, good epidemiologic studies, when available, are generally considered to be the best source of data for use in quantitative risk assessment (Smith, 1988; Hertz-Picciotto, 1995). There are a number of advantages and disadvantages in using epidemiologic studies for risk assessment. One advantage is that they provide direct evidence for carcinogenic or other health effects in humans, thus avoiding the uncertainty of interspecies extrapolation. However, epidemiologic studies do not show cause-and-effect relationships with the same ease as do experimental studies in animals. Another disadvantage to using epidemiologic data for risk assessment is that most studies are retrospective and most persons are exposed to a wide variety of potentially hazardous agents. This makes it difficult to identify with certainty the critical exposures that may have occurred 20 to 40 years in the past. Furthermore, epidemiologic studies are subject to a number of biases and potential confounders that may make their interpretation complex and controversial.

Perhaps the most common statement made about the use of epidemiologic studies for health risk assessment is that they lack adequate exposure data. This has sometimes led to the rejection of human studies for risk assessment purposes, with reliance placed on animal data instead. Exposure data in animal bioassays are, by comparison, more accurate. However, the main sources of error in utilizing animal data for human health risk assessment is the high-to-low dose extrapolation and the animal-to-human extrapolation. It follows that the use of epidemiologic data in health risk assessment should not be based on merely contrasting the quality of available exposure data with that for animal studies. In fact, the uncertainties inherent in human exposure data are usually very small when contrasted to the uncertainties inherent in rodent-to-human risk extrapolation.

Risk assessments based on human data may involve meta-analysis, particularly in the hazard identification and dose-response assessment phases. Meta-analysis is the qualitative and quantitative analysis of a collection of epidemiologic study results (Berlin et al., 1993). Some controversy surrounds the use of meta-analysis of observational epidemiologic studies.

Although there are a number of advantages in doing meta-analysis in risk assessment, the approach can result in inaccurate conclusions if not properly conducted.

This chapter focuses on the hazard identification and dose-response assessment phases of health risk assessment. An example of the use of meta-analysis in hazard identification will be presented as well as a dose-response assessment utilizing data from occupational epidemiologic studies.

Hazard Identification

Hazard identification involves determining if adverse health effects are caused by a particular exposure. Its purpose in environmental epidemiology and health risk assessment is to conclude whether a chemical or physical agent is a human carcinogen or causes other types of adverse health effects. Hazard identification typically includes a review of the physical–chemical properties of the chemical and routes and patterns of exposure; structure–activity relationships; metabolic and pharmacokinetic properties; toxicologic effects other than cancer; short-term tests; long-term animal studies; and human studies. Evidence of possible carcinogenicity in humans comes primarily from long-term animal tests and epidemiologic studies.

Using animal data for hazard identification

In the absence of adequate human evidence, evidence from animal experiments is used to identify chemical hazards. Criteria for the technical adequacy of animal carcinogenicity studies have been published by the NTP (National Toxicology Program, 1984) and the EPA (Environmental Protection Agency 1983a,b,c). The weight of evidence that an agent is potentially carcinogenic for humans increases (1) with the increase in number of tissue sites affected by the agent; (2) with the increase in number of animal species, strains, sexes, and number of experiments and doses showing a carcinogenic response; (3) with the occurrence of clearcut dose-response relationships (malignant and benign tumors combined) in treated compared with control groups; (4) when there is a dose-related shortening of the time-to-tumor occurrence or time to death with tumor; and (5) when there is a dose-related increase in the proportion of tumors that are malignant (EPA, 1989).

A number of factors need to be considered when reviewing the weight of evidence in long-term animal studies. For example, long-term animal studies are typically conducted at or near the maximum tolerated dose (MTD) level to ensure adequate statistical power for the detection of carcinogenic activity. However, the applicability of these bioassay results to human conditions has been questioned because qualitatively different biologic responses may occur at very high exposure levels. Critics have argued that the testing of animals at the MTD and at one-half the MTD causes inflammation and cell proliferation that does not occur at low exposures and that elevated rates of cell mitosis increase the opportunities for spontaneous mutations, thereby contributing to carcinogenic development (Ames and Gold, 1990a, b, 1991). Advocates of the testing protocol state that: (1) toxicity, although frequently observed at the MTD, is usually not observed at one-half MTD even though increased tumor incidence usually is and (2) 90% of the carcinogens identified by the NTP induced tumors in organs that showed no evidence of cellular toxicity (Infante, 1991; Perera, 1990; Huff and Haseman, 1991; Rall, 1991; Cogliano et al., 1991).

Tumor data from sites with high spontaneous background rates also require special consideration. For example, there are widely diverging scientific views about the validity of mouse liver tumors as an indication of potential carcinogenicity in humans when such tumors occur in strains with high spontaneous background incidence and when they constitute the only tumor response to an agent (EPA, 1989).

Using epidemiologic studies for hazard identification

The decision as to whether an epidemiologic study is appropriate as the basis for hazard identification involves judgments about both the qualitative and quantitative nature of the data. Qualitative factors that should be considered include the appropriate selection of the exposed and comparison groups, the reliability of exposure ascertainment, the completeness of follow-up, and the potential biases. If a study meets the minimum criteria for acceptance on qualitative grounds, its appropriateness for quantitative risk assessment depends on its ability to yield reasonably reliable information on doses, time and duration of exposure, and magnitude of response. Unfortunately, the magnitude of past exposure often has to be estimated from fragmentary information. The reliability of quantitative information on the magnitude of response depends on the statistical power of the study, on the completeness and reliability of the information on disease incidence, and on the ability to control for confounding factors, such as cigarette smoking. These qualitative and quantitative criteria are more likely to be met for occupational epidemiologic studies than for environmental epidemiologic studies. For these reasons, quantitative risk assessment using human data is largely based on occupational studies.

In hazard identification, epidemiologic data are used to infer causal associations. The key factors to consider in determining causality from epidemiologic studies are chance, bias, consistency, strength, dose response, temporality, and plausibility.

Chance: How likely is it that the findings in all available studies are due to chance?

Bias: Potential sources of bias should be identified, including selection bias, information bias, and confounding bias. Then, the direction and magnitude of the bias should be determined to assess their effects on study findings. Many potential biases in epidemiological studies may be quite small and of known direction, so it is not appropriate to dismiss a study merely because of the possibility of a particular bias.

Consistency: Studies should demonstrate similar associations that persist despite differing circumstances. This does not mean that studies should produce identical findings, because fluctuations may be caused by chance. In addition, fluctuations are expected because of differences in the durations and intensities of exposure, differences in length of follow-up, and variation in susceptibility between populations.

Strength: Strength of association is an important criterion, because the greater the estimate of risk and the more precise (narrow confidence limits), the more credible the causal association.

Dose response: Dose response is observed if the increase in the measure of effect is positively correlated with an increase in the exposure or estimated dose. A strong dose-response relationship across several categories of exposure supports a causal relationship. However, the absence of a dose-response relationship should not be construed by itself as evidence of a lack of a causal relationship.

Temporality: A temporal relationship must be present if causality is to be considered. This means that the disease occurs within a biologically reasonable time frame after the exposure to account for the specific health effects. Some cancers, for example, have latency periods ranging from 20 to 40 or more years from initial exposure.

Biological plausibility: The association should make sense in terms of biological knowledge. Information from toxicology, pharmacokinetics, genotoxicity and in vitro studies should be considered.

All the above factors should be considered in making causal inference from epidemiologic studies. Causal inference can usually be made only when each of these criteria is met by at least some of the studies. However, inferring causation may be reasonable even in the absence of dose-response information. There should always be a degree of consistency between studies, but it is quite common to see the conclusion made that there is a lack of consistency when, in fact, there is a good explanation for apparent inconsistency. In particular, one should not expect consistency in relative risk estimates when there is wide variation in intensity and duration of exposure between studies.

Dose-Response Assessment

Dose-response assessment is the process of characterizing the relationship between the exposure to an agent and the incidence of an adverse health effect in exposed populations. In quantitative cancer risk assessment, the dose-response relationship is expressed in terms of a linear slope (called a potency slope), which is used in the risk characterization phase to calculate the probability or risk of cancer associated with a given exposure level. One of the primary differences in assessing the dose response for cancer vs. noncancer health outcomes is that carcinogens are commonly assumed to have no threshold whereas noncancer effects are assumed to have a threshold. These assumptions are made by regulatory bodies performing a health risk assessment unless evidence suggests otherwise. The focus of this section is dose-response assessment for carcinogenic effects. Methods for noncancer dose-response assessment have been described by the EPA (1993).

Dose-response assessment using animal data

In the absence of appropriate human studies, data from an animal species that responds most like humans can be used in the dose-response assessment. The EPA (1989) has established guidelines for selecting the appropriate set of data for the assessment, assuming several studies are available to choose from. First, the tumor incidence data are separated according to organ site and tumor type. Second, all biologically and statistically acceptable data sets are presented. Third, the range of the risk estimates is presented with consideration of the biological relevance and appropriateness of route of exposure. Finally, because it is possible that human sensitivity is as high as the most sensitive responding animal species, the biologically acceptable data set from long-term animal studies showing the greatest sensitivity (i.e., the highest potency) is generally given the greatest emphasis.

Low-dose estimates derived from experimental animal data extrapolated to humans are complicated by a variety of factors that differ among species and potentially affect the response to carcinogens. Included among these factors are differences between humans and experimental test animals with respect to life span, body size, genetic variability, population homogeneity, existence of concurrent disease, pharmacokinetic effects such as metabolism and excretion patterns, and the exposure regimen. Extrapolations may also be necessary for route of exposure when the exposure route in the animal study selected for dose-response assessment differs from the route of exposure expected in humans (EPA, 1989).

Equivalent doses between species (animal-to-human dose conversions) may be expressed as mg/kg/body weight/day, parts per million (ppm) in diet or water, mg/m² surface area per day, or mg/kg/body weight/lifetime. The equivalent dose generally used by the EPA is mg/m² surface area/day (EPA, 1987). The reason for selecting the surface area conversion is that certain pharmacologic effects, particularly metabolic rate, commonly vary according to surface area (EPA, 1987). The comparison of an effect between species is proportional to dose/body surface, and body surface is proportional to an animal's weight to the two-thirds power. Thus, $mg/weight^{2/3}/day$ is considered an equivalent dose between mammalian species in the absence of better information on pharmacokinetic differences between animals and humans (EPA, 1987). For example, if a rat is exposed to 100 mg/day, then an equivalent dose for a human for the same exposure would be:

$$100 \ / \ 0.35^{2/3} \text{ kg} = X \ / \ 70^{2/3} \text{ kg}$$

Where:

$$X \ = \ \text{equivalent human dose (mg / day)}$$
$$0.35 \ = \ \text{weight of rat (kg)}$$
$$70 \ = \ \text{weight of human (kg)}$$

Solving for X gives:

$$100 \ / \ 0.49 \ = \ X \ / \ 17$$
$$X \ = \ 3500 \text{ mg / day}$$

Because risks at low exposure levels cannot be directly measured by high-dose animal experiments, mathematical models are used that specify the form of the dose-response relationship at low doses. The choice of model can have a large impact on the final risk estimate, particularly if the human exposures of interest are as much as 100 or 1000 times lower than the doses used in the animal experiments. The discrepancies resulting from the use of different models can be 1000-fold or greater.

Biologically based models, particularly models based on the Armitage-Doll (1954) multistage theory of carcinogenesis, have generally been used for producing low-dose risk estimates from animal bioassay data. The multistage theory asserts that in order for a cell to become cancerous it must progress through a series of ordered, independent, and irreversible stages. This model is approximately linear in the low dose region of the dose-response curve and is therefore thought to be relatively conservative (EPA, 1993). The version of the linearized multistage model most commonly employed by the EPA was developed by Crump et al. (1977) and is expressed as follows:

$$P(d) = 1 - \exp[-(q_0 + q_1 d + q_2 d^2 + \ldots + q_k d^k)], K \geqslant 1$$

where:

$P(d)$ = the probability of cancer at dose d;
k = the number of stages, or k may also be assumed to be equal to the number of dose levels minus one;
q_k = coefficients fitted to the data, and;
d^k = the applied dose raised to the kth power.

The upper 95% confidence interval (CI) estimate for q_1 is then used in calculating comparable human risk. More recently, another biologically based model that takes into account effects on cell proliferation, called the two-stage clonal expansion model, has been increasingly used (Moolgavkar and Knudson, 1981). These and other dose-response models have been described in more detail by the EPA (1993).

Dose-response assessment based on epidemiologic studies

Dose-response estimates based on adequate positive epidemiologic data are preferred over estimates based on animal data. The criteria for selecting an epidemiologic study for dose-response assessment includes (1) consistency of findings with other studies, (2) quality of exposure data for relevant period, (3) statistical precision of the risk estimates, (4) dose-response data, (5) data concerning major confounding factors, and (6) adequacy of follow-up in cohort studies.

The use of epidemiologic data in risk assessment should not be based solely on comparison of the quality of available human exposure data to that in animal studies (Smith, 1988). Even if the exposure data are poor, the fact that no species extrapolation is necessary makes the use of human data preferable over animal data. There are, in fact, surrogate measures for exposure that can be used, such as duration of exposure where data on mean exposure levels are available (Shore et al., 1992; Enterline, 1987).

Epidemiologic studies used in risk assessment generally involve high exposures to the agents of concern, thus requiring extrapolation to risks at low exposure levels. Linear dose-response assumptions for low doses have been used extensively for cancer risk assessment from epidemiologic data.

One simple method for modeling dose response when no dose-specific data are available is to plot exposure versus a relative risk estimate such as the standardized mortality ratio (SMR) by assigning a single average exposure level for the entire cohort and drawing a line from the observed SMR to the origin (SMR = 1) (Smith, 1988). This approach is essentially equal to fitting the model SMR = 1 + xβ, where x = exposure and β = the change in the SMR per unit of exposure (i.e., the slope).

When dose-specific data are available, such as when SMRs are presented for different levels of cumulative exposure, a simple model is to fit the data with weighted least squares regression, forcing the line to go through an SMR of 1 for zero exposure. This model may also be represented as SMR = 1 + xβ, where β is obtained from weighted least squares regression.

It is also possible to apply large numbers of different statistical models each with different assumptions. Normally, however, very few data points are available, and because extrapolations have to be made far below the observed data points, different models can obviously produce markedly different results. Some investigators propose using a variety of different models and giving a range of results (Stayner et al. 1994). However, this approach creates serious problems in the use of human data for health risk assessment (as it does for use of animal studies). In our view, linear regression of relative risk estimates, such as the SMR, forced through a relative risk of 1 for zero exposure, provides stable reproducible results, and is the preferred method for regulatory purposes unless there is clear nonlinearity in the data.

There are a number of reasons for proposing the relative risk model. First, relative risk estimates are usually given in published studies. This means that risk assessments can be conducted without getting the original study data. Second, relative risk estimates in the published literature have already been adjusted for age. All diseases are strongly related to age, therefore modeling risk estimates by other approaches such as additive risk models ($\lambda_x = \lambda_o + x\beta$, where λ_x = rate at exposure x, and λ_o = rate in unexposed) need to incorporate complex functions of age. Another reason is that when relative risk estimates are plotted against cumulative exposure, the relationship is usually linear or close to it. There are not usually sufficient data points to reject linearity. It should be noted that apparent nonlinearity at low exposure points in cohort studies can be fitted with statistical models that have a profound impact on risk extrapolations to lower doses. However, the empirical evidence for nonlinearity may be extremely weak. Finally, there are often no good biological reasons for rejecting linearity. For these reasons it would seem preferable to use the linear relative risk model for quantitative risk assessment using epidemiologic data, *unless there are good reasons to reject it* (i.e., clear evidence of nonlinearity). This does not mean that we criticize the investigation of other models for research purposes. However, for regulatory purposes we believe that this model should be the first choice.

There is one situation in which the relative risk model cannot be used. This occurs when the background rate of the disease in question is extremely low. In these cases, relative risk estimates are very unstable. For example, asbestos is by far the main cause of mesothelioma in adults. The background rates without asbestos exposure are extremely low. SMR estimates are therefore very large, and they are unstable because the expected numbers of cases for a cohort are very small (usually a small fraction of 1). In these settings, additive risk models need to be used, but they will not be discussed here.

An example of dose-response assessment for airborne nickel and lung cancer using published epidemiologic data is presented below. This is an example where one study proved superior to others for dose-response assessment, as opposed to the combining of several study findings by meta-analysis.

Example: Dose-response assessment for airborne nickel and lung cancer using published epidemiologic data

In the following example of risk assessment, published data on occupational cohorts exposed to airborne nickel were used to determine the risk of lung cancer in nickel-exposed communities. This dose-response assessment involves linear regression on SMRs and cumulative exposure estimates. The ultimate goal of this dose-response assessment is to establish a unit risk estimate (URE) that can be used to estimate the cancer risk to any community exposed to nickel in air. The unit risk estimate is currently defined as an estimate of the increased cancer risk from a lifetime (70-year) exposure to a concentration of one unit exposure (EPA, 1993). The URE for inhalation is expressed as risk per $\mu g/m^3$ for air contaminants.

Based on the criteria described earlier in this chapter, four published cohort studies of nickel refinery workers were considered candidates for risk assessment purposes (Enterline and Marsh 1982; Magnus et al., 1982;

Table 3-1. Studies considered for quantitative risk assessment

Study	Cohort Size	Lung Cancer Deaths	Lung Cancer SMR	90% CI	Index of Precision[a]
West VA (Enterline and Marsh, 1982)	259	8	1.12	0.56–2.02	0.12
Norway (Magnus et al., 1982)	2247	82	3.73[b]	3.08–4.48	0.77
Wales (Morgan, 1985)	967	145	5.28	4.58–6.06	0.83
Ontario (Chovil et al., 1981)	495	37	8.71	6.49–11.45	0.71

[a] Ratio of (SMR-1) to upper confidence limit of (SMR-1), where (SMR-1) is an estimate of excess relative risk.

[b] SIR (standardized incidence ratio)

Morgan, 1985; Chovil et al., 1981). Table 3-1 summarizes data from the four studies. The ratio of the excess relative risk point estimate (SMR − 1) divided by the excess relative risk at the upper confidence limit of the SMR gives an "index of precision" by which studies can be compared for use in risk assessment. The West Virginia study (Enterline and Marsh, 1982) was found to be unsuitable for risk estimation because of a low index of precision. The Norwegian (Magnus et al., 1982) and Welsh (Morgan, 1985) studies, although having high indices of precision, were found to be unsuitable because of their lack of exposure data.

The Ontario cohort study was determined to be the most appropriate for cancer risk estimation (Chovil et al., 1981). Exposure measures were available for the whole period of operation of the plant from 1948 to 1963, and the index of precision was high (Table 3-1). A weakness of this study was the incomplete follow-up (75%) which has led some to reject the study from serious consideration (Grandjean et al., 1988). However, bounds can be put on the uncertainty in risk estimation due to incomplete follow-up. The overall strengths of this study led to its choice for lung cancer risk estimation. Although more than one study can be used in a dose-response analysis, in this case only the one study had acceptable data.

The Ontario cohort involved refinery workers at Copper Cliff. Follow-up of this cohort, including the group of sinter plant workers used in this risk assessment, was continued to 1984 (ICNCM, 1990). This plant is unique in that there were measurements relating to airborne nickel made back to 1948 when the plant was opened. Levels of nickel in air escaping from the roof monitors of this plant are available for the period 1948 to 1962 (Warner, 1985).

Table 3-2. Observed and expected numbers of deaths and standardized mortality ratios for the Ontario nickel refinery cohort by cumulative exposure

Cumulative Exposure (mg/m³) × Years	Observed Lung Cancer Deaths	Expected Lung Cancer Deaths	Standardized Mortality Ratios (SMR)
40	0	0.47	0.0
150	0	0.36	0.0
300	3	0.54	7.5
490	4	0.60	8.9
710	6	0.68	11.7
940	13	0.76	22.8
1200	11	0.84	17.5

DOSE-RESPONSE CALCULATIONS FOR THE ONTARIO COHORT STUDY

The next step in the risk assessment is to determine the quantitative relationship between the estimated dose of nickel and lung cancer relative risk (i.e., the response) for the Ontario cohort. The SMR data for the Ontario cohort study are presented in Table 3-2. The expected numbers of deaths were calculated by Chovil et al. (1981) from age-specific rates for males in Ontario. The cumulative exposure data in the first column of Table 3-2 were derived by the EPA (1986) from exposure duration data (Chovil et al., 1981) incorporating a level of 200 mg/m³ for work prior to 1952, and 100 mg/m³ for 1952 and thereafter (Warner, 1985). Reexamination of the Warner data led us to the conclusion that the average exposure level was actually around 75 mg/m³ from 1952 on, and about 150 mg/m³ before 1952. To account for this difference we multiplied the cumulative exposure estimates by an adjustment factor of 0.75. These adjusted cumulative exposures are shown in Table 3-2.

One criticism of the Chovil et al. (1981) study has been that the 25% of the cohort lost to follow-up were counted as survivors to the end of the study in 1978, thereby leading to a potential underestimation of the SMR. To avoid this potential bias, we adjusted the SMRs with the assumption that the rate of lung cancer in those lost to follow-up is the same as in those successfully followed up to the end of 1978. It is generally more difficult to verify survivorship in cohort studies than to identify deaths, thus it is likely that the actual cancer mortality would be less than that estimated by this method. The SMRs were therefore adjusted by multiplying by 1/0.75 because the initial slope was based on cases observed with 75% follow-up of the cohort.

The relative risk model (described earlier) is then utilized in the dose-

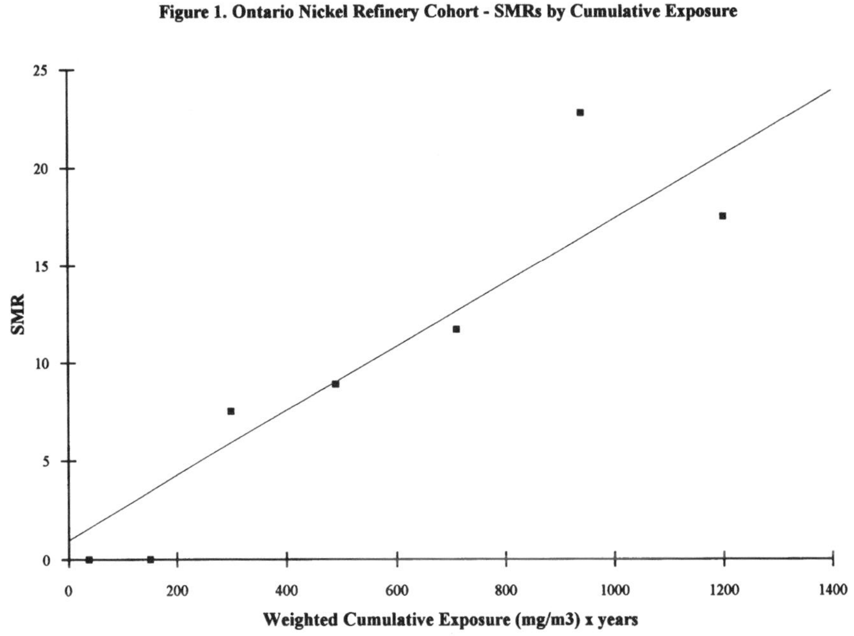

Figure 1. Ontario Nickel Refinery Cohort - SMRs by Cumulative Exposure

Figure 3-1. Ontario Nickel Refinery Cohort: SMRs by cumulative exposure.

response assessment. The SMR values from Table 3-2 were plotted against cumulative exposure (Fig. 3-1). A weighted least squares linear regression analysis using the expected numbers of lung cancer deaths as weights for each exposure category, and forcing an intercept of 1, produced a slope of 16.39 with an upper 95% CI of 20.02 (Table 3-3). This means that for the cohort under study, the upper confidence limit of the excess relative risk is 20.02 for every 1000 (mg/m^3) years. The upper confidence limit is used to yield an estimate of risk that is unlikely to be exceeded.

When using SMRs, one can determine directly lifetime excess cancer risk for a population of workers exposed to nickel through inhalation, using the following model:

$$R_x = R_o(x\beta)$$

where R_x represents the predicted risk to persons with exposure level x, R_o represents the background lifetime risk of dying from lung cancer without nickel exposure, and β represents the upper 95% CI of the slope from the linear relative risk model.

This model is also used to calculate the unit risk estimate (URE) for community exposures. However, a number of additional steps are neces-

Table 3-3. Dose-response calculations for lung cancer mortality based on the Ontario nickel refinery cohort study

Slope of lung cancer SMR versus exposure	16.39
Upper 95% confidence limit on slope	20.02
Unit cumulative exposure level in Figure 3-1	1000 (mg/m^3) × years
Exposure adjustment for 24 hr/day (8/24)	0.33
Adjustment for days per week (5/7)	0.71
Adjustment for weeks per year (48/52)	0.92
Adjusted units of cumulative exposure	216 (mg/m^3) × years
Equivalent lifetime (70-year) exposure level	3.08 mg/m^3
Adjusted upper 95% CI on slope (20.02/3.08 mg/m^3)	6.5
Background lifetime lung cancer mortality risk	0.049
Lifetime added risk for exposure to 1 µg/m^3 (0.049 × 6.5/1000)	0.00032

Note: The calculations are explained in the text.

sary in the linear extrapolation from the unit cumulative exposure of 1000 (mg/m^3) years (Fig. 3-1) for the nickel cohort to a lifetime environmental exposure to 1 µg/m^3. As shown in Table 3-3, adjustments are made for a 24-hour environmental exposure day versus an 8-hour workday, a 7 days per week environmental exposure versus a 5-day work week, and 52 weeks' environmental exposure versus a 48-week work year. The adjusted unit of cumulative exposure was determined to be 216 (mg/m^3) years. Thus, for an environmentally exposed population, the excess relative risk would be 20.02 for each 216 (mg/m^3) yr. In regulatory settings, environmental risk assessment is often based on a 70-year (lifetime) exposure duration. Therefore, the next adjustment in our extrapolation (i.e., 216 [mg/m^3]yr/70 yr = 3.08 mg/m^3) determines that an annual average lifetime exposure to 3.08 mg/m^3 nickel yields an excess relative risk of 20.02. Next we will calculate the URE, or the excess cancer risk associated with a lifetime exposure to 1 µg/m^3 nickel. The background lifetime lung cancer mortality risk for Canada in the years 1963 to 1978 was estimated to be 0.049, or 49 per thousand for males (WHO, 1966–1982). We derived this rate by dividing the total number of lung cancer deaths for the years 1963 to 1978 by the total number of deaths from all causes in those years. Using the model $R_x = R_o(x\beta)$, R_x is the URE, R_o = the background lifetime lung cancer mortality rate of 4.9% (or 0.049), x = 1 µg/m^3, and β = the adjusted slope of 20.02/3.08 mg/m^3, or 6.5 per mg/m^3. Therefore, the excess number of lung cancers expected for a lifetime exposure to 1 µg/m^3 is:

$$\text{unit risk estimate} = 0.049 \times 1 \text{ µg/m}^3 \times 6.5/\text{mg/m}^3 \times 1 \text{ mg/1000 µg}$$
$$= 3.2 \times 10^{-4}$$

or 320 additional lung cancer cases per million people exposed for a lifetime to 1 $\mu g/m^3$ nickel in the air. Calculations of lifetime risks can be made more precise by adjusting for competing causes of death, as described by Gail (1975), but such adjustments usually have negligible effects.

The URE can then be used in the risk characterization phase of environmental risk assessment. For example, the lifetime risk of lung cancer for a community exposed to 0.01 $\mu g/m^3$ nickel in air (a typical air concentration in urban settings), is calculated as follows:

$$\text{excess risk} = 3.2 \times 10^{-4} \; (\mu g/m^3)^{-1} \times 0.01 \; \mu g/m^3$$
$$= 3.2 \times 10^{-6}$$

or 3.2 extra cases of cancer for every million persons exposed to 0.01 $\mu g/m^3$ for a lifetime.

The URE we have derived above for nickel exposure in Canada will be applicable to any other population if the lung cancer risks due to nickel are independent of background causes of lung cancer, particularly smoking. However, if the effects of nickel are synergistic with smoking, then the risks attributable to nickel would be partly dependent on the background rates of lung cancer in other populations of interest, because the effect of nickel exposure would be enhanced by smoking. Thus, if there was little smoking and therefore low background rates of lung cancer, then the risk of exposure to nickel would be lower in that population than if there were a lot of smoking and a high background rate of lung cancer. However, our assessment of the available evidence (Magnus et al., 1982) suggests that the effects of nickel and smoking are additive or close to it, and are therefore independent of background causes of lung cancer. Thus, the URE calculated here can be directly applied when characterizing the lung cancer risk to other populations.

SOURCES OF UNCERTAINTY

Quantitative cancer risk estimation for low-level environmental exposure to carcinogens involves many uncertainties. Nevertheless, systematic, logical, and informed approaches to decision making about carcinogens in the environment calls for quantitative assessments. The real problem with quantitative risk assessment is that findings are sometimes put forward with a degree of implied certainty that has no scientific basis. The estimate of cancer potency for environmental exposure levels must include zero in the range because it is possible that thresholds are present. Thus, the estimate that lifetime exposure to 1 $\mu g/m^3$ nickel might increase cancer risks by as much as 320 per million should be qualified by stating that the increased lung cancer risks may be zero, or they could fall somewhere in the range from zero to 320 per million, but are unlikely to be higher.

The major single source of uncertainty in the above risk assessment is the shape of the dose-response curve, which is based on sparse data. A linear relationship between exposure levels and relative risk was assumed because this fits the data well, and because we know of no evidence to suggest that the relationship is nonlinear.

The second major source of uncertainty involves the adjustment of workplace exposures to equivalent lifetime exposures. The assumption here is that relative risk at a given age relates to cumulative lifetime exposure, whatever the pattern of the exposure in terms of the age at which it was experienced. Thus it is implicitly assumed that someone experiencing continuous exposure from age 0 to age 50 would have the same relative risk as a worker with the same cumulative exposure measure also attained by age 50, but perhaps occurring over only 10 years and confined to the workday. On the one hand, it might be proposed that the lifetime exposure would carry a higher risk because it includes exposure as a child and it is possible that children are more susceptible to carcinogens in the environment. However, this seems unlikely on the basis of epidemiologic data showing very low lung cancer risks under the age of 40. In addition, reductions in cancer risks following cessation of exposure to carcinogens, for example the rapid reduction in lung cancer relative risk after stopping smoking (Office of Smoking and Health, 1982), provides evidence that equating cumulative lifetime risks to shorter-term workplace cumulative exposures should overestimate environmental carcinogen risks. Taken overall, it seems unlikely that the approach adopted leads to an underestimation of cancer risks from lifetime environmental exposures.

The third source of uncertainty involves the workplace exposure estimates themselves. Although it is possible exposures were higher or lower, it seems unlikely that actual exposures would be more than five times higher or five times lower than estimated. In the context of cancer risk assessment, the degree of uncertainty involved here is quite low. It might be noted that animal cancer bioassay studies have more accurate exposure data than occupational epidemiology studies, but the uncertainties in extrapolating risks to humans may involve an order of magnitude or more (Smith, 1988). Use of human data with a two- to fivefold uncertainty in exposure estimation involves less uncertainty overall.

Meta-Analysis in Risk Assessment

Meta-analysis is the structured and systematic qualitative and quantitative integration of the results of several independent studies. As stated earlier, meta-analysis may be a useful tool in the hazard identification and dose-response phases of health risk assessments based on epidemiologic data. Meta-analysis, for which studies are the units of analysis, is different from pooled-data analysis, a method by which raw data from multiple studies of a single topic are combined in a single analysis. Although pooled-data analysis is preferable to meta-analysis in general (Freidenreich, 1993), it is limited by the availability of raw data and is harder to do than meta-analysis. The focus of this section is the use of meta-analysis in hazard identification. Berlin et al. (1993) provide a discussion of the meta-analysis of dose-response data.

The use of meta-analysis in assessing weak causal associations is controversial, especially for observational studies versus clinical trials. A recent group of articles has been published on this controversy (Shapiro, 1994 a,b; Petitti, 1994; Greenland 1994). Shapiro, a strong opponent of meta-analysis of observational studies, stated the opinion that "meta-analysis offers the Holy Grail of attaining statistically stable estimates for effects of low magnitude. In so doing, it ignores what is an absolute limit to epidemiological inference." He proposed that meta-analysis of published non-experimental data should be abandoned.

Greenland (1994) argues that Shapiro's criticisms apply to a prevalent and unsound form of meta-analysis that focuses on synthesis of study results into a single "conclusive" summary estimate. He believes the solution is to adopt a comparative approach in which meta-analysis is used as an aid in comparing studies and identifying patterns among study results. Greenland (1994) states that, "In the absence of ideal studies, there is a potential advantage of meta-analysis (and pooled-data analysis) over any single large study: When used to compare results from different studies meta-analysis can test hypotheses of biases. In contrast, inference from a single study is trapped within the framework of the study design." He does agree, however, that there are problems with synthetic meta-analyses that ignore heterogeneity and report only a single fixed-effects summary.

Despite the controversy surrounding meta-analysis of observational studies, careful and critical application of appropriate meta-analytical techniques facilitates the quantitative exploration of heterogeneities and (where appropriate) syntheses of study results. Methods of quantitative meta-analysis have been reviewed in detail by Greenland (1987), Berlin et al. (1993), and DerSimonian and Laird (1986). The methodology of Greenland (1987) is emphasized here.

The first step in a well-designed meta-analysis is to define the objective—that is, formulate specific goals for the meta-analysis. In epidemiology, this usually means defining the measure of effects to be estimated, or defining the parameters to be estimated within some model for effects (Greenland, 1987). This step also involves the identification of study variables to be included in the meta-analysis, including outcome and exposure.

The second step is to conduct a thorough literature search to gather all relevant published studies. It is possible that published studies are systematically different (more positive) from unpublished studies and therefore meta-analysis based on literature searches alone may lead to "publication bias." This source of bias is discussed further in the example presented later in this chapter. After one has gathered all the relevant published literature, and precisely specified the study exposure and outcome, the next step in the meta-analysis is to identify potential confounders. Some confounders may be generally recognized as so important that any report that fails to fully adjust for them will be immediately suspect (Greenland, 1987). An example of this is cigarette smoking in the study of asbestos and lung cancer.

At this stage of the meta-analysis, inclusion/exclusion criteria should be developed. Inclusion criteria should depend on the specific objectives of the analysis. Some of the variables on which inclusion criteria can be based are the study design, sample size, the outcome of interest, and whether or not the study is published (L'Abbe et al., 1987). Using these criteria, the reviewer should then list the papers to be included and excluded from the meta-analysis.

The next step in the meta-analysis is to record study characteristics for those studies to be included in the analysis. For example, the type of study (cohort, case-control), cohort size, record source, industry, number of deaths from the cause of interest (i.e., lung cancer deaths), the effect measure (i.e., SMR), and the confidence intervals. Extraction of study-specific effect measures and their standard errors from published studies may involve no more than copying it out of the report. Greenland (1987) has reviewed computations that may be necessary to calculate standard errors should only confidence limits or P values be presented rather than standard errors. One may also find that published results are partially or completely unadjusted for known or suspected important confounders, selection bias, and misclassification. Methods for making external adjustments to the effect measures are also described by Greenland (1987).

Once the review and reanalysis of the individual studies are completed, the statistical meta-analysis can be performed. The fundamental meta-analytic approach described by Greenland (1987) is a "fixed-effect" model and is based on weighted regression that treats each study result as the dependent variable with an accompanying weight. The weighted mean of the study results is then calculated. The appropriateness of the weighted mean as a meta-analytic summary of the effect under study depends on a very stringent homogeneity assumption. This assumption states that the studies are estimating the same value for the effect (i.e., "fixed effect"). In other words, after consideration of the extent of real effect and bias in each study, the studies should on average yield the same value, so that differences between the estimates are entirely due to random error. This will clearly not be true if the studies have different average doses, and if a greater dose causes a greater effect. In fact, one should regard any homogeneity assumption as extremely unlikely to be satisfied, because of the differences in covariates, bias, and exposure variables among the studies (Greenland, 1987).

An important aspect of meta-analysis is to qualitatively and quantitatively analyze any heterogeneity that may be present. For multiple studies, the chi-squared test can be employed as basic statistical test of the homogeneity assumption; it is included in the example presented below. If a large amount of unexplained heterogeneity remains, one may consider turning to "random-effect" models (Colditz et al., 1995; Greenland, 1987; DerSimonian and Laird, 1986). With this approach, both random variation within studies and heterogeneity between studies is taken into account. When heterogeneity is present, the estimated confidence interval is more conservative (i.e., wider) than it would have been on the fixed-effect assumption. Criticism of the random-effect approach is that it is based on the assumptions that the studies are representative of some hypothetical population of studies and that heterogeneity between the studies can be represented by a single variance (Thompson and Pocock, 1991). Thompson and Pocock also note that undue weight may be given to small studies that themselves are the most likely to be influenced by publication bias. A number of investigators believe that a more useful approach is to focus on possible reasons for heterogeneity (Thompson and Pocock, 1991; Greenland, 1987). Colditz et al. (1995) have recently reviewed various approaches taken to identify, deal with, and interpret heterogeneity in meta-analysis of epidemiologic data and suggest methods that may be used in future studies. Berlin (1995) has supplemented the Colditz et al. (1995) review by commenting on the benefits of heterogeneity in meta-analysis of epidemiologic data. These and other issues arising from the application of meta-analytic methods will be discussed further in the example presented below.

The steps described earlier were undertaken in the following example of a simple meta-analysis using the fixed-effect model. We use as an example the possible association of silicosis and lung cancer. Although this example is not environmental, it nonetheless illustrates the basic principles of meta-analysis. This example is based on the more detailed meta-analysis performed by Smith et al. (1995).

Example: Is silicosis a risk factor for lung cancer?

Interpretation of the literature concerning the carcinogenicity of silica and an association between silicosis and lung cancer has been controversial. Studies among silicotics tend to demonstrate an excess risk of lung cancer but have been criticized because of possible selection and confounding biases. Other complications affecting the interpretation of the results arise from competing risks from other causes of death, such as silicosis and tuberculosis. In this example of meta-analysis in hazard identification, published data of lung cancer mortality among silicotics were combined to evaluate quantitatively the possible association of silicosis and an increased risk of lung cancer.

METHODS

This meta-analysis was conducted following general principles such as those outlined by L'Abbe et al. (1987). The epidemiologic literature was searched for all studies giving data concerning silicosis and lung cancer. When a study had been published in different articles, only the most recent report was included in the analysis.

The effect measures (relative risks, odds ratios, etc.) for lung cancer mortality among silicotics and their confidence intervals were extracted from each study for use in the meta-analysis. Missing confidence intervals were estimated by Byar's approximation (IARC, 1987) for cohort studies or by the "test-based method" described by Miettinen (1976) for case-control studies. If information on lung cancer mortality was not provided then total respiratory cancer mortality was used. When an SMR analysis used both national and regional populations to calculate expected deaths, the results based on regional disease rates were used in the meta-analysis.

The method of weighting by precision described by Greenland (1987) was used for the meta-analysis. The weight or inverse variance ($w=1/SE^2$) of each study was calculated using a standard error (SE) equal to the natural log of the ratio of the upper to lower 95% confidence intervals divided by 3.92 ($SE=\ln(RR_{upper}/RR_{lower})/3.92$). The weight (w) was then multiplied by the natural log of the effect measure (b). A weighted mean or pooled summary ($\bar{b}$) was then calculated by dividing the sum of the weighted results (Σwb) by the sum of the weights (Σw).

Pooled summaries were estimated for all studies combined, and separately for cohort studies, case-control studies, and studies giving mortality odds ratios (MOR) or standardized incidence ratios (SIR). All pooled summaries were converted into rate ratios ($RR=\exp \bar{b}$) and 95% confidence intervals were estimated. A statistical test of heterogeneity was applied to all pooled summaries where $X^2 = \Sigma w(b - \bar{b})^2$ has a chi-squared distribution with degrees of freedom one less than the number of studies.

RESULTS

Twenty-nine studies were found in the published literature with data concerning lung cancer and silicosis. Information on the industry and record sources for the study participants, number of lung cancer deaths, effect measures and confidence intervals are detailed in Table 3-4. The study weights and any corrections are also given. Twenty-three of the 29 studies found were used in the meta-analysis.

Fourteen of the studies were cohort studies involving SMRs for lung cancer that ranged from 1.1 to 4.4. Armstrong et al. (1979) reported results for all respiratory cancers combined.

Four case-control studies included in the meta-analysis involved odds ratios ranging from 1.8 to 3.9 for lung cancer death. Additional studies included three cohort studies of lung cancer incidence (SIRs range from 1.7 to 2.9) and two studies that calculated mortality odds ratios (MOR=1.5 and 2.2).

Six studies were excluded from the meta-analysis because they suffered from biases that clearly underestimated or overestimated the risk of lung cancer for silicotics. For example, the proportionate mortality study of Rubino et al. (1990) underestimated the lung cancer mortality because the PMR was calculated without regard to competing causes of death for silicosis. The findings of the autopsy-based case-control studies of Hessel and Sluis-Cremer (1986), Hessel et al. (1990), and Hnizdo and Sluis-Cremer (1991) were also found to have underestimated the risk of lung cancer from silicosis. The controls in these autopsy studies may have had other diseases associated with silicosis.

Also excluded from the meta-analysis are two studies based on hospital records that gave SMRs of 5.0 (Chiyotani et al., 1990) and 6.0 (Merlo et al., 1990). The findings from these studies are likely to be biased upward because silicotics with lung cancer are more likely to be admitted to hospitals than silicotics without lung cancer.

The pooled relative risk (RR) for all studies combined (excluding those with competing risk problems and studies based on hospital records) was 2.2 ($P < .001$) with a 95% confidence interval of 2.1–2.4 (Table 3-5). The highest pooled RR of 2.7 was found for the set of studies of lung cancer incidence (CI 2.3–3.2; $P < .001$). Combination of cohort, case-control studies, and MORs yielded pooled RRs of 2.0 (CI 1.8–2.3; $P < .001$), 2.5 (CI 1.8–3.3; $P < .001$), and 2.0 (CI 1.7–2.4; $P < .001$), respectively.

Table 3-4. Summary of studies of silicosis and lung cancer with effect measures, 95% confidence intervals (CI) and weightings (W) for meta-analysis

Reference	Record Source/ Industry	Lung Cancer Deaths	Effect Measure	CI	W
Cohort Studies			*SMR*		
Amandus and Costello (1991)	Medical exam/mining	14	1.7	0.9–2.9	11.2
Amandus et al. (1991)	Medical exam/misc.	33	3.0	2.0–4.2	27.9
Armstrong et al. (1979)	Medical exam/mining	21	1.1	0.6–2.0	10.6
Carta et al. (1991)	Medical exam/misc.	22	1.3	0.8–2.0	18.3
Chen et al. (1992)	Silicosis registry/misc.	?	1.2	0.9–1.6	46.4
Finkelstein et al. (1987)	Compensation/mining and surface workers	78	2.4	1.8–3.2	46.4
Infante-Rivard et al. (1989)	Compensation/misc.	83	3.5	2.8–4.3[a]	83.5
Mehnert et al. (1990)	Compensation/quarry	9	1.8	0.8–3.5	7.1
Neuberger et al. (1986)	Compensation/misc.	42	1.4	1.0–1.9	37.3
Ng et al. (1990)	Compensation/misc.	28	2.0	1.4–2.9	29.0
Puntoni et al. (1988)	Compensation/ refractory brick	6	1.7	0.7–3.6	5.7
Tornling et al. (1990)	Pneumo. registry/ misc.	9	1.9	0.8–3.6	6.8

Study	Comparison	N	Ratio	CI	
Westerholm et al. (1986)	Pneumo. registry/misc	17	4.4	2.0–8.3	7.6
Zambon et al. (1986)	Compensation/misc.	49	2.3	1.7–3.0	47.6
Case-control Studies			*OR*		
Cocco et al. (1990)	Medical exam/misc.	15	2.4	1.0–6.2	4.6
Lagorio et al. (1990)	Compensation/misc.	15	3.9	1.8–8.3	6.6
Mastrangelo et al. (1988)	Compensation/misc.	50	1.8	1.1–2.8	17.6
Steenland & Beaumont (1986)	Silicosis on death certificate/granite	26	3.2	1.6–6.3[b]	8.2
Standardized Incidence Ratios			*SIR*		
Chia et al. (1991)	Silicosis registry/misc.	9	2.0	0.9–3.9	7.1
Partanen et al. (1994)	Silicosis registry/misc.	101	2.9	2.4–3.5	107.9
Sherson et al. (1991)	Medical exam/foundry	11	1.7	0.9–3.1	10.0
Mortality Odds Ratios			*MOR*		
Forastiere et al. (1989)	Compensation/ceramic	64	1.5	1.1–1.9	51.4
Schuler and Ruttner (1986)	National Accident Ins. Fund/misc.	180	2.2	1.8–2.7[b]	93.5

[a] Confidence intervals calculated based on Byar's approximation.

[b] Test-based confidence intervals based on Miettinen, 1976.

Table 3-5. Statistics for meta-analysis of silicosis and lung cancer studies: analysis of all studies combined and by study design

	All Studies	Cohort	Case-control	MOR	SIR
Weighted sum ($\sum wb$)[a]	544.3	286.5	33.7	95.4	128.7
Sum of weights ($\sum w$)	692.3	385.4	37.0	144.9	125.0
Summary $\bar{b}$ ($\sum wb / \sum w$)	0.8	0.7	0.9	0.7	1.0
RR = exp $\bar{b}$	2.2	2.0	2.5	2.0	2.7
Standard error s of $\bar{b}$ ($1/\mathrm{sqr}\sum w$)	0.04	0.06	0.16	0.08	0.09
95% confidence intervals for RR[b]	2.1–2.4	1.8–2.3	1.8–3.3	1.7–2.4	2.3–3.2
Z statistic ($\bar{b}/s$)	20.0	11.7	5.6	8.8	11.1
Homogeneity chi-squared	89.1	57.7	4.0	5.6	4.2
Homogeneity degrees of freedom	22	13	3	1	2

[a] b = log (effect measure)
[b] exp(b ± 1.96s)

The results of the test of homogeneity were statistically significant (i.e., the studies are considered heterogeneous) for all studies combined and for the set of cohort studies (Table 3-5). A heterogeneity P value of 0.3 was estimated for the four case-control studies. The three studies of lung cancer incidence yielded a P value of approximately 0.1.

DISCUSSION

The results of this meta-analysis suggest that there is approximately a two-fold increase in the risk of lung cancer for patients with silicosis. The pooled RRs are consistent across study type. When considered individually, all of the studies found in the literature demonstrated effect measures greater than 1.0. Fifteen of these studies reported confidence intervals that exclude 1.0. Consequently, it is extremely unlikely that the increased lung cancer risk is attributable to chance.

One potential bias affecting the relationship between silicosis and lung cancer is confounding by cigarette smoking. Data on smoking have not been consistently available, and some studies relied on indirect methods of controlling for smoking (Ng, 1990; Forastiere et al., 1989; Merlo et al., 1990). However, four studies included in the meta-analysis did adjust for smoking in their analysis of lung cancer risk among silicotics (Amandus and Costello, 1991; Amandus et al., 1991; Cocco et al., 1990; Lagorio et al., 1990). The smoking-adjusted effect measures were found to be higher than the unadjusted results for all four studies. These findings suggest that the increased risk of lung cancer among silicotics is not attributable to smoking. In fact, there is little consistent evidence that smoking is a risk factor for silicosis, and therefore confounding by smoking would not be expected, or would at best be a very weak confounder in the relationship between lung cancer and silicosis.

Another question concerns whether or not silicosis can lead to lung cancer in the absence of smoking. Elevated lung cancer risks were apparent in two studies that calculated expected deaths from lung cancer based on nonsmokers (Amandus et al., 1991; Mastrangelo et al., 1988). An SMR of 8.6 (CI 3.6–20.5) was calculated in the study by Amandus et al., and an OR of 5.3 (CI 0.5–43.5) was obtained in the Mastrangelo et al. study. Thus, the overall evidence supports increased risks of lung cancer in silicotics who do not smoke.

Other possible biases might result from the choice of external referent populations based on other lifestyle or socioeconomic differences between occupational groups and national populations. In addition, studies based on compensation for silicosis could be biased toward a silicosis–lung cancer relation if diagnosis of lung cancer affected detection of silicosis. Selection bias might also result if cases of silicosis were determined by voluntary medical examination. Smith et al. (1995) discuss these potential biases in greater detail.

The studies of lung cancer risk among silicotics have also been criticized because they often include workers from industries where exposure to other lung carcinogens would have occurred (i.e., PAHs in foundries; radon and arsenic in mines). However, elevated lung cancer risks have been demonstrated in silicotics from granite and stone industries where the principal risk factor is exposure to silica and exposure to other potential carcinogens is unlikely (Finkelstein et al., 1987; Infante-Rivard et al., 1989; Mehnert et al., 1990; Zambon et al., 1986; Steenland and Beaumont, 1986; Kurppa et al., 1986).

Publication bias is a potential limitation in any meta-analysis. Although a tendency to report and publish positive results has been well documented, results of large studies generally approximate the results of all studies published and unpublished (Felson, 1992). Moreover, large studies are generally published whether or not their results are "positive" (Begg and Berlin, 1989). Of the 29 studies found in the peer-reviewed literature, seven studies examined cohorts of over 1000 silicotics (Chen et al., 1992; Finkelstein et al., 1987; Infante-Rivard et al., 1989; Ng et al. 1990; Zambon et al., 1986; Schuler & Ruttner, 1986; Chiyotani et al., 1990). All of the lung cancer relative risk estimates were greater than 1.0. Six of the seven studies were included in the meta-analysis. The pooled effect measure for these studies is 2.2 (95% CI, 2.0–2.5). Ten of the 29 studies reported results for 50 or more lung cancer deaths or cases (Finkelstein et al., 1987; Infante-Rivard et al., 1989; Mastrangelo et al., 1988; Partanen et al., 1994; Forastiere et al., 1989; Schuler & Ruttner, 1986; Rubino et al., 1990; Hessel and Sluis-Cremer, 1986; Hessel et al., 1990; Hnizdo & Sluis-Cremer, 1991). Six of these studies were included in the meta-analysis. The pooled RR was estimated at 2.5 (95% CI, 2.2–2.7). Thus, publication bias is unlikely in this meta-analysis.

Heterogeneity among studies is another problem in many meta-analyses, as discussed earlier. Any group of epidemiologic studies is likely to be heterogeneous by virtue of differences in exposure level, in study design, variation in background rates and differences in length of follow-up, case identification, and so on. The advantage of the weighting method applied in the present analysis is that effect measures from studies with small sample sizes contribute less to the pooled estimate. Possible reasons for heterogeneity particular to studies among silicotics include differences between countries in defining silicosis and possible differences in disease detection methods, patterns of smoking, and choice of referent population. The form of crystalline silica (for example, quartz and cristobalite) to which individuals are exposed would also vary. Because the fibrogenic potential of the various forms differs, so might the potential carcinogenicity. The sources of heterogeneity in this meta-analysis are analyzed in greater detail by Smith et al. (1995).

Finally, the basic hypothesis of this review, that silicosis may lead to lung cancer, is biologically plausible. Silica-induced carcinogenesis has been demonstrated based on studies in the rat (Dagle et al., 1986; Groth et al., 1986; Holland et al., 1983; Holland et al., 1986; Muhle et al., 1989; Spiethoff et al., 1992). However, neither fibrosis nor carcinogenesis has been demonstrated in silica-exposed hamsters (Holland et al., 1983; Renne et al., 1985; Saffiotti, 1992). Silica has been shown to induce fibrotic lesions in the mouse although the carcinogenicity of silica has not been adequately tested in this species (Holland, 1990).

The results of this meta-analysis demonstrate that there are, indeed, increased risks of lung cancer among persons diagnosed with silicosis. It remains unclear whether silicosis itself is involved in lung cancer etiology or whether it is instead an indicator of heavy exposure to silica.

CONCLUSIONS

Environmental risk assessment is the quantification of potential adverse health effects of human exposure to environmental hazards. Good epidemiologic studies, when available, are generally considered to be the best source of data for use in risk assessment. One advantage is that they provide direct evidence for carcinogenic or other health effects in humans, thus avoiding the uncertainty of interspecies extrapolation. However, epidemiologic studies do not show cause-effect or dose-response relationships with the same ease as do experimental studies in animals. Clearly, more can be learned from available epidemiologic studies by a careful, critical, and comprehensive review. Because of the rapid growth of epidemiology over the past decades, the traditional narrative literature review is not always the simplest method of summarizing the results of a collection of studies. Meta-analysis, if appropriately conducted, is an alternative approach to the qualitative and quantitative analysis of a collection of epidemiologic study results, and it can be a valuable tool in the risk assessment process.

References

Allen BC, Crump KS, Shipp AM. 1988. Correlation between carcinogenic potency of chemicals in animals and humans. Risk Analysis 8(4): 531–561.

Amandus HE, Costello J. 1991. Silicosis and lung cancer in U.S. metal miners. Arch Environ Health 46(2): 82–89.

Amandus HE, Shy C, Wing S, Blair A, Heineman EF. 1991. Silicosis and lung cancer in North Carolina Dusty Trades workers. Am J Ind Med 20: 57–70.

Ames BN, Gold LS. 1990a. Too many rodent carcinogens: mitogenesis increases mutagenesis. Science 249: 970.

Ames BN, Gold LS. 1990b. Carcinogens and human health: Part 1 (Letter). Science 250: 1645.

Ames BN, Gold LS. 1991. Carcinogenesis mechanisms: the debate continues (Letter). Science 252: 902.

Armitage P, Doll R. 1954. The age of distribution of cancer and a multi-stage theory of carcinogenesis. Br J Cancer 8: 1–12.

Armstrong BK, McNulty JC, Levitt LJ, Williams KA, Hobbs MS. 1979. Mortality in gold and coal miners in Western Australia with special reference to lung cancer. Br J Ind Med 36: 199–205.

Begg CB, Berlin JA. 1989. Publication bias and dissemination of clinical research. J Natl Cancer Inst 81: 107–114.

Berlin JA, Longnecker MP, Greenland S. 1993. Meta-analysis of epidemiologic dose-response data. Epidemiology 4: 218–228.

Berlin JA. 1995. Invited commentary: benefits of heterogeneity in meta-analysis of data from epidemiologic studies. Am J Epidemiol 142: 383–387.

Bernstein L, Gold LS, Ames BN, Pike MC, Hoel DG. 1985a. Some tautologous aspects of the comparison of carcinogenic potency in rats and mice. Fundam Appl Toxicol 5: 79–86.

Bernstein L, Gold LS, Ames BN, Pike MC, Hoel DG. 1985b. Toxicity and carcinogenic potency. Risk Analysis 5: 263–264.

Carta P, Cocco PL, Casula D. 1991. Mortality from lung cancer among Sardinian patients with silicosis. Br J Ind Med 48: 122–129.

Chen J, McLaughlin JK, Zhang J-Y, Stone BJ, Luo J, Chen R, Dosemeci M, Rexing SH, Wu Z, Hearl FJ, McCawley MA, Blot WJ. 1992. Mortality among dust-exposed Chinese mine and pottery workers. J Occup Environ Med 34(3): 311–316.

Chia S-E, Chia K-S, Phoon W-H, Lee HP. 1991. Silicosis and lung cancer among Chinese granite workers. Scand J Work Environ Health 17: 170–174.

Chiyotani K, Saito K, Okubo T, Takahashi K. 1990. Lung cancer risk among pneumoconiosis patients in Japan, with special reference to silicotics. In: Simonato L, Fletcher AC, Saracci R, Thomas TL, eds. Occupational Exposure to Silica and Cancer Risk. IARC, Lyon, France: 95–104.

Chovil A, Sutherland RB, Halliday M. 1981. Respiratory cancer in a cohort of nickel sinter plant workers. Br J Ind Med 38: 327–333.

Cocco P, Carta P, Bario P, Manca P, Casula D. 1990. Case-control study on silicosis and lung cancer. In: Sakurai H, et al, eds. Occupational Epidemiology. Excerpta Medica, Amsterdam 79–82.

Cogliano VJ, Farland WH, Preuss PW, Wiltse JA, Rhomberg LR, Chen CW, Mass MJ, Nosnow S, White PD, Parker JC, Wuerthele SM. 1991. Carcinogens and human health: Part 3 (Letter). Science 251: 606.

Coldidtz GA, Burdick E, Mosteller F. 1995. Heterogeneity in meta-analysis of data from epidemiologic studies: a commentary. Am J Epidemiol 142: 371–382.

Crouch E, Wilson R. 1979. Inter-species comparison of carcinogenic potency. J Toxicol Environ Health 5: 1095–1118.

Crump KS, Guess HA, Deal KL. 1977. Confidence intervals and test hypotheses concerning dose response relations inferred from animal carcinogenicity data. Biometrics 33: 437–451.

Dagle GE, Wehner AP, Clark ML, Buschbom RL. 1986. Chronic inhalation exposure of rats to quartz. In: Goldsmith DF, Winn DM, Shy CM, eds. Silica, Silicosis, and Cancer. Praeger, New York: 255–266.

DerSimonian R, Laird N. 1986. Meta-analysis in clinical trials. Control Clin Trials 7:177–188.

Enterline PE. 1987. A method for estimating lifetime cancer risks from limited epidemiologic data. Risk Analysis 7(1): 91–96.

Enterline PE, Marsh GM. 1982. Mortality among workers in a nickel refinery and alloy manufacturing plant in West Virginia. J Natl Cancer Inst 68: 925–933.

Environmental Protection Agency. 1993. A Descriptive Guide to Risk Assessment Methodologies for Toxic Air Pollutants. Environmental Protection Agency, Office of Air Quality Planning and Standards, EPA-453/R-93-038. PB94-181880, Research Triangle Park, NC.

Environmental Protection Agency. 1983a. Good laboratory practices standards—toxicology testing. Environmental Protection Agency. Federal Registar 48, 53922.

Environmental Protection Agency. 1983b. Hazard Evaluations: Humans and Domestic Animals. Environmental Protection Agency, PB 83-153916.

Environmental Protection Agency. 1983c. Health Effects Test Guidelines. Environmental Protection Agency, PB 83-232984.

Environmental Protection Agency. 1986. Health Assessment Document for Nickel and Nickel Compounds. Environmental Protection Agency, PB 86-232212.

Environmental Protection Agency. 1987. Qualitative and Quantitative Carcinogenic Risk Assessment. Environmental Protection Agency, Office of Air Quality Planning and Standards. Research Triangle Park, NC.

Environmental Protection Agency. 1989. Workshop Report on EPA Guidelines for Carcinogen Risk Assessment: Use of Human Evidence. Environmental Protection Agency, Risk Assessment Forum.

Felson DT. 1992. Bias in meta-analytic research. J Clin Epidemiol 45(8): 885–892.

Finkelstein M, Liss GM, Krammer F, Kusiak RA. 1987. Mortality among workers receiving compensation awards for silicosis in Ontario 1940–85. Br J Ind Med 44: 588–594.

Forastiere F, Lagorio S, Michelozzi P, Perucci CA, Axelson O. 1989. Mortality pattern of silicotic subjects in the Latium region, Italy. Br J Ind Med 46: 877–880.

Freedman DA, Gold LS, Slone TH. 1993. How tautological are interspecies correlations of carcinogenic potencies? Risk Analysis 13: 265–272.

Freidenreich C. 1993. Methods for pooled analyses of epidemiologic studies. Epidemiology 4: 295–302.

Gail M. 1975. Measuring the benefits of reduced exposure to environmental carcinogens. J Chronic Dis 28: 135–147.

Grandjean P, Andersen O, Nielsen GD. 1988. Carcinogenicity of occupational nickel exposures: an evaluation of the epidemiological evidence. Am J Ind Med 13(2): 193–209.

Greenland S. 1994. Can meta-analysis be salvaged? Am J Epidemiol 140(9): 783–787.

Greenland S. 1987. Quantitative methods in the review of epidemiologic literature. Epidemiol Rev 9: 1–30.

Groth DH, Stettler LE, Platek SF, Lal JB, Burg JR. 1986. Lung tumors in rats treated with quartz by intratracheal instillation. In: Goldsmith DF, Winn DM, Shy CM, eds. Silica, Silicoses, and Cancer. Praeger, New York: 243–253.

Haseman JK, Lockhart A-M. 1993. Correlations between chemically related site-specific carcinogenic effects in long-term studies in rats and mice. Environ Health Perspect 101(1): 50–54.

Hertz-Picciotto I. 1995. Epidemiology and quantitative risk assessment: a bridge from science to policy. Am J Public Health 85(4): 484–493.

Hessel PA, Sluis-Cremer GK. 1986. Case-control study of lung cancer and silicosis. In: Goldsmith DF, Winn DM, Shy CM, eds. Silica, Silicosis, and Cancer. Praeger, New York: 351–355.

Hessel PA, Sluis-Cremer GK, Hnizdo E. 1990. Silica exposure, silicosis, and lung cancer: a necropsy study. Br J Ind Med 47: 4–9.

Hnizdo E, Sluis-Cremer GK. 1991. Silica exposure, silicosis, and lung cancer: a mortality study of South African gold miners. Br J Ind Med 48: 53–60.

Holland LM. 1990. Crystalline silica and lung cancer: a review of recent experimental evidence. Regul Toxicol Pharmacol 12: 224–237.

Holland LM, Gonzales M, Wilson JS, Tillery MI. 1983. Pulmonary effects of shale dusts in experimental animals. In: Wagner WL, Rom WN, Merchant JA, eds. Health Issues Related to Metal and Nonmetallic Mining. Butterworth, Boston, MA: 485–496.

Holland LM, Wilson JS, Tillery MI, Smith DM. 1986. Lung cancer in rats exposed to fibrogenic dusts. In: Goldsmith DF, Winn DM, Shy CM, eds. Silica, Silicosis, and Cancer. Praeger, New York: 267–279.

Huff JE, Haseman JK. 1991. Exposure to certain pesticides may pose real carcinogenic risk. Chem Eng News 69: 33.

Huff J, Hoel D. 1992. Perspective and overview of the concepts and value of hazard identification as the initial phase of risk assessment for human health. Scand J Work Environ Health 18(suppl 1): 83–89.

IARC. 1987. Statistical Methods in Cancer Research, Volume II: The Design and Analysis of Cohort Studies. IARC Scientific Publications No. 82, International Agency for Research on Cancer, Lyon, France.

Infante PF. 1991. Prevention versus chemophobia: a defence of rodent carcinogenicity tests. Lancet 337: 538.

Infante-Rivard C, Armstrong B, Petitclerc M, Cloutier L-G, Theriault G. 1989. Lung cancer mortality and silicosis in Quebec, 1938–85. Lancet 23(30): 1504–1507.

ICNCM. 1990. Report of the International Committee on Nickel Carcinogenesis. Scand J Work Environ Health 10(1 Special Issue): 9–81.

Kreyberg L. 1978. Lung cancer in workers in a nickel refinery. Br J Ind Med 35: 109–116.

Kurppa K, Gudbergsson H, Hannunkari I, Koskinen H, Hernber S, Koskela R-S, Ahlman K. Lung cancer among silicotics in Finland. In: Goldsmith DF, Winn DM, Shy CM, eds. Silica, Silicosis and Cancer. Praeger, New York: 311–319.

L'Abbe KA, Detsky AS, O'Rourke K. 1987. Meta-analysis in clinical research. Ann Intern Med 107: 224–233.

Lagorio S, Forastiere F, Michelozzi P, Cavariani F, Perucci CA, Axelson O. 1990. A case-referent study on lung cancer mortality among ceramic workers. In: Simonato L, Fletcher AC, Saracci R, Thomas TL eds. Occupational Exposure to Silica and Cancer Risk. International Agency for Research on Cancer, Lyon, France: 21–28.

Magnus K, Andersen A, Hogetveit AC. 1982. Cancer of respiratory organs among workers at a nickel refinery in Norway. Int J Cancer 30: 681–685.

Mastrangelo G, Zambon P, Simonato L, Rizzi P. 1988. A case-referent study investigating the relationship between exposure to silica dust and lung cancer. Int Arch Occup Environ Health 60: 299–302.

Mehnert WH, Staneczek W, Mohner M, Konetzke G, Muller W, Ahlendorf W, Beck B, Winkelmann R, Simonato L. 1990. A mortality study of a cohort of slate quarry workers in the German Democratic Republic. In: Simonato L, Fletcher AC Saracci R, Thomas TL, eds. Occupational Exposure to Silica and Cancer Risk. International Agency for Research on Cancer, Lyon, France: 55–64.

Merlo F, Doria M, Fontana L, Ceppi M, Chesi E, Santi L. 1990. Mortality from specific causes among silicotic subjects: a historical prospective study. In: Simonato L, Fletcher AC Saracci R, Thomas TL, eds. Occupational Exposure to Silica and Cancer Risk. International Agency for Research on Cancer, Lyon, France: 105–111.

Miettinen OS. 1976. Estimability and estimation in case-referent studies. Am J Epidemiol 103: 226–235.

Moolgavkar S, Knudson A. 1981. Mutation and cancer: a model for human carcinogenesis. JNCI 66: 1037–1052.

Morgan LG. 1985. Atmospheric monitoring of nickel-containing dusts at the INCO refinery in Clydach, Wales. In: Brown SS, Sunderman FW Jr, eds. Progress in Nickel Toxicology: Proceedings of the Third International Conference on Nickel Metabolism and Toxicology; Paris 4–7 September 1984. Blackwell Scientific Publications, Oxford: 183–186.

Muhle H, Takenaka S, Mohr U, Dasenbrock C, Mermelstein R. 1989. Lung tumor induction upon long-term low-level inhalation of crystalline silica. Am J Ind Med 15: 343–346.

National Toxicology Program. 1984. Report of the Ad Hoc Panel on Chemical Carcinogenesis Testing and Evaluation of the National Toxicology Program, Board of Scientific Counselors. US Government Printing Office, Washington, DC 1984-421-132:4726.

Neuberger M, Kundi M, Westphal G, Grundorfer W. 1986. The Viennese dusty worker study. In: Goldsmith DF, Winn DM, Shy CM, eds. Silica, Silicosis and Cancer. Praeger, New York: 415–422.

Ng TP, Chan SL, Lee J. 1990. Mortality of a cohort of men in a silicosis register: further evidence of an association with lung cancer. Am J Ind Med 17: 163–171.

Office on Smoking and Health. 1982. The Health Consequences of Smoking: Cancer. A report of the Surgeon General, US Department of Health and Human Services, Public Health Service, Maryland.

Partanen T, Pukkala E, Vainio H, Kurppa K, Koskinen H. 1994. Increased incidence of lung and skin cancer in Finnish silicotic patients. J Occup Environ Med 36(6): 616–622.

Perera FP. 1990. Carcinogens and human health: Part 1 (Letter). Science 250: 1644.

Petitti DB. 1994. Of babies and bathwater. Am J Epidemiol 140(9): 779–782.

Piegorsch W, Carr G, Portier C, Hoel D. 1992. Concordance of carcinogenic response between rodent species: potency dependence and potential underestimation. Risk Analysis 12: 115–121.

Puntoni R, Goldsmith DF, Valerio F, Vercelli M, Bonassi S, Di Giorgio F, Ceppi M, Stagnaro E, Filiberti R, Santi L, Merlo F. 1988. A cohort study of workers employed in a refractory brick plant. Tumori 74: 27–35.

Rall DP. 1991. Carcinogens and human health: Part 2 (Letter). Science 251: 10.

Renne RA, Eldridge SR, Lewis TR, Stevens DL. 1985. Fibrogenic potential of intratracheally instilled quartz, ferric oxide, fibrous glass, and hydrated alumina in hamsters. Toxicol Pathol 13(4): 306–314.

Rothman KJ. 1986. Modern Epidemiology. Little, Brown and Company, Boston.

Rubino GF, Scansetti G, Piolatto G, Coggiola M, Giachino GM. 1990. Cancer mortality among silicotic cases. In: Marconi A, ed. Pneumocomioses Conference Poster Session IV. National Health Institute, Rome, Italy: 1509–1513.

Saffiotti U. 1992. Lung cancer induction by crystalline silica. In: Relevance of Animal Studies to the Evaluation of Human Cancer Risk. Wiley-Liss, Inc: 51–69.

Schuler G, Ruttner JR. 1986. Silicosis and lung cancer in Switzerland. In: Goldsmith DF, Winn DM, Shy CM, eds. Silica, Silicosis and Cancer. Praeger, New York: 357–366.

Shapiro S. 1994a. Meta-analysis of observational studies: meta-analysis/shmeta-analysis. Am J Epidemiol 140(9): 771–778.

Shapiro S. 1994b. Is there is or is there ain't no baby: Dr Shapiro replies to Drs Petitti and Greenland. Am J Epidemiol 140(9): 788–791.

Sherson D, Svane O, Lynge E. 1991. Cancer incidence among foundry workers in Denmark. Arch Environ Health 46(21): 75–81.

Shore RE, Iyer Vaidyanath, Altshuler B, Pasternack B. 1992. Use of human data in quantitative risk assessment of carcinogens: impact on epidemiologic practice and the regulatory process. Regul Toxicol Pharmacol 15: 180–221.

Smith AH. 1988. Epidemiologic input to environmental risk assessment. Arch Environ Health 43(2): 124–127.

Smith AH, Lopipero PA, Barroga VR. 1996. Meta-analysis of studies of lung cancer among silicotics. Epidemiology 6: 617–625

Spiethoff A, Wesch H, Wegener K, Klimisch H-J. 1992. The effects of thorotrast and quartz on the induction of lung tumors in rats. Health Phys 63(1): 101–110.

Stayner L, Smith R, Bailer J, Luebeck EG, Moolgavkar SH. 1994. Modeling epidemiologic studies of occupational cohorts for the quantitative assessment of carcinogenic hazards. Am J Ind Med 27: 155–170.

Steenland K, Beaumont J. 1986. A proportionate mortality study of granite cutters. Am J Ind Med 9: 189–201.

Thompson SG, Pocock SJ. 1991. Can meta-analyses be trusted? Lancet 338: 1127–1130.

Tornling G, Hogstedt C, Westerhom P. 1990. Lung cancer incidence among Swedish ceramic workers with silicosis. In: Fletcher AC, Saracci R, Thomas TL, eds. Occupational Exposure to Silica and Cancer Risk. Lyon, France: IARC Scientific Publications No. 97; 113–119.

Warner JS. 1985. Estimating past exposures to airborne nickel compounds in the Copper Cliff sinter plant. In: Brown SS, Sunderman FW Jr, eds. Progress in Nickel Toxicology: Proceedings of the Third International Conference on Nickel Metabolism and Toxicology, Paris 4–7 September 1984. Blackwell Scientific Publications, Oxford: 203–206.

Westerholm P, Ahlmark A, Maasing R, Segelberg I. 1986. Silicosis and lung cancer—a cohort study. In: Goldsmith DF, Winn DM, Shy CM, eds. Silica Silicosis and Cancer. Praeger, New York: 327–333.

World Health Organization. 1966–1982. World Health Statistics, 1963–1978 Vol 1: Vital Statistics and Causes of Death. WHO, Geneva.

Zambon P, Simonato L, Mastrangelo G, Winkelmann R, Saia B, Crepet M. 1986. A mortality study of workers compensated for silicosis during 1959 to 1963 in the Veneto region of Italy. In: Goldsmith DE, Winn DM, Shy CM, eds. Silica, Silicosis and Cancer. Praeger, New York: 367–374.

Diet and Food Contaminants

4

MANUEL POSADA DE LA PAZ

DISEASES caused by food have long been a major concern of humankind and have also been a major concern of environmental epidemiology. Historically, food contamination by microbial agents has caused most outbreaks. Contamination of food by infectious agents such as cholera continues to be extremely important in developing countries, as witnessed by the cholera outbreak in Peru in 1995, for example.

With the development of refrigeration and better systems of food processing, contamination of food by infectious agents has become less problemmatic in developed countries. Nevertheless, outbreaks continue to occur (e.g., the recent *Escherichia coli* poisoning from poorly cooked hamburgers in the United States and possibly the transmission of "mad cow" disease to humans in England), and even in developed countries most food-borne outbreaks are still due to infectious agents.

Contamination of food by chemicals or metals has become more prevalent in recent years. Examples include cadmium, mercury, and chlorinated hydrocarbons (PCBs, PBBs), agents that have caused neurologic and reproductive damage in exposed populations.

This chapter provides an overview of epidemics caused by food contamination by toxins not present (or present in only trace amounts) in the normal diet and describes the major outbreaks since World War II. The focus is on noninfectious agents. Typically the origins of these food-borne epidemics are not initially understood; the diseases that occur are often new and misdiagnosed. Parallel epidemiologic and toxicologic investigations usually then uncover the food contaminant likely to be responsible. Identification of the specific causal agent is often not straightforward, however. In some instances, despite great efforts, the causal agent has not yet been fully ascertained. Examples include the 1981 outbreak of toxic oil syndrome in Madrid and the recent epidemic of optic and neurologic disease in Cuba. In Madrid, epidemiologic investigations identified contaminated cooking oil as the problem, but the exact agent involved is still unknown. The 1991–1993 outbreak of optic and peripheral neuropathy in Cuba is thought to have been caused by a combination of poor nutrition and tobacco smoking.

Although this chapter is primarily concerned with epidemics, endemic disease caused by an imbalance of nutrients in the normal diet is also briefly discussed. The example presented here is diet and cancer, which has been the subject of much epidemiologic research in recent decades. While this is part of a specialized field known as nutritional epidemiology, the role of diet in causing cancer can also be seen as part of environmental epidemiology, defined as the involuntary and widespread exposure of large populations to agents that may cause disease. In the case of diet and cancer, there has been as much emphasis on prevention of cancer (by diets high in fruits and vegetables, or in vitamins) as on cancer causation (by diets high in red meat). Specific antioxidant agents, such as beta-carotene, have been proposed as important nutrients that prevent cancer, but early epidemiologic evidence in favor of this hypothesis has not been supported by later and more rigorous studies.

Diseases resulting from environmental agents can appear either in an epidemic or an endemic manner. Diet is an environmental exposure that can produce both kinds of epidemiologic phenomena. Epidemiologists are more inclined to think of a dietary factor as the cause of an epidemic outbreak. However, in the past years there are many studies addressing the role that diet plays in some of the diseases of an endemic character (cancer, cardiovascular disorders, etc.) (Department of Health and Human Services, 1988). This chapter will review some of the most recent food-borne epidemics, as well as briefly review our current knowledge on diet and cancer.

Food contaminated by microbes is still the most frequent cause of food-borne outbreaks. It has been estimated that more than two-thirds of these outbreaks are produced by infectious agents, namely bacteria and viruses (Roberts, 1982). Preparation too far in advance, storage at ambient temperature, and inadequate cooling are the most frequent causes of contamination (Marwick, 1990). Hygienic and preventive measures have lessened the appearance of these episodes. Nevertheless, other kind of risks cannot be controlled by these measures, such as intoxications caused by natural food toxicants (e.g., mushrooms), or overnesting of fungi or bacteria capable of producing toxins such as aflatoxins and enterotoxins. Descriptions of potential outbreaks from this kind of intoxication date back centuries. The Salem witchcraft crisis in Massachusetts in 1692 may have been the result of women eating grain contaminated by fungi (ergotism) (Caporael, 1976).

Industrial processing has provided a better quality life but has brought about the possibility of chemical contamination of food. Although this type of contamination causes only a minority of food-borne outbreaks, such outbreaks can be severe. Also, many chemically induced food-borne diseases probably either pass unnoticed or are badly classified (Marwick 1990). Reporting of food-borne diseases in the United States between 1970 and 1974 demonstrated that from a total of 1747 outbreaks, 139 (7.9%) episodes had been caused by chemical food contamination (Hughes et al., 1977). Another study performed in England and Wales between 1970 and 1979 demonstrated that of 1,044 outbreaks, only 54 proved to be chemically related (Roberts, 1982).

Japan has been particularly affected by contamination of food by chemicals, probably because of the density of its population as well as changes in its industrial and agricultural production since the end of World War II. The Yusho, Itai-Itai, and Minamata epidemics are the best known outbreaks caused by food contamination. Other serious events have been the result of the use of agricultural chemicals (Japan uses more pesticides than any other country). For example, in rice paddies, the amounts of pesticides applied in order to maintain constant levels of insect damage nearly tripled between 1956 and 1970 (Commoner, 1976; Oiso and Suzue, 1972).

Although some of food's natural compounds could potentially produce injury in experimental models, their effects may not be harmful to human beings, because (a) there are low concentrations of those substances that would be hazardous only if consumed in large quantities or if consumed by persons susceptible to specific diseases (favism or sensitivity to gluten), (b) the toxicities of the thousands of different chemicals present in our daily diet do not appear to have additive effects, and (c) antagonistic interactions occur when the toxicity of one element is offset because of the presence of an adequate amount of another (e.g., cadmium and zinc) (Coon, 1974).

On the other hand, changes resulting from alimentary patterns in Western countries during the past 20 years (Raithel, 1988) and the abundance of food supplies in the international market have led to an increase of chronic exposure to additives in food. An estimate of over 2,000 additive substances involved are present in today's food in industrialized countries. Most of these additives have previously been assessed by laboratory tests or have been used for years without any toxic effects. However, unknown interactions with other substances in the diet may result in risks that have not been detected in the laboratory.

In this chapter we limit our discussion of the health effects of the diet to a review of some of the most recent epidemics in which food has proven to be the main vehicle, as well as some comments on current knowledge on diet and cancer.

Epidemics Due to Food Contamination

Table 4-1 provides a relatively complete list of known food-borne disease outbreaks. Here we discuss a few of the best-known examples of recent outbreaks; most are caused by food contamination by chemicals or metals.

Cadmium and Itai-Itai disease

The disease known as Itai-Itai obtains its name from the Japanese word "itai," which means "ouch" or "painful." The disease was recognized and described in 1955. It occurred primarily among multiparous women in the Toyama Prefecture in Japan and was characterized by pains in the extremities and difficulty in walking, sometimes accompanied by bone fractures (Tsuchiya, 1978). X-rays and pathological findings suggested a diagnosis of osteomalacia, a weakening of bones usually caused by calcium deficiency. Further records review revealed that since the beginning of the 20th century, similar cases of bone pathology appeared in the Toyama Prefecture. Further studies carried out in this prefecture revealed the presence of an endemic situation characterized by osteomalacia associated with nutritional problems. In 1961 the environmental pollution along the Jinzu River was reported, particularly the damage to vegetation caused by waste water from a lead and zinc mine near the river. Three years later, high concentrations of cadmium in the area were first associated with Itai-Itai disease. From 1929 till 1990, one hundred and fifty females over 50 years of age were recognized as "Itai-Itai" cases in the prefecture of Toyama (one of the nine cadmium-polluted districts). Cases increased gradually to the peak of 1955–1959 and decreased thereafter.

In 1965 the Japanese Ministry of Health and Welfare recognized that the disease known as Itai-Itai was caused by intoxication by cadmium with renal tubular dysfunction, causing loss of calcium, and secondary osteomalacia. Further studies found that the contamination by cadmium was

Table 4-1. Food-borne epidemics

Agent	Reference	Location	Date
Natural Toxicants			
Lathyrism	Ludolph, 1987	Many countries	Since 1920
Konzo (cassava)	Tylleskar, 1991	Zaire	1975–88
Mantakassa (cassava)	Ministry of Health, 1984a, b	Mozambique	1981
Red kidney beans	Rodhouse, 1990	United Kingdom	1976–89
Natural Contaminants			
Micotoxins			
Ergostism	King, 1979	Russia, Ethiopia	1926, 1977
Aflatoxins	Krishmamachari, 1975	India	1975
	Ngindu, 1982	Kenya	1981
Trichocemes	Bhat, 1989	India	1987
Veno-occlusive disease (Alkaloids)	Mohabbat, 1976	India	1975
	Tandon, 1976	Afghanistam	1970–72
Marine food products			
Paralytic shellfish poisoning	Gessner, 1995	Alaska	1973–1992
Neurotoxic shellfish poisoning	Hughes, 1976	Gulf of Mexico	*
	Bagnis, 1970	Pacific Islands	*
	Ariño-Moneva, 1993		
Ciguatera fish poisoning	Merson, 1974	USA	1973
Scombroid fish poisoning	Gilbert, 1980	Britain	1976–79
Domoic acid	Perl, 1990	Canada	1987
Environmental Pollution			
Packaging materials	Barker, 1972	USA	1969
Metals			
Itai-Itai (e.g., cadmium)	Tsuchiya, 1978	Japan	Since 1950
Methylmercury (fish)			
Minamata and Niigata	WHO, 1990	Japan	1953–65
Cree Indians, Quebec	McKeown-Eyssen, 1983	Canada	1975
Methylmercury (seed grain)	Bakir, 1973	Iraq, Pakistan, Ghana, Guatemala	1956–71

	Location	Reference	Year
Accidental Contaminants			
Pesticides			
Misuse (e.g., Aldicarb)	Many countries	Ferrer, 1991	1931–86
Seed dressing (e.g. Hexachlorobenzene)			
Handling (e.g., Endrin)			
Confusion (e.g., sodium fluoride)			Since 1969
Yusho (PCBs)	Japan	Urabe, 1979	
Yu-Cheng (PCBs)	Taiwan	Hsu, 1985	1979
Michigan (PBBs)	USA	Landrigan, 1979	1973
Epping jaundice	UK	Kopelman, 1966	1965
Toxicants Added to Food			
Additives			
Margarine disease	Holland	Doeglas, 1961	1960
TOCP			
Ginger jake paralysis	USA	Smith, 1930	1930
Morocco episode	Morocco	Smith, 1959	1959
Hormonal and related products added cattle feed			
Thyroid derivatives	USA	Hedberg, 1987	1985
Steroid derivatives	Italy	Fara, 1979	1977
	Puerto Rico	Sáenz de Rodriguez, 1985	1976–84
Analogous (clembuterol)	Spain	Martinez-Navarro, 1990	1990
Toxic oil syndrome	Spain	Tabuenca, 1981	1981
Unknown Origin			
Cuba episode	Cuba	Tucker, 1993	1991–93

* These epidemics have been reported worldwide for a long time.

mainly produced through mining and refining activities that led to contamination of food and drinking water. Estimates made in 1973 showed that the daily amount of cadmium ingested was 50 to 60 µg, with only about 6 µg coming from sources other than food. Rice was the most polluted food.

A large number of studies on cadmium pollution and its association with Itai-Itai in different districts of Japan have since been published. Dose-response relationships have been established between cadmium concentration in urine and the amount of glucose and proteins excreted (Nogawa et al., 1978). Other scientists suggested that cadmium is one risk factor and concomitant exposure to other metals or nutrional deficits cannot be excluded as contributory causes (Editorial, 1971).

The main reasons for considering cadmium as the cause of the Itai-Itai disease are as follows (Tsuchiya, 1978): (1) In the Jinzu River Basin, rice and river waters were polluted by cadmium. In this area, the prevalence of renal tubular changes is much higher than in other areas (Nogawa et al., 1979). (2) The disease called Itai-Itai was limited to this area and there was a relationship between the level of cadmium pollution and prevalence of the illness. (3) The highest prevalence of the disease was estimated to have occurred immediately after World War II, at which time environmental pollution by cadmium was at its highest. (4) Cadmium concentration levels are higher in urine samples from both patients and healthy inhabitants of this area. These levels are also elevated in liver tissues from Itai-Itai patients. (5) In experimental animal models, bone changes similar to osteomalacia are detected when submitted to cadmium poisoning under special conditions such as malnutrition.

It is now generally accepted that cadmium, probably accompanied by nutritional deficiencies after World War II, was responsible for Itai-Itai disease via damage to the renal tubules and subsequent loss of calcium and osteomalacia. Apparent discrepancies generally have had other explanations. For example, the decrease in osteomalacia prior to the adoption of measures against cadmium exposure, seemingly paradoxical, may have been due to increased intake of vitamin D.

Intoxications due to methylmercury

One of the earliest cases of poisoning by methylmercury was probably that of Isaac Newton. Newton exhibited signs of mental illness in 1692 that reached a peak during the following year. Four hairs from his head kept as relics were subjected to laboratory tests and the results revealed elevated concentrations of mercury, a substance he frequently used in alchemical experiments (Broad, 1981).

The first reported outbreaks associated with methylmercury occurred during 1953 and 1960 in the city of Minamata, Japan (WHO, 1990). More than 700 people presented neurologic features such as constriction of the visual field and neurologic motor-sensitive impairment. The epidemic was centered in fishermen settlements near the mouth of a river that received mercury-containing effluents from an industrial plant. Fish ingestion appeared to be the main causative agent for the intoxication; further laboratory studies revealed high concentrations of methylmercury in fish. During 1964–65 a new outbreak similar to that in Minamata, also due to the consumption of contaminated fish, was detected in Niigata, Japan (WHO, 1990).

A total of eight epidemic episodes associated with this product have been reported from 1953 to 1972 (Clarkson et al., 1976). With the exception of the Minamata and Niigata outbreaks, the rest of the epidemics were caused by seeds treated with mercury derivatives.

Yusho (polychlorinated biphenyls or PCBs)

In October 1968, an outbreak erupted in Fukuoka Prefecture, Japan. Its clinical features consisted of acneiform eruptions and pigmentation of the face, eyelids, gingivae, and nails as well as hypersecretion from the eyes (Kuratsune et al., 1972; WHO, 1993). Mucocutaneous symptoms were accompanied by other systemic signs, such as loss of appetite, nausea, vomiting, malaise, and numbness of the extremities. From October 1968 to January 1969, a total of 325 cases were reported. The disease developed in family clusters; the 325 patients belonged to 112 families. The examinations indicated that both sexes were equally affected and more than 90% of the patients were younger than 50 years. Two case-control studies were done, comparing affected subjects to healthy controls. These studies implicated either eating fried foods or consuming rice-bran oil (Yoshimura and Hayabuchi, 1985).

A thorough investigation was undertaken to determine which factories and oil brands might have been implicated as a possible cause of the disease. A group of experts concluded that the intoxication had been produced by a batch of oil produced by a specific company. Chemical studies demonstrated that suspect bottled oils from that factory contained Kanechlor 400 (polychlorinated biphenyl, PCB). Subsequently, it was discovered that Kanechlor had been used at the oil company in the equipment for heating the processed oil and presumably had contaminated the oil. This new disease was called "Yusho" (oil disease). Similar cases were later detected in the Nagasaki Prefecture. By the end of 1977, a total of 1,665 cases from both prefectures were reported (Urabe et al., 1979).

From 1969 to 1975, clinical status improved substantially in 64% of the patients, but clinical signs persist to date for many.

Yu-Cheng (PCBs)

Another outbreak similar to Yusho occurred in Taiwan in May 1979 (Hsu et al., 1985). Health authorities were informed by a school for the blind that a strange cutaneous disease had been occurring among students and staff. Unfortunately, the studies undertaken did not identify the etiology of the disease. At the same time, 85 of 150 workers from a nearby factory also suffered from the same symptoms. After an extensive epidemiologic investigation, the victims in both outbreaks were found to have consumed the same brand of rice oil manufactured by a specific company. On September 1979, two more companies reported that their workers had the same problems related to the consumption of rice oil. The laboratory analysis showed that the rice oil from both the school and the F-H Stores (the company from which the oil consumed at the factory had been purchased) contained a Kanechlor 400–500 mixture at concentrations of 65 and 108 ppm, respectively (Masuda, 1985).

Further analysis from both the Taiwan and the Japan outbreaks revealed that contaminated oils contained components not only of PCBs (62 ppm), but also polychlorinated dibenzofurans (PCDFs—0.14 ppm) and polychlorinated quaterphenyls (PCQs—20 ppm).

In the Taiwan outbreak, over 4 years, 2,060 individuals were affected and 24 of them died of the poisoning. More than half of those who died presented with severe hepatic disorders such as hepatoma, liver cirrhosis, or liver disease (Jones, 1989).

Babies born to Taiwanese mothers who had ingested PCB-contaminated oils during pregnancy presented with clinical features that consisted of growth retardation, dark brown pigmentation of skin and mucous membranes, exophthalmic edematous eye, gingival hyperplasia, and abnormal calcification of the skull. Severity of these symptoms was correlated with the quantities of oil ingested by women during pregnancy. The presence of PCBs was detected in the skin and adipose tissue of stillborn fetuses. These findings indicated that transplacental feeding was the vehicle of this toxin.

The exact causal agent of the two epidemics in Japan and Taiwan has not yet been ascertained. Determinations in blood samples from affected by the two epidemics have shown a close relationship between concentrations of PCDF and severity of the illness that suggests a strong association of PCDF with the development of the disease, although PCDFs were a relatively minor contaminant of the oils.

Polybrominated byphenyls or PBBs

In September 1973, a farmer in Michigan noticed a decrease in milk production of his dairy cows. At the same time he also noted increased lacrimation in the animals. Some of them developed abscesses, hematomas, and thickening of the skin and others lost weight and suffered from an acute disease characterized by severe cutaneous manifestations leading to death (Landrigan et al., 1979). A year later, the feed company—after undertaking its own chemical analysis—found the presence of an unexpected chemical compound corresponding to the family of polybrominated biphenyls (PBBs). Subsequently, an FDA inspector discovered that bags containing PBBs had been mixed with bags meant to feed cattle in May 1973; an estimated 10–15 bags of Firemaster containing PBBs were mistakenly shipped as Nutrimaster (an animal feed). The farmers did not notice any difference as the product was similar in both consistency and colour. In May 1974 the Michigan Department of Public Health was contacted because of concerns regarding possible human health problems due to PBB contamination of meat, dairy products, and eggs. Studies of farm residents showed no clinical evidence of disease, although high PCB and PBB levels were found in blood and adipose tissue of the exposed population (Wolff et al., 1982). Control measures were taken by the Michigan Agriculture Department on more than 300 farms; over 30,000 dairy cattle, 3,500 swine, 500 sheep, and 1,500,000 chickens as well as 5 million eggs were destroyed. Today, few if any clinical long-term health effects have been observed in this population. One recent report, based on small numbers, has found that women with higher PBB serum levels are more likely to get breast cancer (Henderson et al., 1995).

Toxic oil syndrome

In the spring of 1981, a sudden and massive epidemic struck Spain (Tabuenca, 1981; Ross 1981; Aldridge 1992a). On May 1, 1981, an 8-year-old boy suffering from a strange pulmonary disease was admitted to a hospital and died of acute respiratory insufficiency. Within the next weeks, thousands of cases were recorded and a total of 20,643 persons were affected, of whom more than 60% had to be admitted to hospitals; 313 people died during the first year. Initially, an infectious origin was suspected, but a month after the first case, surveys had shown a clear-cut relationship between the illness and intake of a rapeseed oil denatured with 2% aniline that had been imported for industrial use and then diverted for human consumption. Oils for human consumption do not contain aniline. In 1983 the World Health Organization (WHO) officially designated this new disease as toxic oil syndrome (TOS) (Grandjean and Tarkowski, 1984).

The disease developed in three clearly differentiated phases, presenting a great variety of symptoms (Abaitua and Posada, 1992; Alonso-Ruíz et al., 1993; Ortega-Benito, 1992). The features of the acute phase were alveolar-interstitial infiltration often accompanied by pleural effusion, peripheral eosinophilia, myalgias, cramps, rash, and fever not exceeding 30°C. Approximately, 70% of the patients presented with a combination of these symptoms. The intermediate phase comprised many syndromes and symptoms, with a fast development that merged into the chronic phase. The most frequent clinical features observed were pulmonary hypertension, thromboembolic phenomena of large vessels, dysphagia, skin infiltrates, hepatic cholestasis, and marked weight loss (Abaitua and Posada, 1992). About 59% of the affected individuals developed symptoms of the chronic phase characterized by peripheral neuropathy, scleroderma, neuropathy, pulmonary hypertension, and involuntary muscular activity. The main causes of death were respiratory insufficiency by noncardiogenic pulmonary edema in the acute phase; pulmonary hypertension and vascular thrombosis in the intermediate phase; and respiratory insufficiency by neuromuscular weakness and pulmonary hypertension in the chronic phase. A recent 10-year mortality study of the cohort has shown a 6.2% crude mortality rate. The highest standard mortality ratio (SMR) corresponded to 1981 (4.91, 95% CI 4.38–5.48) (Abaitua et al., 1995).

The disease developed in family clusters. Gender and age were not significant risk factors, although females were more frequently affected than males (1.5:1). Low and medium socioeconomic groups were mainly affected, probably because the oil was sold as olive oil at a cheap price. The geographic distribution of the epidemic was closely linked to the secondary road-network in Spain's central and northwestern areas where itinerant salesmen in local *mercadillos* (open air markets) sold the oil (Cañas, 1987). The epidemic curve showed a monophasic character (Fig. 4-1) suggestive of a point source epidemic.

Within the first months after the epidemic onset, several case-control studies were performed that uncovered evidence of a strong association between the illness and the ingestion of oils sold in 5-liter plastic containers without sanitary control. Other analytical studies carried out in two convents of nuns supported this association (Díaz de Rojas et al., 1987). The study of isolated cases of potential epidemiologic importance due to their unusual temporal and geographic distribution provided no evidence against this association (Posada et al., 1987, 1989).

A case-control study conducted 4 years after the outbreak, using stored

EPIDEMIC CURVE FOR TOS

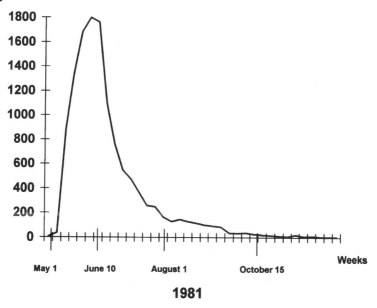

Figure 4-1. Epidemic curve for toxic oil syndrome.

oil samples from case and non-case families, showed a dose-response relationship between the amount of an aniline-derivative chemical compound (oleyl-anilide) and the risk of becoming ill (Kilbourne et al., 1988)
(Fig. 4-2). This study, carried out in two locations in the Madrid province,
was replicated 2 years later by a similarly designed study that covered all
the areas affected by the epidemic (Posada et al., 1994).

In vivo and in vitro studies have shown some toxic effects of these
aniline-derivative compounds but they have failed to reproduce the clinical or pathological feature of TOS as expressed in humans (Aldridge,
1992b).

Two large families of chemical compounds have been identified in the
ingested toxic oil: fatty acid anilides (Bernert et al., 1987) and propanediol derivatives. Each of these two groups contains around 14 compounds
with different oil concentrations. The oleic acid anilide and the dioleyl
ester of 3-(N-phenylamino) 1,2-propanediol (DEPAP) are the most representative compounds of these two families. DEPAP appears to be the

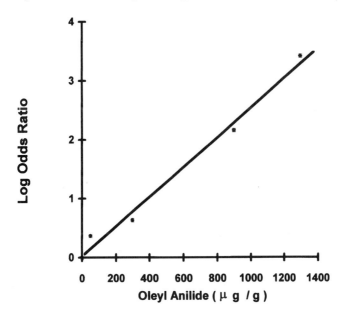

Figure 4-2. The natural log of the odds ratio plotted as a function of oil oleyl anilide concentration study of oil specimens from Alcorcón and Leganés (Madrid Province). Spain related to epidemic of Toxic Oil Syndrome in 1981. The line is fitted to the points by eye.

most probable causal agent (Hill et al., 1995). Toxicologic studies of these substances are ongoing.

In 1989 a disease outbreak linked to ingestion of L-tryptophan, which came to be called the eosinophilia-myalgia syndrome (EMS), was recognized in the United States. Pathogenesis of this disease shares very close features with TOS, although this epidemic was neither caused by food nor was any oil involved as a vehicle of the toxic agent. The close similarity between these two diseases emphasizes the importance of updating knowledge of new disease entities (Philen and Posada, 1993, Hertzman and Abaitua, 1993).

Neuropathy epidemic in Cuba

An epidemic of optic and peripheral neuropathy affected more than 50,000 persons in Cuba from late 1991 through the fall of 1993 (Tucker and Hedges, 1993; Cuban National Operative Group on Epidemic Neuropathy, 1993). Symptoms of the optic form of the neuropathy included a decreased visual acuity and color vision, central and cecocentral scotomas, optic disk pallor, and a wedge-shaped temporal defect of the maculo-papillary bundle fibers. A peripheral form was reported as characterized by diminished sensation to vibration, pinprick, and light touch, more severe distally and in the lower extremities, along with diminished ankle reflexes (Lincoff et al., 1993; Centers for Diseases Control and Prevention, 1994). Patients presented with characteristics of either one or both forms. A case-control study of the optic form of the disease examined a wide variety of potential risk factors for disease, and the investigators concluded that the epidemic involved both nutritional and toxic factors (Cuban Neuropathy Field Investigation Team, 1995). The most strongly associated factors included tobacco use, particularly cigar smoking, and a high cassava consumption relative to total energy intake. In contrast, the risk of optic neuropathy was reduced among persons with relatively high serum concentrations of antioxidant carotenoids, in particular lycopene, or relatively high dietary intakes of nutrients from animal products and B-complex vitamins. In this study, reduced risk of disease was also associated with characteristics such as raising chickens or having relatives overseas, features that were considered to be surrogates for increased access to food.

Visual loss due to poor nutrition or other toxins (amblyopias) have been reported previously, with clinical pictures similar to that in Cuba (Miller, 1982). Tobacco, particularly cigar smoking, has been shown to cause amblyopia, with a clear dose response (Lessell, 1977). B-complex vitamins, in particular vitamin B_{12}, and improved diet are accepted as important in the treatment of tobacco amblyopia, and patients who continue to smoke have been reported to recover their vision with nutritional therapy alone (Rizzo and Lessell, 1993). Cyanide exposure from tobacco smoke has been hypothesized to be toxic to the optic nerve, especially when inadequate intakes of B vitamins and sulfur-containing amino acids (methionine and cystine) impair the body's ability to detoxify cyanide through the transulfuration pathway (Dang, 1981; Chisholm and Pettigrew, 1970). High cyanide exposure combined with dietary inadequacy could enhance cyanide toxicity.

Cyanide exposure from cassava has also been implicated in epidemics of neurologic disease in Africa that include a component of visual impairment as in Konzo and Mantakassa diseases (Tylleskar et al., 1992; Ministry of Health Mozambique, 1984a); however, these have generally been described as a spastic paraparesis, whereas the clinical picture seen in Cuba was predominantly an optic and peripheral sensory neuropathy. Although cassava consumption may have contributed to the Cuban epidemic, its role is less important than cigar smoking, carotenoids, or B-complex vitamins.

Although the report does not assign a definitive "cause" for this epidemic, the investigators concluded that it may have been linked to a deterioration in diet specifically affecting nutrients such as methionine, B-complex vitamins, and carotenoids, in conjunction with a high prevalence of tobacco use, in which the balance of these factors, as well as individual susceptibility, may have determined who developed disease.

Endemics: Diet and Cancer

Experimental studies have for years tested the possible relationship between nutritional factors and tumor incidence. The possibility that diet may play an important role in cancer in human beings has been a major subject of epidemiology in the past 20 to 30 years. Early data collected from ecologic studies across countries suggested that high dietary fat intake increased the risks of both breast and colon cancers. Change in cancer rates for immigrants suggested that genetic predisposition could not account for the geographic variations in incidence rates and that environmental risks might influence cancer occurrence. In 1981 Doll estimated that 35% (range 10% to 70%) of cancer incidence in the United States was potentially avoidable by dietary factors (Doll and Peto, 1981). Since then, many observational studies have been undertaken to test nutritional factors. Overall, the evidence of a large causal role for diet in cancer still has not been well established (Comstock et al., 1992), but small effects can have large public health impact. Willett (1995) has recently estimated that 32% (range 20% to 42%) of cancer in the United States is potentially avoidable by dietary changes, a figure similar to Doll's.

One difficulty has been in accurately assessing exposure. Food-frequency questionnaires have been used (Rimm et al., 1992) to assess the intake of the different components of diet, but intra-individual variability of diet over time hampers the capacity to obtain accurate exposure data. In addition environmental measurements do not always reproduce the real biological dose that an individual receives.

Some natural components of food have been shown to cause cancer in animals and humans. The association between aflatoxins and hepatocellular carcinoma (Geng-Sun Qian et al., 1994; Harris, 1994) appears to be well established. Other factors, such as the ingestion of bracken fern (common only in Japan) and the consumption of herbal *mate* in South America, appear to be associated with the development of esophageal cancer (Castelleto et al., 1994; De Stefani et al., 1990). Other possible mechanisms that are not substantiated include the formation of carcinogens in the body by providing substrates (e.g., nitrites and nitrosamines)

(Ramón et al., 1993), or alteration of the bacterial flora of the bowel, which may be related to colon cancer.

Food additives may also influence cancer development. For example, artificial sweeteners such as saccharin have been linked to bladder cancer in animal studies involving large doses (Carlborg, 1985). However, observational studies in humans have been negative (Morgan and Wong, 1985; Hoover and Strosser, 1980; Editorial, 1980). Direct extrapolation of data collected from a study performed on rats found no expected increased risk for humans exposed to this substance (Hertz-Picciotto and Neutra, 1994). There have also been suggested associations between nitrite additives and cancers (Valle-Vega, 1986), but the evidence is weak.

Besides natural components and additives, environmental agents enter the food chain. Pesticides, vinyl chloride (PVC), cadmium, and benzopyrenes are several examples of environmental toxins that may enter the human organism through food. Cancer incidence caused by such agents has not been established, although some of these same agents can cause cancer in animals or in humans when inhaled or absorbed at high doses. Studies to evaluate low-level risks from low exposures via the diet are difficult to conduct. Of recent interest are some organochlorines (eg, DDT, PCBs) that have long half-lives in fatty tissues in the body. These chemicals are capable of exerting estrogen-like effects, and recent studies have considered their serum levels in relation to breast cancer. A prospective breast cancer incidence study (Wolff et al., 1993) showed that higher baseline levels of serum DDE (a metabolite of DDT) were associated with breast cancer, but follow-up time was short and some cancers occurred shortly after baseline, raising the issue of temporal sequence. A recent nested case-control study on a cohort of 57,040 women, using serum samples stored many years earlier, did not support the hypothesis that exposure to DDE and PCBs increased risk of breast cancer (Krieger et al., 1994).

Perhaps the largest body of evidence relating diet and cancer relates to hypotheses about meat intake, fruit and vegetable intake, and fat intake. Meat intake has been hypothesized to be positively associated, and fruit and vegetable intake negatively associated, with a variety of cancers. Fat intake has been hypothesized to increase risk of breast cancer, but recent meta-analyses do not support this claim.

Willett (1995) has reviewed the colon cancer studies to date, and concluded that red meat consumption increases risk of colon cancer, and that fiber consumption (chiefly fruits and vegetables) may have a protective effect, but the evidence is not consistent. Studies in recent years point to a protective effect of physical activity on colon cancer, and this variable may have acted as a confounder in some of the dietary studies.

Studies of immigrants from countries where low-fat diets are common to ones with high-fat diets (Japan to the United States) suggest that fatty diets may increase the risk of breast cancer. Information gathered from case-control studies designed to evaluate the hypothesis that dietary fat intake increases risk of breast cancer has suggested a weak increase in risk (Howe et al., 1992). In recent years, at least 10 different prospective studies have been published. Reviews of these studies provided no evidence of an increased risk due to fat intake (Hunter and Willett, 1993; Willett, 1995). On the other hand, there is strong animal and human evidence that overall energy restriction (decreased calories) decreases breast cancer risk (Willett, 1995). However, it is not clear whether practical public health benefits can be derived from this finding, because the required caloric restriction may be too severe to be practical or even desirable.

A 1992 review of the epidemiologic evidence concluded that fruit and vegetable consumption was protective against a number of cancers. Most studies demonstrated a protective effect, particularly for lung, esophagus, oral cavity and larynx. Suggestive evidence of this effect has also been observed in pancreas, stomach, colorectal, and bladder cancers (Block et al., 1992).

The protective effect of fruit and vegetable consumption has been often attributed to antioxidant vitamins (vitamins C and E, as well as beta-carotene, a precursor of vitamin A) which are found at high levels in these foods. Antioxidant vitamins are scavengers of free radicals, which damage DNA. Observational studies have studied intake of these vitamins or have measured their levels in the blood. Small protective effects have been found, with perhaps the most consistent effects seen between beta-carotene and lung cancer. However, cross-sectional measurements of beta-carotene in the blood reflects exposure over the prior weeks to months; what may be of interest is long-term exposure. Furthermore, studies based on food intake cannot easily distinguish effects of correlated nutrients. The best study design to evaluate antioxidants is a randomized clinical trial in which participants are randomly assigned antioxidant supplements. Three such studies have recently been completed; none has shown a protective effect for beta-carotene, beta-carotene combined with vitamin A, or vitamin E. One study included 29,000 middle-aged male smokers followed up for 6 years, who received randomly supplements of vitamin E and/or beta-carotene (20 mg/day of beta-carotene) sufficient to raise blood levels one-third and 10-fold, respectively. (The Alpha-Tocopherol, Beta Carotene Cancer Prevention Study Group, 1994). Neither supplement reduced cancer rates. A second large 12-year clinical trial studied 22,000 male physicians who took either daily doses of 50 mg beta-carotene or a placebo. No effect was seen on cancer rates (New York Times, 1996). Finally, a third study of 18,000 men and women at high risk of lung cancer (smokers, ex-smokers, asbestos-exposed) involved a combined supplement of vitamin A and 30 mg beta-carotene versus a placebo. This study was stopped after 4 years when the data indicated that the supplements were providing no benefit and might indeed be causing some harm (New York Times, 1996).

Conclusion

Diets in our industrialized societies are increasingly based on packaged foods and fast food restaurants. The demands of the large cities entail an increase in food production, leading to a massive handling of foodstuffs and the use of additives to preserve them. Chemicals added to foods are usually thoroughly tested to evaluate their acute and chronic effects in human beings. This testing may not always be adequate if chemicals are transformed during long storage periods before consumption, of if chronic effects such as human cancer cannot be detected by conventional testing procedures. In addition, industrial processing may produce accidental contamination with harmful health effects (Philen and Posada, 1993).

Synthetic compounds are not inherently toxic; the potential toxicity of natural compounds is often higher than that observed in man-made products. Man-made additives are essential for preservation of food and also give it consistency and flavor. Technology may also be used to eliminate natural products that are potentially toxic, such as the erucic acid in rapeseed oil.

Dietary contamination results in epidemic and possibly endemic effects. Epidemics due to contamination, such as those described here for contaminated oil, are likely to continue to occur. In less developed countries, epidemics linked to dietary insufficiencies (e.g., the Cuban neuropathy epidemic) are also likely to continue. Both types of epidemics may or may not be recognized as such, depending on whether an abnormally high number of cases of an apparently unusual disease occur.

The study of endemics and the chronic effects of diet will require evermore sophisticated use of biomarkers closely related to real doses received by the individuals. Most biomarker measurements, however, are only single cross-sectional observations at baseline rather than a true reflection of levels over time. Furthermore, the wrong biomarkers may be chosen. Food intake of complete foods such as fruits and vegetables involve thousands of chemicals, and we are by no means sure which ones are important in exerting protective effects. Exposure assessment in nutritional epidemiology therefore represents one of the biggest challenges in epidemiology.

References

Abaitua I, Posada M. 1992. Clinical Findings. Toxic Oil Syndrome: Current knowledge and future perspectives. WHO Regional Publications. European Series 42:27–38.

Abaitua I, Posada M, Diez M, Gomez de la Cámara, Philen RM, Kilbourne EM. 1996. Mortality by specific causes in a cohort of toxic oil syndrome (TOS) victims (1981–1994). The XIV International Scientific Meeting of the International Epidemiological Association. August 27–30, 1996. Nagoya, Japan.

Aldridge WN. 1992a. The toxic oil syndrome (TOS, 1981): from the disease towards a toxicological understanding of its chemical aetiology and mechanism. Toxicol Lett. 64/65:59–70.

Aldridge WN. 1992b. Experimental studies. Toxic oil syndrome: Current knowledge and future perspectives. WHO Regional Publications. European Series 42:6797.

Alonso-Ruiz A, Calabozo M, Pérez-Ruiz F, Mancebo L. 1993. Toxic oil syndrome: a long-term follow-up of a cohort of 332 patients. Medicine 72(5): 285–295.

Ariño Moneva A, Herrera Marteache A. 1993. Biotoxins in marine foods: II. Shellfish poisonings. Alimentaria 30 (248): 43–47.

Bagnis R, Berglund F, Elias PS, Van Esch J, Halstead BW., Kojima K. 1970. Problems of toxicants in marine food products. I. Marine biotoxins. Bull WHO 42: 69–88.

Bakir F, Al-Damluji SF, Amin-Zaki L, Murtadha M, Khalidi A, Al-Rawi NY, Tikriti S, Dhahir HI. 1973. Methylmercury poisoning in Iraq: an interuniversity report. Science 181:230–41.

Barker WHJr., Runte V. 1972. Tomato juice-associated gastroenteritis, Washington and Oregon, 1969. Am J Epidemiol 96(2): 219–226.

Bernert JT, Kilbourne EM, Akins JR, Posada M, Meredith NK, Abaitua I. 1987. Compositional analysis of oil samples implicated in the Spanish toxic oil syndrome. J Food Sci 52 (6):1562–1569.

Bhat RV, Beedu, SR, Ramakrishna, Y, Munshi, KL. 1989. Outbreak of trichothecene mycotoxicosis associated with consumption of mould-damaged wheat products in Kashmir Valley, India. Lancet 1(8628): 35–37.

Block G, Patterson B., Subar A. 1992. Fruit, vegetables, and cancer prevention: a review of the epidemiological evidence. Nutr Cancer 18(1):1–29.

Broad WJ. 1981. Sir Isaac Newton: mad as a hatter. Science 213: 1341–4.

Cañas R, Kilbourne EM. 1987. Oil ingestion and toxic oil syndrome: Results of a survey of residents of the Orcasur neighbourhood in Madrid, Spain. Int J Epidemiol 16(1): 3–6.

Caporael LR. 1976. Ergotism: the satan loosed in Salem? Science 192(4234): 21–26.

Carlborg FW. 1985. A cancer risk assesment for saccharin. Food Chem Toxicol 23: 499–506.

Castelletto R, Castellsague X, Munoz N, Iscovich J, Chopita N, Jmelnitsky A. 1994.

Alcohol, tobacco, diet, mate drinking, and esophageal cancer in Argentina. Cancer Epidemiol Biomarkers Prev 3(7): 557–564.

Chisholm IA, Pettigrew AR. 1970. Biochemical observations in toxic optic neuropathy. Trans Ophthalmol Soc UK 90:827–38.

Centers for Disease Control and Prevention. 1994. Epidemic Neuropathy—Cuba, 1991–1994. MMWR 43: 183, 189–92.

Clarkson TW, Amin-Zaki L, AL-Tikriti SA. 1976. An outbreak of methylmercury poisoning due to consumption of contaminated grain. Fed Proc 35(12): 2395–2399.

Commoner B. 1976. What price productivity. Hosp Pract 11(1): 101–102.

Coon JM. 1974. Natural food toxicants—a perspective. Nutr Rev 32(11): 321–332.

Comstock GW, Bush TL, Helzlsouer K. 1992. Serum retinol, beta-carotene, vitamin E, and selenium as related to subsequent cancer of specific sites. Am J Epidemiol 135 (2):115–121.

Cuban National Operative Group on Epidemic Neuropathy. 1993. Epidemic neuropathy in Cuba. Cuban Ministry of Public Health, Havana, Cuba, July 30.

Cuban Neuropathy Field Investigation Team. 1995. Epidemic optic neuropathy in Cuba: Clinical characterization and risk factors. N Engl J Med 333:1176–82.

Dang CV. 1981. Tobacco-alcohol amblyopia: a proposed biochemical basis for pathogenesis. Med Hypotheses 7:1317–1328.

Diaz de Rojas F, Abaitua I, Castro M, Alonso JM, Posada M, Kilbourne EM. 1987. The association of oil ingestion with Toxic Oil Syndrome in two convents. Am J Epidemiol 125 (5):907–911.

Department of Health and Human Services 1988. The Surgeon General's Report on Nutrition and Health, DHHS (PHS) Publication No. 88–50211.

De Stefani E, Munoz N, Esteve J, Vasallo A, Victora CG, Teuchmann S. 1990 Mate drinking, alcohol, tobacco, diet, and esophageal cancer in Uruguay. Cancer Res 50(2): 426–431.

Doeglas HM, Huisman J. 1961. The margarine disease. Arch Dermatol 83: 837–843.

Doll R, Peto R. 1981. The causes of cancer: quantitative estimates of avoidable risk of cancer in the United States today. J Natl Cancer Inst 66(6): 1192–1308.

Editorial. 1971. Cadmium pollution and Itai-Itai disease. Lancet vol i: 382–383.

Editorial. 1980. Saccharin and bladder cancer. Lancet vol i: 855–856.

Fara GM, Del Corvo G, Bernuzzi S, Bigatello A, Di Pietro C, Scaglioni S, Chiumello G. 1979. Epidemic of breast enlargement in an Italian school. Lancet 2: 295–297.

Ferrer A, Cabral R. 1991. Toxic epidemics caused by alimentary exposure to pesticides: a review. Food Addit Contam 8(6):755–776.

Geng-Sun Quian, Ross RK, Yu MC, Yuan J-M, Gao Y-T, Henderson BE, Wogan GN, Groopman JD. 1994. A follow-up study of urinary markers of aflatoxin exposure and liver cancer risk in Shanghai, People's Republic of China. Cancer Epidemiol Biomarkers Prev 3:3–10.

Gessner BD, Middaugh JP. 1995. Paralytic shellfish poisoning in Alaska: a 20-year retrospective analysis. Am J Epidemiol 141(8): 766–770.

Gilbert RJ, Hobbs G, Murray CK, Cruickshank JG, Young SE. 1980. Scombrotoxic fish poisoning: features of the first 50 incidents to be reported in Britain (1976–9). Br Med J 281(6232):71–72.

Grandjean P, Tarkowski S. 1984. Toxic Oil Syndrome: mass food poisoning in Spain. World Health Organization. Regional Office for Europe. Copenhagen.

Harris CC. 1994. Solving the viral-chemical puzzle of human liver carcinogenesis. Cancer Epidemiol Biomarkers Prev 3:1–2. Editorial.

Hedberg CW, Fishbein DB, Janssen RS, Meyers B, McMillen JM, MacDonald KL, White KE, Huss LJ, Hurwitz ES, Farhie JR, Simmons JL, Braverman LE, Ingbar SH, Schonberger LB, Osterholm MT. 1987. An outbreak of thyrotoxicosis caused by the consumption of bovine thyroid gland in ground beef. N Engl J Med 316(16): 993–998.

Henderson AK, Miller GL, Figgs LW, Zahm SH, Sieber SM, Rothman N, Humphrey HEB, Sinks T. 1995. Breast cancer among women exposed to polybrominated biphenyls. Epidemiol 6: 544–546.

Hertzman PA, Abaitua I. 1993. The toxic oil syndrome and the eosinophilia-myalgia syndrome: pursuing clinical parallels. J Rheumatol 20(10):1707–1710.

Hertz-Picciotto I, Neutra RR. 1994. Resolving discrepancies among studies: the influence of dose on effect size. Epidemiology 5(2): 156–163.

Hill RHJr., Schurz H, Posada M, Abaitua I, Phillen RM, Kilbourne EM, Head SL, Bailey SL, Driskell WJ, Barr JR, Needham LL. 1995. Possible etiologic agents for toxic oil syndrome: fatty acid esters of 3–(N-Phenylamino)–1, 2–propanediol. Arch Environ Contam Toxicol 28:259–264.

Howe G, Hirohata T, Hislop T, Iscovich I, Yuan J, Katsoouyanni K, Lubin F, Marubini E, et al. 1992. Dietary factors and risk of breast cancer: combined analysis of 12 case-control studies. J Natl Cancer Inst 58: 774–780.

Hoover RN, Strasser PH. 1980. Artificial sweeteners and human bladder cancer. Lancet Apr, 19: 837–840.

Hsu ST, Ma CI, Hsu SK, Wu SS, Hsu NH, Yeh CC, Wu SB. 1985. Discovery and epidemiology of PCB poisoning in Taiwan: a four-year followup. Environ Health Perspect 59: 5–10.

Hughes JM, Horwitz MA, Merson MH, Barker WH Jr., Gangarosa EJ. 1977. Foodborne disease outbreaks of chemical etiology in the United States, 1970–1974. Am J Epidemiol 105(3): 233–244.

Hughes JM, Merson MH. 1976. Fish and shellfish poisoning. N Engl J Med 295(20): 1117–1120.

Hunter DJ., Willett WC. 1993. Diet, body size, and breast cancer. Epidemiol Rev 15(1):110–132.

Jones GR. 1989. Polychlorinated biphenyls: where do we stand now? [see comments]. Lancet 2:791–794.

Kilbourne EM, Bernert JT, Posada M, Hill RH, Abaitua I, Kilbourne BW et al. 1988. Chemical correlates of pathogenicity of oils related to TOS epidemic in Spain. Am J Epidemiol 127 (6):1210–1227.

King B. 1979. Outbreak of ergotism in Wollo, Ethiopia [letter]. Lancet 1: 1411.

Kopelman H, Robertson MH, Sanders PG, Ash I. 1966. The Epping jaundice. Br Med J vol no 1:514–516.

Krieger N, Wolff MS, Hiatt RA, Rivera M, Vogelman J, Orentreich N. 1994. Breast cancer and serum organochlorines: a prospective study among white, black and Asian women. J Natl Cancer Inst 86 (8):589–599.

Krishnamachari KAVR, Bath RV, Nagarajan V, Tilak TBJ. 1975. Hepatitis due to aflatoxicosis. Lancet May 10: 1061–1063.

Kuratsune M, Yoshimura T, Matsuzaka J, Yamaguchi A. 1972. Epidemiologic study on Yusho, a poisoning caused by ingestion of rice oil contaminated with a commercial brand of polychlorinated biphenyls. Environ Health Perspect 1: 119–128.

Landrigan PJ, Wilcox KR Jr., Silva J Jr., Humphrey HEB, Kauffman C, Heath CW Jr. 1979. Cohort study of Michigan residents exposed to polybrominated biphenyls: epidemiologic and immunologic findings. Ann NY Acad Sci 320: 284–294.

Lessell S. 1977. Comment: What is the cause of alcohol and tobacco amblyopia? In: Brockhurst RJ, Boruchoff SA, Hutchinson BT, Lessell S, eds. Controversy in Ophthalmology. Philadelphia, Saunders: 873–874.

Lincoff NS, Odel JG, Hirano M. 1993. 'Outbreak' of optic and peripheral neuropathy in Cuba. JAMA 270(4): 511–518.

Ludolph AC, Hugon J, Dwivedi MP, Schaumburg HH, Spencer PS. 1987. Studies on the aetiology and pathogenesis of motor neuron diseases. I. Lathyrism: Clinical findings in established cases. Brain 110: 149–165.

Martinez-Navarro JF. 1990. Food poisoning related to consumption of illicit-agonist in liver. Lancet 336: 1311.

Marwick C. 1990. Disease pattern changes with food system [news]. JAMA 264 (22): 2858–2859.

Masuda Y. 1985. Health status of Japanese and Taiwanese after exposure to contaminated rice oil. Environ Health Perspect 60: 321–325.

McKeown-Eyssen GE, Ruedy J. 1983. Methyl mercury exposure in Northern Quebec I. Neurologic findings in adults. Am J Epidemiol 118(4): 461–469.

Merson MH, Baine WB, Gangarosa EJ, Swanson RC. 1974 Scombroid fish poisoning. Outbreak traced to commercially canned tuna fish. JAMA 228(10): 1268–1269.

Miller NR. 1982. Retrobulbar toxic and deficiency optic neuropathies. In: Miller NR, ed. Walsh and Hoyt's Clinical Neuro-Ophthalmology. Baltimore. Williams and Wilkins :289–307.

Ministry of Health, Mozambique. 1984a. Mantakassa: an epidemic of spastic paraparesis associated with chronic cyanide intoxication in a cassava staple area of Mozambique. 1. Epidemiology and clinical and laboratory findings in patients. Bull WHO 62(3): 477–484.

Ministry of Health, Mozambique. 1984b. Mantakassa: an epidemic of spastic paraparesis associated with chronic cyanide intoxication in a cassava staple area of Mozambique. 2. Nutritional factors and hydrocyanic acid content of cassava products. Bull WHO 62(3): 485–492.

Mohabbat O, Younos MS, Merzad AA, Srivastava RN, Sediq GG, Aram GN. 1976. An outbreak of hepatic veno-occlusive disease in northwestern Afghanistan. Lancet 2(7980) 269–271.

Morgan RW, Wong O. 1985. A review of epidemiological studies on artificial sweeteners and bladder cancer. Food Chem Toxicol 23(4/5): 529–533.

New York Times, Studies find beta-carotene taken by millions can't forestall cancer or heart disease, January 19, 1996.

Ngindu A, Johnson BK, Kenya PH, Ngira JA, Ocheng DM, Nandwa H, Omondi TN, Jansen AJ, Ngare W, Kavati JN, Gatei D, Siongok TA. 1982. Outbreak of acute hepatitis caused by aflatoxin poisoning in Kenya. Lancet vol i: 1346–1348.

Nogawa K, Ishizaki A, Kawano S. 1978. Statistical observations of the dose-response relationships of cadmium based on epidemiological studies in the Kakehashi River Basin. Environ Res 15: 185–198.

Nogawa K, Ishizaki A, Kobayashi E. 1979. A comparison between health effects of cadmium and cadmium concentration in urine among inhabitants of the Itai-Itai disease endemic district. Environ Res 18: 397–409.

Ortega-Benito JM. 1992. Spanish toxic oil syndrome: ten years after the disaster. Public Health 106: 3–9.

Oiso T, Suzue R. 1972. Topics of nutrition in Japan. Am J Clin Nutr vol.: 25: 1215–1218.

Perl TM, Bedard L, Kosatsky T, Hockin JC, Todde CD, Remis RS. 1990. An outbreak of toxic encephalopathy caused by eating mussels contaminated with domoic acid. N Engl J Med 322 (25): 1775–1780.

Philen RM Posada M. 1993. Toxic oil syndrome and eosinophilia myalgia syndrome WHO Meeting Report. Semin Arthritis Rheum 23:104–124.

Posada M, Abaitua I, Kilboune EM, Tabuenca JM, Diaz de Rojas F, Castro M, Alonso JM. 1989. Late cases of toxic oil syndrome: evidence that the aetiological agent persisted in oil stored for up to one year. Food Chem Toxicol 27 (8): 517–521.

Posada M, Castro M, Kilboune EM, Diaz de Rojas F, Abaitua I, Tabuenca JM, Vioque A. 1987. Toxic oil syndrome: case report associated with the ITH oil refinery in Sevilla. Food Chem Toxicol 25 (1):87–90.

Posada M, Phillen RM, Abaitua L, Diez Ruiz-Navarro M, Abraira V, Pozo F, Pla R, Pollán M, Sicilia JM, Azpeitia P, Woodruff R, Kilbourne EM. 1994. Factors associated with pathogenicity of oils related to the toxic oil syndrome epidemic in Spain. Epidemiology 5 (4):404–409.

Raithel KS. 1988. Concerns, challenges of keeping nation's food supply safe in 21st century being studied now [news]. JAMA 260(1): 15–16.

Ramón JM, Serra L, Cerdó C, Oromí J. 1993. Dietary factors and gastric cancer risk. A case-control study in Spain Cancer 71(5):1731–1735.

Rimm EB, Giovannucci EL, Stampfer MJ, Colditz GA, Litin LB, Willett WC. 1992. Reproducibility and validity of an expanded self-administered semiquantitative food frequency questionnaire among male health professionals. Am J Epidemiol 135:1114–1126.

Rizzo JF, Lessell S. 1993. Tobacco amblyopia. Am J Ophthalmol 116:84–87.

Roberts D. 1982. Factors contributing to outbreaks of food poisoning in England and Wales 1970–1979. J Hyg (Lond) 89(3): 491–498.

Rodhouse JC, Haugh CA, Roberts D, Gilbert RJ. 1990. Red kidney bean poisoning in the UK: an analysis of 50 suspected incidents between 1976 and 1989. Epidemiol Infect 105 (3): 485–492.

Ross G. 1981. A deadly oil. BMJ 283: 424–425.

Sáenz de Rodriguez CA, Bongiovanni AM, Conde de Borrego L. 1985. An epidemic of precocious development in Puerto Rican children. J Pediatr 107(3): 393–396.

Sinks T, Steele G, Smith AB, Watkins K, Shults RA. 1992. Mortality among workers exposed to polychlorinated biphenyls. Am J Epidemiol 136(4):389–397.

Smith MI. 1930. The pharmacological action of certain phenol esters, with special reference to the etiology of so-called ginger paralysis. Public Health Rep 45 (42): 2509–2524.

Smith HV, Spalding JMK. 1959. Outbreak of paralysis in Morocco due to ortho-cresyl phosphate poisoning. Lancet vol: 1019–1021.

Tabuenca JM. 1981. Toxic-allergic syndrome caused by ingestion of rapeseed oil denatured with aniline. Lancet 2: 567–568.

Tandon BN, Tandon HD, Tandon RK, Narndranathan M, Joshi YK. 1976. An epidemis of veno-occlusive disease of liver in central India. Lancet 2(7980): 271–272.

Tsuchiya K. 1977. Various effects of arsenic in Japan depending on type of exposure. Environ Health Perspect 19: 35–42.

The Alpha-Tocopherol, Beta Carotene Cancer Prevention Study Group. 1994 The effect of vitamin E and beta carotene on the incidence of lung cancer and others cancers in male smokers. N Engl J Med 330:1029–1035.

Tsuchiya K. 1978. Cadmium studies in Japan—a review. Kodansha Ltd. and Elsevier/North-Holland Biomedical Press.

Tylleskart T, Banea M, Bikangi N, Fresco L, Person LA, Rosling H. 1991. Epidemiological evidence from Zaire for a dietary etiology of konzo, an upper motor neuron disease. Bull WHO 69 (5): 581–590.

Tylleskar T, Banea M, Bikangi N, et al. 1992. Cassava cyanogens and konzo, an upper motoneuron disease found in Africa. Lancet 339:208–211.

Tucker K, Hedges TR. 1993. Food shortages and an epidemic of optic and peripheral neuropathy in Cuba. Nutr Rev 51(2): 349–357.

Urabe H, Koda H, Asahi M. 1979. Present state of yusho patients. Ann NY Acad Sci 320: 273–276.

Valle Vega P. 1986. Toxicología de los Alimentos. Centro Panamericano de Ecología Humana y Salud: Organización Panamericana de la Salud. WHO. Mexico.

Willett W. 1995. Diet, nutrition, and avoidable cancer. Environ Health Persp 103 (suppl 8): 166–170.

Wolff MS, Anderson HA, Selikoff IJ. 1982. Human tissue burdens of halogenated aromatic chemicals in Michigan. JAMA 247(15): 2112–2116.

Wolff MS, Toniolo PG, Lee EW, Rivera M, Dubin N. 1993. Blood levels of organochlorine residues and breast cancer. J Natl Cancer Inst 55(8): 648–652.

WHO. 1990. Methylmercury. IPCS. Environmental Health Criteria 101. Geneva.

WHO. 1993. Polychlorinated Biphenyls and Terphenyls (second edition). IPCS. Environmental Health Criteria 140. Geneva.

Yoshimura T, Hayabuchi H. 1985. Relationship between the amount of rice oil ingested by patients with yusho and their subjective symptoms. Environ Health Perspect 59: 47–51.

Water: Chlorinated Hydrocarbons and Infectious Agents

5

DAVID A. SAVITZ
CHRISTINE L. MOE

EPIDEMIOLOGIC studies of drinking water have traditionally been divided into two main classes, those of infectious agents and those of chemical contaminants, such as chlorination by-products and pesticides. The concern in the first instance has usually been with epidemics of infectious disease; in the latter it has most often been cancer. Although these two key areas of investigation appear quite distinct, this chapter will demonstrate that the methods to address them are more closely linked than might have been expected.

As societies have developed, providing a safe water supply ranks high among the requirements for advancing public health. Even in developed countries, provision of a water supply free of microbial pathogens is a constant challenge. The *Cryptosporidium* outbreak in Milwaukee in 1993, described in this chapter, illustrates just how close we are to the threshold of safety. More sophisticated methods of preventing waterborne infectious disease are in part a matter of technology and expense, but the treatment methods themselves may have unintended health consequences. For at least some infectious agents, higher levels of chlorination will reduce the probability of their survival through the treatment process, yet the creation of chlorination by-products argues for using the minimally effective dose. We have entered an era in which fine-tuning of the type of treatment and concentration of the disinfecting agent is required, and epidemiology is needed to supply clear, quantitative dose-response information to help weigh the risks and determine the optimal approach.

Like other environmental media, water raises distinctive issues pertaining to exposure assessment. The distinction between drinking water and surface water used solely for recreation or transportation is crucial. Even though there is a potential for health risks from contaminated recreational water sources, the exposed population is typically much smaller than the population using community drinking water supplies. Similarly, private wells are susceptible to severe chemical contamination, with adverse health consequences to the users of that water, but the greatest potential for adverse effects on large populations comes from public supplies.

The way in which waterborne agents reach humans, primarily through ingestion but also potentially through inhalation and contact, is relevant to the assessment of exposure. In the broadest sense, those who are served by a given drinking water supplier are "exposed," yet there are profound gradations in the degree of exposure depending on such factors as point-of-use water treatments, water consumption habits, and variability within the treatment and distribution system. Estimating the biologically effective dose of microbial pathogens or chemical contaminants acquired through drinking water is an elusive goal.

The distinction between endemic and epidemic health concerns is particularly important with regard to drinking water supplies. Recent research has raised the possibility that chronic exposure to microorganisms in water may contribute significantly to the baseline level of mild gastrointestinal disease, and the potential for a number of "normal" chemical constituents to affect health is the focus of a wide range of ongoing investigations. While epidemiologic evaluation of such endemic concerns has the great advantage of large populations and continuing exposures that are amenable to study, epidemiology is still a rather crude tool for detecting what is likely to be a small, widespread risk, if any increased risk is present at all. In contrast, epidemic situations have complementary advantages and disadvantages for research—often they affect small populations and are isolated in time, requiring ad hoc methods for reconstructing exposure, for example. However, the magnitudes of effect can be substantial and emerge clearly in spite of suboptimal research methods.

Potentially harmful agents in drinking water raise a wide range of health concerns. These concerns vary markedly between developed and developing countries, and this chapter is focused on the former. Discussions of water contamination and health implications in developing countries can be found elsewhere (Esrey et al., 1990). The chapter addresses drinking water and health issues that have been or should be examined by environmental epidemiologists. Many specific agents and health outcomes are of interest, but our goal is not to provide a comprehensive review.

Instead, we have chosen two topics for detailed discussion in order to illustrate an endemic (chlorination by-products and cancer) and an epidemic (*Cryptosporidium* and gastroenteritis) concern, one chemical and the other microbiological. Through these examples, we have tried to illustrate the principles that are applicable to a much wider array of issues regarding drinking water and health. For each extended example, we provide background information, present a specific epidemiologic study in some detail, then discuss the applicable methodological issues, focusing on exposure assessment and the relation of exposure to disease. Finally, we note the methodologic commonalities among studies of waterborne agents that should be addressed and provide some recommendations for improved design of epidemiologic studies of drinking water and health.

Chemical Agents

Many agents and health concerns related to chemical constituents in drinking water have been examined by epidemiologists. These include the effects of naturally occurring chemicals, such as high levels of arsenic, fluoride, and radon; agricultural by-products such as nitrates and pesticides; products of industrial contamination in waste sites, such as solvents and heavy metals; and by-products of water disinfection, such as trihalomethanes (THM). Table 5-1 summarizes the major lines of investigation, indicating the agent or class of agents, potential health consequence of exposure, and a reference. Except for the discussion of chlorination by-products and cancer, only general observations will be made about these other chemical water contaminants. A comprehensive review of potential carcinogens in drinking water is available elsewhere (Cantor et al., 1996).

For a number of natural products in water, including arsenic and fluoride, there is clear evidence of increased risk of disease with markedly elevated levels of exposure. Unusual geological conditions may give rise to high levels of such agents in drinking water, making detection of adverse effects relatively easy. This is particularly the case when some unique health consequence follows exposure, such as Blackfoot disease from arsenic (I'Cheng and Blackwell, 1968) and dental fluorosis from elevated fluoride levels in drinking water (Driscoll et al., 1983). The question that follows, which has proven much more difficult to answer, is whether exposure to lower levels in large populations over long periods of time is also associated with increased risk of disease. The shape of the dose-response curve in the low-dose range is rarely known with sufficient certainty to extrapolate from higher to lower doses; direct epidemiologic observations are needed.

Table 5-1. Examples of chemical agents in drinking water and health concerns

Agent	Source	Health Concern	Illustrative Reference
Arsenic	Natural	Skin cancer Internal cancers	Chen et al., 1985 Bates et al., 1992
Asbestos	Cement pipe	Colon cancer	Polissar et al., 1984
Disinfection by-products	Water treatment	Cancer Reproductive health	Morris et al., 1992 EPA/ILSI, 1993
Fluoride	Natural	Osteoporosis Bone cancer Dental fluorosis	Sowers et al., 1991 Hoover et al., 1976 Driscoll et al., 1983
Minerals (Hardness)	Natural	Cardiovascular disease	Comstock, 1979
Heavy metals	Hazardous wastes	Neurobehavioral	Phillips & Silbergeld, 1985
Nitrates	Fertilizer	Stomach cancer	Beresford et al., 1985
Pesticides	Agriculture	Cancer Reproductive health	Wong et al., 1989 Whorton et al., 1989
Radionuclides	Natural	Cancer	Bean et al., 1982
Sodium	Natural	Hypertension	Hallenbeck et al., 1981
Solvents	Hazardous wastes	Neurobehavioral Cancer Reproductive health	Phillips & Silbergeld, 1985 Griffith et al., 1989 Deane et al., 1989

The mix of agents encountered in drinking water poses another methodological challenge, particularly for agricultural and industrial sources. Farm by-products include nitrates from fertilizer use and runoff and a wide range of agricultural pesticides. The most extreme in diversity are hazardous waste sites, which typically store a mixture of toxic materials that may leak into surface or groundwater supplies. The risk associated with specific agents is extremely difficult to determine, even when an association is found between exposure to waste site contaminants and adverse health outcomes. Whereas linkage of the mix of agents to health harm may be sufficient to justify remediation, without determining which agents or class of agents are responsible, there is little opportunity to apply the knowledge to other settings.

Virtually all of the contaminants encountered in drinking water are encountered to varying degrees through other pathways. For some contaminants, such as nitrates, the amount of exposure through drinking water is normally smaller than dietary exposure, but can constitute a sizable fraction of total intake in rural areas (Chilvers et al., 1984). It is possible (but unlikely) for a small incremental exposure to have discernible health consequences. For other agents, such as THMs, no other common environmental sources exist.

Illness associated with water ranges from rare, severe events such as birth defects or cancer to common, mild symptoms. Research focused on the rare, severe outcomes poses the challenge of finding adequately large exposed populations to conduct informative studies. Extremely high levels of contaminants tend to be concentrated in small geographic areas, thereby exposing relatively small populations. In such circumstances, the failure to observe increased rates of rare health events provides little information to judge whether such exposures cause disease in general, though it does address the specific concerns in the exposed population of interest.

The magnitude of public concern with chemical contamination of drinking water varies markedly. In general, public interest in endemic issues such as arsenic and chlorination by-products in drinking water has not been high. In contrast, water contamination from hazardous waste sites has generated a great deal of public concern.

Chlorination by-Products and cancer

AGENTS OF CONCERN AND EVOLUTION OF RESEARCH

Concern with chlorination by-products began with the recognition that chlorine treatment of waters containing natural organic substances derived from vegetation produced small amounts of halogenated compounds, such as chloroform and other THMs, that are known to be toxic (Rook, 1974). The concentration of THMs and other chlorination by-products, such as haloacetic acids, in the finished water is a complex function of the levels and characteristics of the organic precursors, as well as the exact nature of the water treatment, temperature, and residence time (Kachur, 1994). Nonetheless, measurable levels of these chemicals in the parts per billion range are an inevitable by-product of the chlorination of surface waters, all of which contain some amount of organic precursors. In contrast, groundwater is generally free of such precursors, so that even when treated with chlorine, elevated levels of chlorination by-products are not found.

With the awareness that potentially toxic chemicals were formed by chlorination of drinking water, a series of epidemiologic investigations began in the late 1970s to address the possibility that cancer risk might be increased by chronic exposure to low levels of these chlorination by-products. A compelling consideration that motivates research on this topic is the widespread exposure of large segments of the population, with approximately 75% of U.S. drinking water treated by chlorination (Cantor, 1983), and the consumption of these contaminants over extended periods of time. The cancer sites of particular interest, given the pathway of water ingestion, have been bladder, colon, and rectum (Cantor et al., 1996), though the systemic exposure through inhalation of volatile chlorinated compounds raises concern with other sites such as leukemia and breast cancer (Morris et al., 1992; Cohn et al., 1994).

The evolution of the epidemiologic investigations provides a useful illustration of successive refinements in exposure assessment that continues to the present. The earliest studies consisted of ecologic analyses, in which exposure and cancer rates were characterized on an aggregate (typically county) level (Kuzma et al., 1977). Because chlorination by-products are formed only when there is an organic substrate with which the chlorine can react, communities served by groundwater were considered to be the unexposed referent group. Thus, the division of counties based on the proportion served by surface water was used as a crude marker of exposure potential and examined in relation to readily available cancer mortality rates (Cantor et al., 1996). The results from these studies were mixed with regard to reporting increased cancer mortality in areas served by (chlorinated) surface water; but given the recognized crudeness of exposure assessment, the actual risk associated with this exposure could be much larger than the modest risk ratios of 2 or less that were typically found.

The next major step in evaluating chlorination by-products and cancer was incorporation of individual residential and water use histories, linked with monitoring data from public water supplies. Note that the ecological analyses typically could not consider the duration of individual residence in the service area, such that in-and out-migration would dilute any influence of the local water supply in cancer etiology. Consideration of latency between exposure to the pollutants and development of cancer, which may be on the order of decades, also diminishes the validity of studying current water supply as an exposure marker. Furthermore, among residents, some individuals drink large amounts of cold tap water and others drink only bottled water. By conducting case-control studies in which cancer cases and controls are queried directly about their residence history and water use, exposure estimates can be greatly improved.

Despite the many years of research, the overall conclusion about whether chronic exposure to low levels of chlorination by-products causes cancer in humans is not clear. Studies have clearly improved in the sophistication of their measurement tools, yet the small associations with bladder cancer and rectal cancer have not gone away nor have they reached a magnitude of association at which we can be confident of their existence (Cantor et al., 1996). Perhaps some progress can be noted in that the potential association reported for colon cancer has largely been disproved (Bull et al., 1995). The epidemiologic research can be summarized as a series of studies, with differing strengths and weaknesses, which support in the aggregate a small association between drinking higher levels of chlorination by-products and risk of bladder and rectal cancer. According to the meta-analysis by Morris et al. (1992), the relative risk for bladder cancer was 1.21 and for rectal cancer, 1.38, based on seven and six studies, respectively. There has been much criticism of the legitimacy of aggregating studies of such dissimilar methodologies, but despite lack of agreement over the exact magnitude of association, there is a reasonably high probability that some positive association is truly present. Unfortunately, to reach a high level of confidence that relative risks on the order of 1.2 to 1.4 are likely to be causal will take more large, expensive studies, and even then the potential for such a small amount of bias or confounding will be difficult to disprove. Clarity could also be attained by identifying some exposure circumstances or specially susceptible population in which larger relative risks are present. For the near-term, however, we can only note that chronic exposure to elevated levels of chlorination by-products may be related to cancer, and water treatment policies should and do account for that possibility.

CASE STUDY: BLADDER CANCER AND CONSUMPTION OF CHLORINATED TAP WATER

To illustrate the methods and results of such studies, the report by Cantor et al. (1987) on bladder cancer and drinking water source in a large, well-designed case-control study is described in some detail. Drinking-water assessment was one component of an investigation of bladder cancer in 10 areas of the United States. Using cancer registries, researchers identified and interviewed 2,982 persons with incident bladder cancer. A total of 5782 control subjects were frequency-matched to case subjects on sex, age, and geographic area; control subjects under age 65 were identified through random-digit dialing and those age 65 and older through the Health Care Financing Administration roster.

An extensive interview was administered in person that covered a number of potential bladder cancer risk factors (demographic background, tobacco use, coffee consumption, etc.) as well as a series of items to determine water use and thereby history of chlorination by-product exposure. Lifetime residential history was assessed, with an indication of the water source at each residence (private well, community supply, bottled water, or other). In addition, subjects were asked if they had changed their drinking water source during their time in that residence. These locations and time periods can be viewed as the rows of a residence-exposure matrix. Also, patterns of consumption of cold and hot beverages were examined based on the interview data. (Hot water contains much lower levels of volatile organic compounds than cold tap water.)

The next challenge was to obtain information on the water utilities to supply the exposure information (columns of the residence-exposure matrix). A survey was conducted of 1102 suppliers that served 1,000 or more persons in the geographic areas in which study participants had lived. Information was sought on water sources, treatments, and service area since 1900. Groundwater information was also collected, including origins from springs or wells, and the depth and other characteristics of the wells. A sample of water was also collected for analysis of THMs. Indices of water source and treatment by year were constructed.

Among controls, 20% of the person-years were in residences served by private wells, 30% in residences served by chlorinated surface waters, 13% in residences served by mixed surface and ground water, and 18% percent in residences served by municipal suppliers with unknown chlorination status. The practical problems encountered in obtaining this information are worth noting. Even this extensive effort did not provide a complete inventory of each respondent in each year of residence. Those who lived outside the study area or were served by suppliers of fewer than 1,000 persons had missing information. Some suppliers used mixtures of surface water and groundwater in varying combinations, with some geographic areas receiving only surface water and other areas only groundwater, whereas other suppliers mixed surface and ground waters for all customers. Analyses of duration of chlorinated surface water use were restricted to the 58% of subjects who had at least 50% lifetime coverage, incurring a substantial loss of data.

Regardless of water source, risk of bladder cancer increased with increasing levels of self-reported tap water consumption. Divided into quintiles of tap water consumption, the adjusted odds ratios for both sexes were 1.0 (referent), 1.1, 1.1, 1.3. and 1.4 across the five levels. For the analysis of chlorinated surface water, a referent group was defined consisting of persons who had never used surface water and compared with those with increasing duration of surface water use. Among men, there was no gradient of increasing risk, but among women, the odds ratios were 1.5 for 1–19 years of surface water use (relative to none), 1.2 for 20–39 years of use, 1.5 for 40–59 years of use, and 2.1 for 60+ years of use. The association with years of surface water use occurred only among those with higher levels of consumption and was much stronger among women than among men.

Relative to the previous investigations, the exposure assessment in this study was quite advanced. Many earlier studies were based on ecologic measures of exposure (e.g., percent on surface supplies in county of residence)and some used individual data but only at a single point in time (e.g., time of diagnosis or death). Consideration of a lifetime history of specific community residence and self-reported water use is a major step forward. Nonetheless, as the authors note, misclassification of true exposure to THMs and related chlorination by-products is undoubtedly present. Incomplete or inaccurate data on beverage consumption, water supply information, and specific chemical constituents over the historical periods of interest limit the certainty of conclusions based on specific chemical exposures.

Methodological issues

In evaluating the quality of exposure assessment for chemical contaminants of drinking water, it is useful to consider the ideal but infeasible gold standard measure to which more feasible approaches can be compared. Imagine a personal dosimeter that tabulates every molecule of the relevant chemical(s) of concern that is consumed over the relevant etiologic period. This would provide a perfectly accurate measure of the precisely relevant dose, ignoring such concepts as timing of exposure or biologically effective dose to the target organs. From that point of reference, we can consider the deviations that arise in actual epidemiologic studies.

In practice, there are three approaches to assessing exposure to waterborne chemical or infectious agents. Investigators may attempt to measure the agent of interest in water samples or measure a proxy of the agent of interest. Alternatively, the presence, and possibly the amount, of the agent of interest may be estimated on the basis of characteristics of the water source and treatment processes. Finally, the investigator may estimate individual consumption or exposure to the water supply.

ASSESSMENT OF CHEMICAL AGENTS IN WATER

In the case of chlorination by-products, our ability to specify precisely which agent is of concern is imperfect. Chloroform or total THM is used as a convenient marker of "chlorination by-products," but other compounds such as haloacetic acids are also of possible relevance. Thus, whatever chemical marker is chosen, potential loss of information is incurred relative to the biologically relevant dose. For more clearly defined single agents, such as fluoride or lead, the identity of the important chemical is unambiguous.

The water source is generally treated as stable over time and homogeneous throughout the system. Some level of THM or other marker is typically compared across treatment systems based on a small number of sample points. Typically, a single number is used to characterize the exposure associated with that supplier. However, the number that is assigned is known to be an imperfect indicator of the levels in tap water at a given point in time (Kachur, 1994). Seasonal changes are substantial, with approximately threefold higher levels in warm months than in cold months due to the kinetics of the chemical reactions that produce these agents. Short-term fluctuations are possible within the treatment system itself, as the level of organic precursors or the disinfection process varies. The storage time further influences the levels of by-products present because the chemical reactions continue as long as free chlorine is present, also in the range of a threefold difference from highest to lowest. Even within a given home, the intensity of water consumption in the neighborhood may affect residence time and exposure levels over relatively short periods, e.g., early in the morning versus late afternoon.

CHARACTERIZATION OF WATER SUPPLY
BY SOURCE AND TREATMENT

The water source and methods used to treat the water prior to consumption influence both the chemical and microbial quality. In the case of chlorination by-products, the concentration of THMs and other halogenated compounds is determined by the amount and character of the organic precursors in the source water as well as a number of water treatment and distribution factors. A recent analysis of determinants of THM concentration in a specific water supply in central North Carolina (Kachur, 1994) examined a number of parameters as predictors of tap water THM levels, including pH, chlorine dose, water temperature, residence time in the distribution system, and estimated chlorine consumed. The THM levels at the time the water leaves the treatment plant are obviously a function of the content of organic precursors and the precise methods of treatment, which can be modeled with some accuracy. However, chemical reactions continue while the water is in storage and being distributed, such that intermediate markers such as "residence time" and "chlorine consumed" have substantial predictive value for individual homes beyond knowledge of the treatment methods per se.

ASSESSING INDIVIDUAL EXPOSURE

In addition to the inherent variability introduced from the water supply itself, the user has abundant opportunity to influence exposure to chemical or microbial contaminants for a given quality of water. A variety of devices applied to the tap within the home may influence (reduce) chlorination by-product levels and infectious agents that are ingested. However, it is difficult in studies that rely on self-report to obtain sufficiently accurate reports on the type of home treatment to incorporate the information into assignment of exposure.

Individual consumption patterns are obviously an important determinant of exposure, with substantial variability in the number of glasses of cold tap water consumed daily (Ershow et al., 1991). Even the volume ingested does not fully reflect the chemical content of the water, because volatile agents such as THMs are released from the water during storage. Collection in a closed container would preserve the original THM levels, whereas storage in an open pitcher for some period of time would allow the volatile chemicals to escape. Similarly, products prepared from tap water such as juice concentrates or instant iced tea will contain the tap water levels of chlorination by-products. Depending on how these beverages are stored, ingestion may or may not have the same implications for exposure as drinking tap water directly. For infectious agents, the type of water storage vessel, how it is cleaned, and the method of water abstraction has been shown to greatly influence the microbiological quality of household water (Mintz et al., 1995).

An additional dimension relevant to THM exposure is exposure through inhalation and dermal absorption, which some suggest may be nearly equal in magnitude to ingestion (Andelman, 1985; Jo et al., 1990a). As water is used in the home (bathing, showering, flushing toilets, washing dishes, boiling water, etc.), the agents are volatilized and released into the home. The rate of release and home ventilation determine the contribution from inhaled THMs. Exposures from showering and bathing have been studied intensively (Jo et al., 1990b) including dermal absorption, inhalation within the shower or bath area, and inhalation in the bathroom where the volatile agents concentrate. A wide range of behavioral characteristics help to determine actual exposure such as duration of bath or shower, depth of bath, droplet size of shower, closed or open bath area, and ventilation in the bathroom. Although all of these are subject to assessment, in principle, the feasibility of obtaining adequately precise information is questionable.

Recreational use of water also plays an important role in determining exposure to infectious agents. Whether exposure occurs through swimming, wading, or water sport activities such as water skiing, the duration of water contact, the opportunity for inadvertent ingestion of water, and the type of water (treated swimming pools versus natural surface waters, freshwater or marine water) all affect the type of infectious agents to which an individual may be exposed and the likelihood of acquiring a water-related infection (Dufour, 1986). Some epidemiologic studies of health effects of recreational water exposure have collected detailed information on individual behaviors (e.g., wading, swimming with head above water, swimming with head immersed in water) in order to better assess exposure (Cheung et al., 1990).

Given this array of considerations, research can still be done by ordering or grouping typical chlorination by-product levels of treatment systems, with likely ability to discriminate average levels. However, all these contributors tend to blur the distinctions among them and introduce misclassification in assignment of individual exposures based on the average score for the system.

Infectious Agents

Numerous infectious agents have been associated with waterborne disease through ingestion, contact, or inhalation (Tables 5-2 and 5-3). Disease outcomes associated with waterborne infections include mild to life-threatening gastroenteritis, hepatitis, skin infections, wound infections, conjunctivitis, respiratory infections, and generalized infections. Some agents of waterborne diseases are indigenous aquatic organisms, such as Legionella spp., *Vibrio vulnificus, Vibrio parahemolyticus, Aeromonas hydrophila*, and *Pseudomonas aeruginosa*. However, most microbial waterborne pathogens originate in the enteric tract of humans or animals and enter the aquatic environment via fecal contamination. Control of these diseases depends on sanitation measures and wastewater treatment to prevent the introduction of these organisms into drinking water supplies or recreational waters, and on adequate water treatment to remove or inactivate microbial pathogens in drinking water. Most of these pathogens can also be transmitted person-to-person by contact with fecally contaminated hands or objects or by consumption of fecally contaminated food. In endemic situations with poor sanitation and hygiene, the attributable risk due to water versus other routes of exposure may be difficult to determine.

Techniques have been developed for assessing risks to health from microbes in drinking water (Sobsey et al., 1993). Risk assessment models are based on field data on the occurrence of specific microorganisms in raw and treated water supplies, experimental data on removal or inactivation by various water treatment processes, and experimental dose-response data (Regli et al., 1991; Rose et al., 1991). As with chemical agents, the shape of the dose-response curve, especially in the low-dose region representative of waterborne exposure, is ill-defined. Furthermore, it is difficult to take into account variation in microbial virulence factors and host-specific characteristics (e.g., age, immune status) that may affect susceptibility to infection and disease.

Table 5-2. Illnesses acquired by ingestion of water

Agent	Incubation Period	Clinical Syndrome	Duration
Viruses			
Astrovirus	1–4 days	Acute gastroenteritis	2–3 days; occasionally 1–14 days
Calicivirus	1–3 days	Acute gastroenteritis	1–3 days
Enteroviruses (polioviruses, coxsackie viruses, echoviruses)	3–14 days, (usually 5–10 days)	Febrile illness, respiratory illness, meningitis, herpangina, pleurodynia, conjunctivitis, myocardiopathy, diarrhea, paralytic disease, encephalitis, ataxia	Variable
Hepatitis A	15–50 days (usually 25–30 days)	Fever, malaise, jaundice, abdominal pain, anorexia, nausea	1–2 weeks to several months
Hepatitis E	15–65 days (usually 35–40 days)	Fever, malaise, jaundice, abdominal pain, anorexia, nausea	1–2 weeks to several months
Norwalk and Norwalk-related viruses	1–2 days	Acute gastroenteritis with predominant nausea and vomiting	12–48 hours
Group A rotavirus	1–3 days	Acute gastroenteritis with predominant nausea and vomiting	5–7 days
Group B rotavirus	2–3 days	Acute gastroenteritis	3–7 days
Bacteria			
Aeromonas hydrophila		Watery diarrhea	Avg. 42 days
Campylobacter jejuni	3–5 days (1–7 days)	Acute gastroenteritis, possible bloody and mucoid feces	1–4 days, occasionally >10 days

(continued)

Table 5-2. Illnesses acquired by ingestion of water (*continued*)

Agent	Incubation Period	Clinical Syndrome	Duration
Enterohemorrhagic *Escherichie coli* 0157:H7	3–5 days	Watery, then grossly bloody diarrhea, vomiting, possible hemolytic uremic syndrome	1–12 days (usually 7–10 days)
Enteroinvasive *E. coli*	2–3 days	Possible dysentery with fever	1–2 weeks
Enteropathogenic *E. coli*	2–6 days	Watery to profuse watery diarrhea	1–3 weeks
Enterotoxigenic *E. coli*	12–72 hours	Watery to profuse watery diarrhea	3–5 days
Plesiomonas shigelloides	1–2 days	Bloody and mucoid diarrhea, abdominal pain, nausea, vomiting	Avg. 11 days
Salmonellae	8–48 hours	Loose, watery, occasionally bloody diarrhea	3–5 days
Salmonella typhi	7–28 days (avg: 14 days)	Fever, malaise, headache, cough, nausea, vomiting, abdominal pain	Weeks to months
Shigellae	1–7 days	Possible dysentery with fever	4–7 days
Vibrio cholerae 01	9–72 hours	Profuse, watery diarrhea, vomiting, rapid dehydration	3–4 days
Non-01 *Vibrio cholerae*	1–5 days	Watery diarrhea	3–4 days
Yersinia enterocolitica	2–7 days	Abdominal pain, mucoid, occasionally bloody diarrhea, fever	1–21 days (avg: 9 days)
Protozoa			
Balantidium coli	Unknown	Abdominal pain, occasional mucoid or bloody diarrhea	Unknown
Cryptosporidium species	1–2 weeks	Profuse, watery diarrhea	4–21 days
Entamoeba histolytica	2–4 weeks	Abdominal pain, occasional mucoid or bloody diarrhea	Weeks–months

Table 5-2 (*continued*)

Agent	Incubation Period	Clinical Syndrome	Duration
Giardia lamblia	5–25 days	Abdominal pain, bloating, flatulence, loose, pale, greasy stools	1–2 weeks to months and years
Algae			
Cyanobacteria (*Anabaena, Aphanizomenon,* and *Microcystis* species)	Few hours	Toxin poisoning (blistering of mouth, gastroenteritis, pneumonia)	Variable
Helminths			
Dracunculus medinensis (guinea worm)	8–14 months (usually 12 months)	Blister, localized arthritis of joints adjacent to site of infection	Months

Infectious agents and gastrointestinal disease

RESEARCH APPROACHES IN ENDEMICS

The primary concern with infectious agents in drinking water is acute gastrointestinal illness. In industrialized countries, there have been few studies of endemic gastrointestinal disease associated with the consumption of drinking water. A randomized intervention trial was conducted in Montreal, Canada, to examine the risk of gastrointestinal illness associated with the consumption of treated drinking water that met current microbiological standards (Payment et al., 1991). Gastrointestinal symptoms were recorded in family health diaries. Water samples from the surface water source, treatment plant, distribution system, and study households were analyzed for several indicator bacteria and culturable viruses. Over a 15-month period, a 35% higher rate of gastrointestinal symptoms was observed among 307 study households drinking tap water compared with 299 study households supplied with reverse-osmosis filters. Symptomatology and serologic evidence suggested that much of this increased illness may have been caused by low levels of enteric viruses in the municipal water supply that originated from a river contaminated by human sewage.

A longitudinal study of endemic disease in French alpine villages that used untreated groundwater observed a weak relationship between rates of acute gastrointestinal disease and the presence of fecal streptococci

Table 5-3. Illnesses acquired by recreational contact with water[a]

Agent	Incubation Period	Clinical Syndrome	Duration
Viruses			
Adenovirus (serotypes 1, 3, 4, 7, 14)	4–12 days	Conjunctivitis, pharyngitis, fever	7–15 days
Bacteria			
Aeromonas hydrophila	8–48 hr	Wound infections	Weeks to months
Legionellae	Legionnaires' disease: 2–10 days (usually 5–6 days)	Legionnaires' disease: pneumonia with anorexia, malaise, myalgia and headache, rapid fever and chills, cough, chest pain, abdominal pain and diarrhea	Legionnaires' disease: variable, usually weeks to months
	Pontiac fever: 5–66 hours (usually 24–48 hours)	Pontiac fever: fever, chills, myalgia, headache	Pontiac fever: 2–7 days
Leptospira interrogans	4–19 days, (usually 10 days)	Leptospirosis (headache, chills, fever, severe myalgia, nausea, neck or joint pain)	Few days to 3 weeks or longer
Mycobacterium spp. (*M. marinum, M. balnei, M. platy, M. kansasii, M. szulgai*)	2–4 wk	Lesions of skin or subcutaneous tissues	Months

indicator bacteria in the public water system over a 15-month study period (Zmirou et al., 1987). Illness data were collected by active surveillance of physicians, pharmacists, and schoolteachers. Weekly water samples were collected from frequently used taps in the distribution system of each village and were analyzed for several bacterial indicator organisms.

Ecological studies have attempted to find a relationship between endemic rates of hepatitis A infection and municipal source water quality or treatment (Batik et al., 1980). Other studies have taken advantage of the fact that giardiasis is a reportable disease in some states and have examined the consumption of unfiltered municipal water or shallow well water as a risk factor for endemic giardiasis (Chute et al., 1987; Birkhead and Vogt, 1989; Dennis et al., 1993).

Table 5-3 (*continued*)

Agent	Incubation Period	Clinical Syndrome	Duration
Pseudomonas spp.		Dermatitis, ear infections, conjunctivitis	
Vibrio spp. (*V. alginolyticus, V. parahemolyticus, V. vulnificus, V. mimicus*)	*V. vulnificus:* 24 hours	*V. vulnificus:* acute gastroenteritis, wound infections, septicemia	*V. vulnificus:* septicemia fatal in 2–4 days
	V. parahemolyticus: 4–48 hours	*V. parahemolyticus:* acute gastroenteritis, wound infections	*V. parahemolyticus:* usually 3 days
		Ear infections	
Other			
Cyanobacteria (*Anabaena, Aphanizomenon,* and *Microcystis* species)	Few hours	Dermatitis	
Naegleria fowleri	3–7 days	Meningoencephalitis, headache, anorexia, fever, nausea and vomiting. Usually fatal.	10 days
Acanthamoeba species		Subcutaneous abscesses, conjunctivitis	8 days to several months
Schistosoma species	Few minutes to hours	Dermatitis, prickly sensation, itching	Years

[a] Agents acquired through ingestion of water are not included in this table.

RESEARCH APPROACHES IN EPIDEMICS

Most of the information on the risk factors and etiologic agents of waterborne disease comes from investigations of waterborne disease outbreaks by state and local health departments and the surveillance program maintained by the Centers for Disease Control and Prevention (CDC) and the Environmental Protection Agency (EPA). Most infections caused by waterborne agents are not reportable diseases, so it is difficult to recognize disease clusters. The existing surveillance system is based on voluntary reporting by state health departments and clearly represents only a fraction of the true incidence of waterborne disease outbreaks. However, these data indicate that since the early

1980s, parasitic agents have become the major etiologic agents associated with waterborne disease outbreaks in the United States and that recently recognized etiologic agents such as *Escherichia coli* 0157:H7 and *Cryptosporidium* are being reported more frequently and from new settings, such as outbreaks associated with recreational water use (CDC, 1993).

Still, the vast majority of waterborne outbreaks reported by this surveillance system are classified as "acute gastrointestinal illness of unknown etiology." Stool examinations by hospital laboratories typically include culture for *Salmonella, Shigella,* and *Campylobacter.* In addition, more laboratories now test for rotavirus in specimens from young children and for *Giardia* and, more recently, *Cryptosporidium,* at the request of a physician. Clinical symptoms suggest that many outbreaks of acute gastrointestinal illness may be due to viral agents, such as Norwalk virus and related small, round structured viruses. However, inadequate diagnostic technology has limited the detection of these agents in clinical and environmental samples. Finally, there is some evidence of waterborne disease associated with a number of newly recognized etiologic agents such as *Cyclospora cayetanensis* (Wurtz, 1994), Cyanobacteria (Carmichael et al., 1985), *Helicobacter pylori* (Klein et al., 1991), mycobacteria (Jenkins, 1991), and *Aeromonas* (Schubert, 1991).

CRYPTOSPORIDIUM

Cryptosporidium is a protozoan parasite that was first recognized as a human pathogen in 1976. At the time of the much-publicized Milwaukee outbreak in 1993 (described below), five *Cryptosporidium* outbreaks associated with drinking water had been reported in the United States (Texas, 1984; Georgia, 1987; Pennsylvania, 1991; Oregon, 1992 [two outbreaks]) (CDC, 1993; Hayes et al., 1989; D'Antonio et al., 1985). *Cryptosporidium* is transmitted by the ingestion of oocysts excreted in the feces of infected humans and animals. Because the oocysts are relatively large (3–6 μm diameter), it was initially believed that *Cryptosporidium* would not be able to move into groundwater supplies and would be effectively removed from surface water by conventional coagulation/flocculation and filtration processes. Therefore it was perceived as a threat only to communities that used unfiltered surface water. The EPA responded to the threat of waterborne giardiasis and cryptosporidiosis in 1989 with the Surface Water Treatment Rule (54 FR 27486-27541) that required filtration and disinfection of all surface waters unless they met certain site-specific conditions. However, two reported outbreaks (Georgia, 1987, and Oregon, 1992) have involved municipal filtered surface water supplies (Hayes et al., 1989) and two other outbreaks (Texas, 1984, and Pennsylvania, 1991) were associated with contaminated groundwater (D'Antonio et al., 1985).

Surveys of raw and finished water supplies indicate that the occurrence of *Cryptosporidium* oocysts is widespread. Two surveys of almost 300 surface water supplies in the United States revealed that 55% to 77% of surface water samples were positive for *Cryptosporidium* oocysts (Rose, 1988, Rose et al., 1991). Water analysis at 66 U.S. and Canadian surface water treatment plants demonstrated that up to 27% of drinking water samples had low levels of *Cryptosporidium* oocysts (LeChevallier et al., 1991).

Despite these data, there was not widespread recognition of the threat of waterborne cryptosporidiosis among U.S. water utilities, and several major metropolitan areas were resisting the water filtration requirement. The EPA sponsored a human challenge study to determine the minimum infectious dose of *Cryptosporidium* (DuPont et al., 1995). However, there was little support among government agencies or water utilities for prospective epidemiologic studies of the risk of waterborne cryptosporidiosis.

CASE STUDY: CRYPTOSPORIDIUM OUTBREAK IN MILWAUKEE, WISCONSIN

Because of time limitations and the urgent need to protect public health, epidemiologic field investigations of waterborne disease outbreaks do not allow the same level of advance planning and scientific rigor as other types of epidemiologic research. However, they often provide valuable insights into existing public health hazards, water treatment deficiencies, and disease surveillance. In the spring of 1993, the largest documented outbreak of waterborne disease in U.S. history occurred in Milwaukee, Wisconsin, affecting an estimated 403,000 people (MacKenzie et al., 1994). This outbreak is noteworthy for several reasons: (1) it involved a relatively newly recognized waterborne pathogen, *Cryptosporidium*, (2) *Cryptosporidium* oocysts were detected in historical samples of ice so that past waterborne exposure could be estimated, (3) the drinking water met microbiological quality standards for total coliforms and average turbidity standards, (4) the public water supply used standard water treatment processes of coagulation/flocculation, filtration, and disinfection, (5) routine testing of patients for *Cryptosporidium* in this community was so infrequent that it was not adequate to detect this epidemic.

The outbreak was first recognized around April 5, 1993, after reports of numerous cases of gastroenteritis and high rates of absenteeism in schools and hospital employees. Initially many cases were misdiagnosed as "intestinal flu" on the basis of the clinical symptoms and were not further investigated. Because laboratory testing for *Cryptosporidium* was not a routine procedure, recognition of *Cryptosporidium* as the causative agent of this outbreak was delayed. From March 1 through April 16, a total of 2300 stool specimens were submitted to the 14 clinical laboratories in the Milwaukee area for routine examination of enteric pathogens. Twelve of these laboratories tested for *Cryptosporidium* only at the request of the physician, and by April 6, only 42 stool specimens had been examined for *Cryptosporidium* (12 [29%] were positive). On April 7, two laboratories identified *Cryptosporidium* oocysts in the stools of seven adults in the Milwaukee area and, at the request of public health officials, the other 12 laboratories began to routinely test all stool specimens for *Cryptosporidium*. From April 8 through April 16, *Cryptosporidium* oocysts were detected in 331 of 1009 specimens (33%). Between March 1 and May 30, 739 *Cryptosporidium* infections were detected by the 14 surveillance laboratories.

Persons with laboratory-confirmed cases of *Cryptosporidium* infection with illness between March 1 and May 15 (N=285) were interviewed by telephone and compared with persons who had experienced watery diarrhea (201 cases between March 1 and April 12) that were identified by telephone surveys in the Milwaukee area. The epidemiologic features and dates of illness were similar in both groups and suggested many of the watery diarrhea cases were also caused by *Cryptosporidium*.

The total extent of the outbreak was estimated on the basis of a random-digit dialing telephone survey of 840 households in the greater Milwaukee area. Among the 1663 respondents, 26% reported watery diarrhea in the period from March 1 though April 28. Extrapolation of this rate to the total population of the greater Milwaukee area (1.6 million people) and subtracting a background rate of diarrhea of 0.5% per month (16,000 cases) gives an estimate of 403,000 cases of *Cryptosporidium* associated with this outbreak.

An early survey of nursing home residents, a relatively immobile population, indicated that *Cryptosporidium* infection was significantly higher during the first week of April among nursing homes supplied by water from the southern treatment plant. The household telephone survey provided additional information on the geographic distribution of the cases. The risk (often referred to as "attack rate" in outbreak investigations) of watery diarrhea was 2.7 times higher among residents of the Milwaukee Water Works service area compared to residents outside the service area. Within the service area, the highest risk (52%) was among residents served by the southern water treatment plant, and the lowest risk (26%) was among residents served by the northern water treatment plant. Residents who lived in the middle of the service area and could be exposed to water from either or both treatment plants reported a risk of 33%.

Waterborne transmission was suspected by April 7, when public health officials issued an advisory to boil water and then closed the southern water treatment plant on April 9. The southern plant had noted highly variable turbidity of the treated water since around March 21, with peaks of 1.7 NTU (nephelometric turbidity unit) on March 28 and 30 and 1.5 NTU on April 5. Consumer complaints about poor quality of drinking water were also reported to the Milwaukee Water Works during this period (*Milwaukee Journal,* 6/26/93). At all times during this period, samples of treated water were negative for coliforms and met the Wisconsin regulations for turbidity. Investigation of the water treatment plant determined no evidence of an obvious mechanical breakdown in the flocculation and filtration system. However, difficulty in determining the appropriate dose of coagulant to aggregate particulates, failure to continuously monitor the turbidity from each filter bed, and recycling of filter backwash water were cited as possible contributing factors to this outbreak.

Methods to detect *Cryptosporidium* oocysts in water are laborious and relatively inefficient and are currently limited to research laboratories. In this outbreak investigation, samples of ice made on March 25 and April 9 were melted down and filtered to concentrate *Cryptosporidium* oocysts that were later detected by an immunofluorescent technique. Estimates of oocyst concentrations in these samples ranged from 2.6 to 13.2 oocysts per 100 liters and 0.7 to 6.7 oocysts per 100 liters for March 25 and April 9, respectively. Recent data from human volunteers indicate that the dose at which 50% of subjects become infected with *Cryptosporidium parvum* is 132 oocysts (DuPont et al., 1995). Visitors to the Milwaukee Water Works service area who consumed only very small amounts (< 240 mL) of water still developed laboratory-confirmed cryptosporidiosis. Thus, the epidemiologic data suggested that these estimates of oocyst concentration in ice may have been gross underestimates of the actual contamination, possibly due to the effect of freezing and thawing on the oocysts or poor recovery from the filters.

The source of the *Cryptosporidium* oocysts and the timing of the water contamination are still unknown. The number of cases with onset of illness before March 23 (when the turbidity increases were noted) indicate that oocysts must have entered the water supply before the turbidity rose. Speculation about the effect of heavy rains and runoff from cattle farms and slaughterhouses into nearby rivers and Lake Michigan has yet to be confirmed.

Several public health recommendations came from this investigation. The adequacy of current microbiological water standards and the turbidity standard to protect the public from waterborne transmission of enteric protozoa was questioned. Continuous monitoring of treated water for turbidity and tightening the turbidity standard to 0.1 NTU or lower were recommended. Changes in water treatment procedures related to filter maintenance and backwashing were implemented, and laboratory facilities for routine *Cryptosporidium* monitoring of raw and finished waters were established. MacKenzie et al. (1994) advocated the routine examination for *Cryptosporidium* oocysts in stools even though the infection is self-limited in the immunocompetent host and no effective treatment is available. Furthermore, they advised making *Cryptosporidium* infection a reportable disease to improve the recognition of *Cryptosporidium* outbreaks in the United States.

Assessment of infectious agents in water

MEASURING WATERBORNE ENTERIC PATHOGENS

Exposure assessment for infectious agents in water is simplified by the relatively short incubation period of these diseases relative to chemicals that may cause chronic disease. However, in most epidemic studies of waterborne transmission of infectious agents, water is identified as the vehicle of transmission by epidemiologic evidence rather than by the detection of the infectious agent in water samples. Of the 32 waterborne infectious disease outbreaks reported in the United States between 1991 and 1992, the etiologic agent was detected in the water for only four outbreaks: *Shigella* (one), *Giardia* (two), and *Cryptosporidium* (one) (CDC, 1993). This may be because the contamination of the water supply was temporary and the infectious agent died off or was flushed out of the water system before appropriate water samples were collected, or because of limited laboratory methods.

Many waterborne pathogens are difficult to detect or quantify in water. Because the concentrations of these organisms are much lower in water than in clinical specimens, their detection in water starts with some type of concentration process such as filtration. This is followed by a process to recover the pathogen from the filter and an amplification process either by culture or molecular biology methods. Typically the recovery efficiencies of these procedures are low, making it difficult to estimate the original concentration of the infectious agent in the water. Failure to detect a pathogen in a water sample does not prove that the water was free from contamination. Furthermore, as demonstrated in the Milwaukee outbreak, many of these laboratory techniques are limited to specialized research or reference laboratories and are not done on a routine basis.

INDICATORS OF MICROBIAL WATER QUALITY

Both epidemic and endemic studies of infectious agents and waterborne disease frequently rely on proxy measures of microbiological water quality.

EPA and WHO guidelines for microbiological water quality are expressed in terms of "total coliforms" and "fecal coliforms," which are groups of bacteria excreted by healthy humans and animals that serve as indicators of fecal contamination (US EPA, 1994; WHO, 1993). Laboratory assays for total and fecal coliforms in water are much easier to perform than tests to detect pathogenic microorganisms in water. Because these indicator organisms are excreted in high numbers by all individuals, they are consistently found in high concentrations in community fecal waste. By contrast, specific pathogens are only excreted by infected individuals and their numbers in the community fecal waste "pool" depend on excretion level of the particular pathogen and on the number of infected individuals in the community.

Total and fecal coliforms have many limitations as predictors of risk of waterborne disease. Because of their shorter survival times in water and their greater susceptibility to water treatment processes, these indicator organisms tend to be poor models for many waterborne pathogens—especially enteric protozoa and viruses. Outbreaks of waterborne disease, particularly protozoal outbreaks such as the Milwaukee epidemic, have been associated with water that met total and fecal coliform standards. Moreover, there are nonfecal sources for these indicator organisms and, in contrast to most enteric pathogens, total and fecal coliforms may multiply in aquatic environments with sufficient nutrients and optimal temperatures. Such characteristics may result in false-positive reports of water contamination and consequent misclassification of exposure.

Many alternative indicator organisms have been proposed. Enterococci and E. *coli* were included in the revision of the EPA recreational water standards (US EPA, 1986). *Clostridium perfringens* and male-specific coliphage have been proposed as potential indicators of drinking water quality that may better model the survival and disinfection resistance of enteric protozoa and viruses (Payment and Franco, 1993). There is increasing recognition that no single organism can serve as an adequate indicator for all types of water and all routes of exposure.

Physical parameters, such as turbidity and particle counts, have also been used as indicators of microbiological water quality. Marked increases in turbidity of water from Milwaukee's southern water treatment plant was the only indication that the quality of the water was compromised in the 1993 epidemic.

WATER SAMPLING ISSUES

Depending on the type of water system involved in the outbreak, it may be very difficult to obtain representative samples of the microbiological water quality that caused illness. For infectious agents, the exposure of concern is less likely to be chronic exposure to low levels of a microbial pathogen but rather short-term exposure to a "slug" of fecal contamination in the water system. Untreated and unprotected water supplies, such as those used in many developing countries, can have tremendous variability in microbiological water quality. Seasonal changes in rainfall and water temperature influence the introduction of fecal contamination into water sources and the survival characteristics of microbial pathogens in water.

Risk assessment models have considered Poisson, negative binomial, and log-normal distributions to describe the spatial occurrence of microorganisms in water (Regli et al., 1991; Haas, 1993). However, this information has rarely been used to design systematic water sampling schemes to optimize the number of samples, volume of samples, and frequency of sampling for epidemic or endemic studies of waterborne disease. Critical points for microbiological monitoring in the chain of source water, treatment, and distribution, and the performance of different methods to assess pathogens and indicator organisms in drinking water have been reviewed by Havelaar (1993). EPA and WHO guidelines for sampling are based primarily on the size of the population served (WHO, 1993). For persistent microorganisms, epidemic studies have attempted to obtain "historical" samples from ice, toilet tanks, or dead ends in distribution lines.

CHARACTERIZATION OF WATER SUPPLY
BY SOURCE AND TREATMENT

Studies of water quality and health in developing countries have frequently used type of water source as a proxy for microbiological water quality, which can lead to serious misclassification of exposure because some traditional water sources (deep wells) may be of higher microbiological quality than some intervention water supplies (piped water) that become contaminated in the distribution system. In industrialized countries, water source (groundwater versus surface water) and type of treatment (coagulation/flocculation [chemical aggregation of particulates], filtration, disinfection) give some indication of the likelihood of the presence of certain types of infectious agents such as enteric protozoa. Epidemiologic studies have been proposed in the United States to compare *Cryptosporidium* infection rates in communities that use groundwater supplies with those of communities that use surface water supplies (CDC, 1995).

Discussion and Recommendations

The demands of perfectly accurate exposure assessment could mistakenly lead to the pessimistic conclusion that assessment of exposure to drinking water contaminants is hopelessly complex and little can be done to improve upon it. Certainly, no approach suitable for epidemiologic application could be as accurate as those used in laboratory settings in which exposures are experimentally manipulated and thus known with certainty. However, consideration of the sources of uncertainty has several direct and immediate benefits and suggests several avenues of methodologic research.

We need to examine the extent to which the relatively crude exposure measures traditionally used adequately capture inter-individual differences in exposure. Even though precise quantitative exposure indicators may be beyond our reach, the available markers may perform quite well for identifying broader categories of exposure. In the case of THM exposure, for example, simple dichotomies based on consumption of water from groundwater supplies versus surface water supplies may well provide a meaningful distinction but must be examined in comparison to more precise measures. Quantitative risk assessment, of course, requires more detailed information. Similarly, though there are clear limitations in the use of indicator organisms as proxies for specific pathogens such as *Cryptosporidium*, the conventional measures presumably do provide some information on the presence of fecal contamination. The question for any indicator is whether it is adequate for a specific purpose. Identification of deficiencies in the routinely used measures points toward specific avenues for improvement. Given sufficient importance, almost any one of the sources of uncertainty is amenable to further study and incorporation, at least to some extent, in epidemiologic studies. For example, if duration of showering or the time of the day that water is ingested is a factor in determining THM exposures, those questions can be asked. What is missing in many cases is an understanding of which of the many potential sources of uncertainty is most important and what strategies will be most effective in refining epidemiologic studies.

In addition to the logistical issues in assessing waterborne exposures, some of the attributes of the exposure–disease relationship of interest must be taken into account. A particular concern is with the expected time course relating exposure to disease. In the case of chemical agents and cancer, the presumed course is one of prolonged exposure and prolonged latency, whereas for birth defects, the same agent may be of interest in a brief time window in early pregnancy. Infectious agents, while generally following an acute time course between exposure and disease, follow a variable response course that depends on dose of the agent, prior exposure to the agent, and specific host factors.

The ability to attribute disease to a waterborne agent is in part a function of the specificity of the exposure–disease relationship. Multifactorial diseases such as acute diarrhea or bladder cancer have many known and potential causes, only one of which may be the agent of concern. Thus, among all cases with a particular set of symptoms or disease, only a subset is even potentially attributable to the particular exposure. Infectious disease may be refined by analyzing clinical specimens collected from cases to subdivide the disease of interest by etiologic agent or by identifying a set of symptoms pathognomic for the organism of concern. In contrast, the ability to subdivide chronic diseases such as cancer based on the etiologic agent is at a very early stage. Related to specificity is vulnerability to confounding. Where there are important causes of the disease other than the one of interest, there is the potential for distortion of the effects of exposure. Although it may seem initially that exposure to water contaminants is essentially random, correlates of water source such as geographic location and health habits are quite plausible as sources of confounding.

More work in this area is likely, given the regulatory and public health concerns with drinking water. Perhaps more important than any specific technical refinement is the need for collaboration of epidemiologists with experts in exposure assessment, including engineers, microbiologists, and chemists. Among epidemiologists concerned with waterborne exposures, there appears to be some fragmentation based on the class of agent (infectious, chemical) or even the type of outcome (gastrointestinal disease, cancer, birth defects), which may impede the appreciation of the issues involving exposure assessment that cut across such boundaries.

References

Andelman JB. 1985. Inhalation exposure in the home to volatile organic contaminants of drinking water. Sci Total Environ 47:443–460.

Bates MN, Smith AH, Hopenhayn-Rich C. 1992. Arsenic ingestion and internal cancers: a review. Am J Epidemiol 135:462–476.

Batik O, Craun GF, Tuthill RW, Kraemer DF. 1980. An epidemiologic study of the relationship between hepatitis A and water supply characteristics and treatment. Am J Public Health 70:167–168.

Bean JA, Isacson P, Hahne RMA, Kohler J. 1982. Drinking water and cancer incidence in Iowa: II. Radioactivity in drinking water. Am J Epidemiol 116: 924–932.

Beresford SAA. 1985. Is nitrate in the drinking water associated with the risk of cancer in the urban UK? Int J Epidemiol 14:57–63.

Birkhead G, Vogt RL. 1989. Epidemiologic surveillance for endemic Giardia lamblia infection in Vermont. Am J Epidemiol 129:762–768.

Bull RJ, Birnbaum LS, Cantor KP, Rose JB, Butterworth BE, Pegram R, Tuomisto J. 1995. Water chlorination: essential process or cancer hazard? Fund Appl Toxicol 28:155–166.

Cantor KP. 1983. Epidemiologic studies of chlorination by-products in drinking water: an overview. In: Jolley RL, ed. Water Chlorination: Environmental Impact and Health Effects, 4th Ed. Ann Arbor, MI, Ann Arbor Scientific Publishers, 1381–1397.

Cantor KP, Shy CM, Chilvers C. 1996. Water pollution. In: Schottenfeld D, Fraumeni JF Jr, eds. Cancer Epidemiology and Prevention, 2nd ed. New York, Oxford University Press, in press.

Cantor KP, Hoover R, Hartge P, Mason TJ, Silverman DT, Altman R, Austin DF, Child MA, Key CR, Marrett LD, Myers MH, Narayana AS, Levin LI, Sullivan JW, Swanson GM, Thomas DB, West DW. 1987. Bladder cancer, drinking water source, and tap water consumption: a case-control study. J Natl Cancer Inst 79:1269–1279.

Carmichael WW, Jones CLA, Mahmood NA, Theiss WC. 1985. Algal toxins and water-based diseases. CRC Crit Rev Environ Control 15:275–313.

Centers for Disease Control and Prevention. 1993. Surveillance for waterborne disease outbreaks—United States, 1991–1992. MMWR 42:1–22.

Centers for Disease Control and Prevention. 1995. Assessing the public health threat associated with waterborne cryptosporidiosis: report of a workshop. MMWR 44:1–19.

Chen C-J, Chuang Y-C, Lin T-M, et al. 1985. Malignant neoplasms among residents of a blackfoot disease endemic area in Taiwan: high arsenic artesian well water and cancers. Cancer Res 45:5895–5899.

Cheung WHS, Chang KCK, Hung RPS. 1990. Health effects of beach water pollution in Hong Kong. Epidemiol Infect 105:139–162.

Chilvers C, Inskip H, Caygill C, Bartholomew B, Fraser P, Hill M. 1984. A survey of dietary nitrate in well-water users. Int J Epidemiol 13: 324–331.

Chute CG, Smith RP, Baron JA. 1987. Risk factors for endemic giardiasis. Am J Public Health 77:585–587.

Cohn P, Klotz J, Bove F, Berkowitz M, Fagliano J. 1994. Drinking water contamination and the incidence of leukemia and non-Hodgkin's lymphoma. Environ Health Perspect 102:556–561.

Comstock GW. 1979. Water hardness and cardiovascular disease. Am J Epidemiol 110:375–400.

D'Antonio RG, Winn RE, Taylor JP, Gustafson TL, Current WL, Rhodes MM, Gary GW, Zajac RA. 1985. A waterborne outbreak of cryptosporidiosis in normal hosts. Ann Intern Med 103:886–888.

Deane M, Swan SH, Harris JA, Epstein DM, Neutra RR. 1989. Adverse pregnancy outcomes in relation to water contamination, Santa Clara County, California, 1980–1981. Am J Epidemiol 129:894–904.

Dennis DT, Smith RP, Welch JJ, Chute CG, Anderson B, Herndon JL, von Reyn CF. 1993. Endemic giardiasis in New Hampshire: a case-control study of environmental risks. J Infect Dis 167:1391–1395.

Driscoll WS, Horowitz HS, Meyers RJ. 1983. Prevalence of dental caries and dental fluorosis in areas with negligible, optimal, and above-optimal water fluoride concentrations. J Am Dent Assoc 107: 42–47.

Dufour AP. 1986. Diseases caused by water contact. In: Craun GF, ed. Waterborne Disease in the United States. Boca Raton, FL. CRC Press: 23–41.

DuPont HL, Chappell CL, Sterling CR, Okhuysen PC, Rose JB, Jakubowski W. 1995. The infectivity of Cryptosporidium parvum in healthy volunteers. N Engl J Med 332:855–859.

Ershow AG, Brown LM, Cantor KP. 1991. Intake of tapwater and total water by pregnant and lactating women. Am J Public Health 81:328–334.

Esrey SA, Potash JB, Roberts L, Shiff C. 1990. Health benefits from improvements in water supply and sanitation: survey and analysis of the literature on selected diseases. WASH Technical Report No. 66.

Gallaher MM, Herndon JL, Nims LJ, Sterling CR, Grabowski DJ, Hull HF. 1989. Cryptosporidiosis and surface water. Am J Public Health 79:39–42.

Griffith J, Duncan RC, Riggan WB, Pellom AC. 1989. Cancer mortality in U.S. counties with hazardous waste sites and ground water pollution. Arch Environ Health 44:69–74.

Haas CN. 1993. Quantifying microbiological risks. In: Craun GF, ed. Safety of Water Disinfection: Balancing Chemical and Microbial Risks. Washington, DC: ILSI Press 389–398.

Hallenbeck WH, Brenniman GR, Anderson RJ. 1981. High sodium in drinking water and its effect on blood pressure. Am J Epidemiol 114:817–826.

Havelaar AH. 1993. The place for microbiological monitoring in the production of safe drinking water. In: Craun GF, ed. Safety of Water Disinfection: Balancing Chemical and Microbial Risks. Washington, DC:ILSI Press 127–141.

Hayes EB, Matte TD, O'Brien TR, McKinley TW, Logsdon GS, Rose JB, Ungar BLP, Word DM, Pinsky PF, Cummings ML, Wilson MA, Long EG, Hurwitz ES, Juranek DD. 1989. Large community outbreak of cryptosporidiosis due to contamination of a filtered public water supply. N Engl J Med 320:1372–1376.

Hoover RN, McKay FW, Fraumeni JR Jr. 1976. Fluoridated drinking water and the occurrence of cancer. J Natl Cancer Inst 57:757–768.

I'Cheng C'I, Blackwell RQ. 1968. A controlled retrospective study of Blackfoot disease: an epidemic peripheral gangrene disease in Taiwan. Am J Epidemiol 88:7–24.

Jenkins PA. 1991. Mycobacteria in the environment. J Appl Bacteriol; 70 (suppl); 137S–141S.

Jo WK, Weisel CP, Lioy PJ. 1990a. Chloroform exposure and the health risk associated with multiple uses of chlorinated tap water. Risk Anal 10:581–585.

Jo WK, Weisel CP, Lioy PJ. 1990b. Routes of chloroform exposure and body burden from showering with chlorinated tap water. Risk Anal 10:575–580.

Kachur SB. 1994. An evaluation of methods for predicting total trihalomethane concentrations in exposure assessment studies. Thesis for Master of Science in Environmental Engineering, Department of Environmental Sciences and Engineering, University of North Carolina, Chapel Hill, North Carolina.

Klein PD. Gastrointestinal physiology working group. 1991. In: Graham DY, Gaillour A, Opekun AR, Smith EO. Water source as risk factor for Helicobacter pylori infection in Peruvian children. Lancet 337:1503–1506.

Kuzma RJ, Kuzma CM, Buncher CR. 1977. Ohio drinking water source and cancer rates. Am J Public Health 67:725–729.

LeChevallier MW, Norton WD, Lee RG. 1991. Giardia and Cryptosporidium spp. in filtered drinking water supplies. Appl Environ Microbiol 57:2617–2621.

MacKenzie WR, Hoxie NJ, Proctor ME, Gradus MS, Blair KA, Peterson DE, Kazmierczak JJ, Addiss DG, Fox KR, Rose JB, Davis JP. 1994. A massive outbreak in Milwaukee of Cryptosporidium infection transmitted through the public water supply. N Engl J Med 331:161–167.

Milwaukee Journal. 1993. Watering down a disaster (Editorial). June 26.

Mintz ED, Reiff FM, Tauxe RV. 1995. Safe water treatment and storage in the home. JAMA 273:948–953.

Morris RD, Audet A-M, Angelillo IF, Chalmers TC, Mosteller F. 1992. Chlorination, chlorination by-products, and cancer: a meta-analysis. Am J Public Health 82:955–963.

Payment P, Franco E. 1993. Clostridium perfringens and somatic soliphages as indicators of the efficiency of drinking water treatment for viruses and protozoan cysts. Appl Environ Microbiol 59: 2418–2424.

Payment P, Richardson L, Siemiatycki J, Dewar R, Edwardes M, Franco E. 1991. A randomized trial to evaluate the risk of gastrointestinal disease due to consumption of drinking water meeting current microbiological standards. Am J Public Health 81:703–708.

Phillips AM, Silbergeld EK. 1985. Health effects studies of exposure from hazardous waste sites—where are we today? (Editorial). Am J Ind Med 8:1–7.

Polissar L, Severson RK, Boatman ES. 1984. A case-control study of asbestos in drinking water and cancer risk. Am J Epidemiol 119:456–471.

Regli S, Rose JB, Haas CN, Gerba CP. 1991. Modeling the risk from Giardia and viruses in drinking water. J Am Water Works Assoc 83:76–84.

Rook JJ. 1974. Formation of haloforms during chlorination of natural waters. Water Treat Exam 23:234–243.

Rose JB. 1988. Occurrence and significance of Cryptosporidium in water. J Am Water Works Assoc 80:53–58.

Rose JB, Gerba CP, Jakubowski W. 1991. Survey of potable water supplies for Cryptosporidium and Giardia. Environ Sci Technol 25:1393–1400.

Schubert RHW. 1991. Aeromonads and their significance as potential pathogens in water. J Appl Bact 70 (suppl) :131S–135S.

Sobsey MD, Dufour AP, Gerba CP, LeChevallier MW, Payment P. 1993. Using a conceptual framework for assessing risks to health from microbes in drinking water. J Am Water Works Assoc 85:44–48.

Sowers MR, Clark MK, Jannausch ML, Wallace RB. 1991. A prospective study of bone mineral content and fracture in communities with differential fluoride exposure. Am J Epidemiol 133:649–660.

US Environmental Protection Agency. 1986. Ambient water quality criteria for bacteria—1986. EPA 44015-84-002. Washington, DC, Office of Regulations and Standards.

US Environmental Protection Agency. 1994. National Primary Drinking Water Standards. EPA 810-F-94-001A, February 1994. Washington, DC, Office of Water.

Whorton MD, Wong O, Morgan RW, Gordon N. 1989. An epidemiologic investigation of birth outcomes in relation to dibromochloropropane contamination in drinking water in Fresno County, California. Int Arch Occup Environ Health 61:403–407.

Wong O, Morgan RW, Whorton MD, Gordon N, Kheifets L. 1989. Ecological analyses and case-control studies of gastric cancer and leukaemia in relation to DBCP in drinking water in Fresno County, California. Br J Ind Med 46:521–528.

World Health Organization. 1993. Guidelines for drinking-water quality. 2nd ed. Vol. 1. Recommendations. World Health Organization, Geneva. 183 pages.

Wurtz R. 1994. Cyclospora: a newly identified intestinal pathogen of humans. Clin Infect Dis 18: 620–623.

Zmirou D, Ferley JP, Collin JF, Charrel M, Berlin J. 1987. A follow-up study of gastro-intestinal diseases related to bacteriologically substandard drinking water. Am J Public Health 77:582–587.

Outdoor Air I:

Particulates

6

DOUGLAS W. DOCKERY

C. ARDEN POPE III

MANY aspects of the study of health effects of particulate air pollution typify the challenges in environmental epidemiology. The evidence that acute air pollution episodes, consisting primarily of particulate matter and sulfur air pollution, can cause short-term increases in mortality is persuasive. Episodes such as the one in London in 1952 resulted in clear increases in the number of deaths over the period concurrent with the pollution episode. Thus, we have an anchor of certainty that particulate air pollution causes adverse health effects in the high-dose region of the dose-response curve.

A much greater challenge is to determine whether an analogous phenomenon occurs within the much lower range of particulate air pollution routinely experienced in urban areas of the United States and other modern societies. The research question arises directly out of these historical acute episodes—are there increases in the frequency of adverse health outcomes, including mortality, as a result of elevations in particulate air pollution? Some studies have addressed the possible effects of long-term, low-level exposure to particulate air pollution on the development of chronic diseases such as lung cancer and cardiovascular disease, but the current and most intensively pursued research avenue is the short-term effect of pollutant levels on mortality and morbidity, an etiologic process operating on the time scale of days rather than years.

Because the likely magnitude of effect is so much more modest than the levels associated with historical episodes, sophisticated statistical tools are required to make this assessment. Instead of examining one pollution episode and the health effects associated with it, these studies have focused on "normal" fluctuations in pollution on a day-to-day basis, addressing hundreds or thousands of tiny pollution episodes and the consequent health patterns.

The unique aspects of studying a time series in which the exposure and disease are thought to be related over relatively short time intervals presents very different methodological issues than are typically of concern in relation to chronic disease etiology. We are no longer comparing rates of health outcome among subsets of the population that have varying exposure, with the accompanying concerns of long-term exposure assessment or confounding by health behaviors such as tobacco use or diet. Instead, a given community is monitored over a period of time in which everyone's exposure changes over short periods of time and the investigator tries to determine whether there are discernible patterns of disease related to the temporal variation in exposure.

Despite the methodological challenges in distinguishing the absence of any adverse effect of low levels of particulates from a small adverse effect, the question is of critical regulatory and public health importance. By definition, dramatic pollution episodes are rare events, with strong effects over a short period of time. Regulators acknowledge the need to avoid such events with little debate. Repeated, persistent small adverse effects in large populations have the potential for a much more sizable public health consequence, yet there is no piece of evidence that constitutes the "smoking gun." The entire array of evidence is circumstantial, and is persuasive only in its consistency across geographic settings and analytic methods and in the lack of plausible alternative explanations. In a contentious regulatory environment, such a constellation of evidence is much more conducive to debate than a small number of definitive experiments or epidemiologic studies showing dramatic effects.

Even accepting the possible influence of particulates on disease, some have argued that accelerating the onset of an inevitable death or disease by a few days or weeks ("harvesting") is of little public health concern. However, episodes of excess deaths have not been accompanied by corresponding deficits a few days later, suggesting that the "harvesting" effect is small. Furthermore, a few well-designed prospective studies have shown long-term effects of pollution on the development of chronic respiratory and cardiovascular disease.

Another major challenge is the separation of the influence of particulates from that of other closely associated pollutants such as sulfates, as well as from temperature. Efforts to control for these correlated variables have been made both statistically and by identifying unusual geographical areas in which levels of other pollutants are very low.

Air pollution in the United States and many other countries is regulated on the basis of ambient concentrations of specific air pollutants. The United States Environmental Protection Agency has promulgated ambient air quality standards for four specific chemicals—sulfur dioxide (SO_2), nitrogen dioxide (NO_2), carbon monoxide (CO), and ozone (O_3). The World Health Organization (1987) has recommended air quality guidelines for these same pollutants that have been adopted by most other countries. The combined evidence from toxicologic, controlled exposure clinical, and epidemiologic studies provides the basis for these standards or guidelines. There is evidence from the toxicologic and clinical studies of acute health effects following exposure to these specific chemicals. The observed associations from epidemiologic studies do not demonstrate causal relations but support the findings of these controlled exposure studies. In real exposure situations, pollutants always are mixtures, and epidemiologic studies cannot absolutely eliminate the possibility of confounding by other pollutants. On the other hand, epidemiologic studies are very effective at assessing the effects of these combined exposures, an assessment that is very difficult in controlled exposure studies.

Ambient air quality standards have also been promulgated for particulate matter, a complex mixture of multiple pollutants. Particulate air pollution is essentially everything suspended in the air that is not a gas. Particulate matter includes smoke, soot, and other combustion products. It includes wind-blown dust, sea salt, pollens, spores, and insect parts. Toxicologic and clinical studies have not reported adverse health effects from controlled exposures to models of particulate matter except at extremely high concentrations.

The evidence for health effects of particulate air pollution has come almost exclusively from epidemiologic studies. The estimated relative risks associated with particulate matter at concentrations observed in most developed countries are small—1.2 or less. The ability of epidemiology to detect relative risks of this magnitude while excluding bias from confounding has been questioned (Taubes, 1995). Moreover, the lack of supporting toxicologic and clinical evidence has raised questions regarding the validity and generalizability of these epidemiologic findings (Utell and Samet, 1993). Nevertheless, these findings have remained resilient and quantitatively consistent. Thus the experience with the assessment of the health effects of particulate air pollution provides an interesting case study of issues facing environmental epidemiology in general.

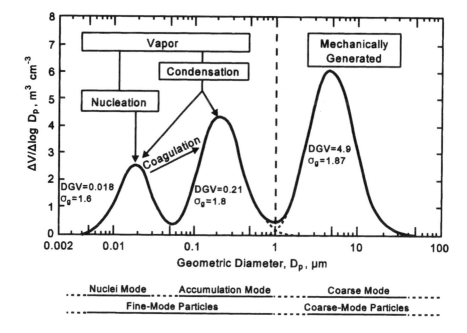

Figure 6-1. Schematic of atmospheric aerosol surface area distribution showing principal modes and main sources of mass for each mode (from Wilson and Suh, 1996.)

Characteristics of Particulate Air Pollution

Particulate air pollution is a mixture of solid, liquid, or solid and liquid particles suspended in the air. These suspended particles vary in size, composition, and origin. It is convenient to classify particles by their aerodynamic properties because (1) the aerodynamics govern the transport and removal of particles in the air, (2) the aerodynamics govern their deposition within the respiratory system, and (3) the chemical composition and sources of particles are associated with their aerodynamic characteristics. The aerodynamic properties are conveniently summarized by the *aerodynamic diameter*—the size of a unit-density sphere with the same aerodynamic characteristics. Particles are sampled and described on the basis of their aerodynamic diameter, usually called simply the particle size.

The size of suspended particles in the atmosphere varies over four orders of magnitude, from a few nanometers to tens of micrometers (Fig. 6-1). The largest particles, called the *coarse fraction* (or *mode*), are mechanically produced by breaking up larger solid particles. These particles can include wind-blown dust from agricultural processes, uncovered soil, unpaved roads, or mining operations. Traffic produces road dust and air turbulence that can re-entrain road dust. Near the coasts, evaporation of sea spray can produce large particles. Pollens, mold spores, and plant and insect parts are all in this larger size range. The amount of energy required to break these particles into smaller sizes increases as the size decreases, which effectively establishes a lower limit for the production of these coarse particles of approximately 1 μm (Friedlander, 1978).

Smaller particles, called the *fine fraction* or *mode*, are largely formed from gases. The smallest particles, less than 0.1 μm, are formed by nucleation, that is, condensation of low-vapor-pressure substances formed by high-temperature vaporization or by chemical reactions in the atmosphere to form new particles (nuclei). Particles in this *nucleation range* or *mode* grow by coagulation, that is, the combination of two or more particles to form a larger particle, or by condensation, that is, condensation of gas or vapor molecules onto the surface of existing particles. Coagulation is most efficient for large numbers of particles, and condensation is most efficient for large surface areas. Therefore, the efficiency of both coagulation and condensation decreases as particle size increases, which effectively produces an upper bound such that particles do not grow by these processes beyond approximately 1 μm. Thus particles tend to "accumulate" between 0.1 and 1 μm, the so-called *accumulation range*.

Submicron-sized particles can be produced by the condensation of metals or organics, which are vaporized in high-temperature combustion processes. Submicron particles can also be produced by condensation of gases that have been converted in atmospheric reactions to low-vapor-pressure substances. For example, sulfur dioxide (SO_2) is oxidized in the atmosphere to form sulfuric acid (H_2SO_4). Nitrogen dioxide (NO_2) is oxidized to nitric acid (HNO_3), which in turn reacts with ammonia (NH_3) to form ammonium nitrate (NH_4NO_3). The particles produced by intermediate reactions of gases in the atmosphere are called *secondary particles*. Secondary sulfate and nitrate particles are the dominant component of fine particles in the United States. Combustion of fossil fuels such as coal, oil, and gasoline can produce coarse particles from the release of noncombustible materials (flyash); fine particles from the condensation of materials vaporized during combustion; and secondary particles through the atmospheric reactions of sulfur oxides and nitrogen oxides initially released as gases.

Deposition, Clearance, and Toxicity

Aerodynamic particle size is the most important characteristic influencing deposition in the respiratory system. Models of inhaled particle deposition

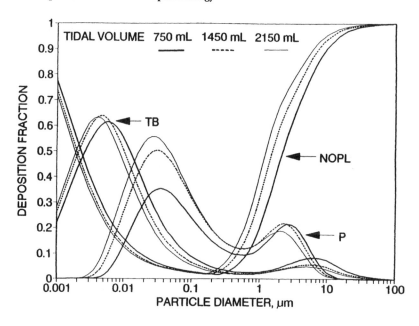

Figure 6-2. Disposition efficiencies in different parts of the respiratory system. "Rest," "Normal," and "Exercise" correspond to tidal volumes of 750, 1450, and 2150 mL, respectively. (After Phalen *et al,* 1991.)

relate aerodynamic particle diameter to the site of deposition within the respiratory system as a function of tidal volume (Fig. 6-2). Particles larger than 10 μm aerodynamic diameter are deposited in the nose and mouth and do not penetrate into the lungs. Particles smaller than 1 μm aerodynamic diameter are more likely to penetrate deeply into the lungs and deposit in the smaller airways and the alveoli. Thus the submicron particles produced by combustion processes are also those particles most likely to be deposited in the lower airways and alveoli of the lungs.

Particles are cleared by several mechanisms specific to the region of deposition. Particles deposited in the bronchi and bronchioles—the ciliated airways—are captured on the layer of mucus lining these airways and are carried out of the lungs on the mucociliary ladder to be expelled by coughing or to be swallowed. In healthy subjects these particles deposited in the ciliated airways are cleared quickly, 90% within the first 6 hours and the remaining 10% between 6 and 24 hours (Pavia et al., 1980). Particles deposited deeper, in the nonciliated airways and alveoli, are engulfed by lung macrophages and cleared more slowly, as macrophages transport the ingested particles onto the mucociliary ladder or into the lymphatic system. Cohen and coworkers (1979) found that 90% of these particles were removed within a year in healthy nonsmokers. Long-term clearance rates are reduced in older adults, in smokers, and in people with chronic respiratory disease (Bates, 1989).

Submicron particles not only penetrate to the alveolar regions but also transport other toxins to these regions of the lung. Soluble gaseous pollutants are effectively removed in the upper airways before they can penetrate to the deep lung. However, if they are adsorbed onto the surface of submicron particles, they can be deposited in the lower airways and alveoli. Thus the large surface area of submicron particles and their ability to penetrate deeply into the lungs make them effective carriers of potentially toxic metals and chemicals into the lower airways and alveolar regions of the lungs, where they may reside for extended periods of time.

Biologic effects of deposited particles are determined by the physical and chemical nature of the particle itself (particularly its solubility), the site of deposition within the lungs, and the physiologic response to the particles. Toxicity of urban particles depends in part on the type of metal compounds they contain and their combustion-derived organic content (Hatch et al., 1985). Particles themselves or the toxic metals and chemicals they carry may not directly produce injury to the lungs or other organ systems. Rather the clearance processes may trigger a chain of physiologic responses that lead to an amplified, potentially injurious response. For some air pollutants, specifically the gaseous pollutants such as sulfur dioxide and ozone, the effects are direct and immediate. For particles, however, it appears that a series of steps may be necessary following deposition in the lungs before overt physiologic or clinical effects can be observed.

In summary, submicron particles penetrate into the lower airways and alveolar regions of the lung where they may reside for extended periods before being cleared. These submicron particles carry soluble gaseous pollutants or metals into the gas-exchange regions of the lung. Direct injury is possible, particularly by contaminants adsorbed to the surface of particles. However, a likely pathway begins with the physiologic process of clearing particles, which starts a chain of events that amplify the response and injury. People with heightened immunologic status, such as asthmatics and patients with chronic obstructive pulmonary disease, may be particularly at risk.

Measuring exposure to particles

In 1987, the U.S. Environmental Protection Agency (EPA) redefined the National Ambient Air Quality Standard (NAAQS) for particles based on particulate matter smaller than 10 μm aerodynamic diameter (PM_{10}) (EPA, 1987). This 10-μm cutoff focused monitoring and regulatory efforts on particles of a size that would be deposited in, and damaging to, the conducting airways and the gas-exchange areas of the respiratory system during mouth breathing (Miller et al., 1979). Recent epidemiologic studies have used PM_{10} measurements as the basis of exposure estimation. Earlier studies, however, used a variety of measures of particle concentration to define exposure.

The EPA's initial reference measure for particles was total suspended particulates (TSP), measured by high-volume samplers. This sampling method has an ill-defined upper size limit between 25 μm and 45μm, which is dependent on wind speed and direction (Lippmann and Lioy, 1985). In addition, TSP measurements are subject to artifactual conversion of SO_2 to sulfate on the filters or to volatilization of nitrate aerosols from sampler filters. Many epidemiologic studies of air pollution in the 1960s and 1970s in the United States used TSP measurements as the indicator of particle exposures. The inclusion of noninhalable particles and chemical artifacts weakens the power of epidemiologic studies based on TSP measures of exposure to detect associations with particulates.

A potentially more specific estimate of the etiologically relevant exposure is given by measurement of particles smaller than 2.5 μm aerodynamic diameter ($PM_{2.5}$). This size cut separates particles on the basis of their characteristic chemical composition and their ability to penetrate into the gas-exchange regions of the respiratory tract (Miller et al., 1979). As noted earlier, a smaller size cut, closer to 1 μm, might be more appropriate to achieve these goals. The continued use of the 2.5-μm cut is a historical artifact of the sampler design in the late 1970s. Smaller size cuts require higher flow rates, and 2.5 μm was effectively the smallest size cut that could be accomplished with the equipment available in the late 1970s. Although better equipment and alternative size cuts are now available, the low number and mass concentrations of particles between 1 and 3 μm implies that there will only be small differences in samples collected within this range.

Studies from Great Britain and other European countries have often used a pseudo-measure of particle mass called British or black smoke (BS). This is a measure of the darkness of particles collected on a filter as determined by reflectance. Mass concentration is estimated on the basis of the reflectance of a standard particle mass. Calibration of reflectance depends on the specific chemical composition of the particles (Lippmann and Lioy, 1985). The upper size limit of the sampler is nominally 4.5 μm aerodynamic diameter, although the penetration of particles through the sampler inlet does not define a sharp size cut-point (Lippmann and Lioy, 1985). Generally, particles in the fine mode tend to be dark whereas those in the coarse mode tend to be lighter in color (Dzubay and Stevens, 1975).

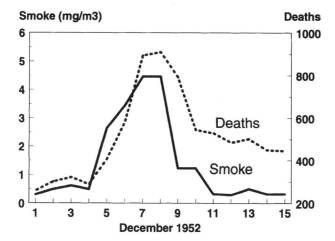

Figure 6-3. Daily mean pollution concentrations and daily number of deaths during the London fog episode of 1952. (After Ministry of Health, 1954.)

Black smoke, therefore, is often considered to be a surrogate measure of fine particle mass concentrations.

Epidemiologic evidence of health effects

The hazard of episodes of high air pollution was recognized in the first half of this century, when episodes of extreme air pollution were associated with increased deaths and morbidity in the Meuse Valley, Belgium, in 1934 (Firket, 1936) and Donora, Pennsylvania, in 1947 (Schrenk, 1949). However, it was the air pollution episodes of December 1952 in London that provided the first quantitative air pollution exposure data and the most convincing evidence of the hazard.

On Thursday, December 4, 1952, a slow-moving anticyclone came to a halt over the city of London (Brimblecombe, 1987). Fog developed over the city, and particulate and sulfur pollution began accumulating in the stagnating air mass. Smoke and sulfur dioxide concentrations built up over the following 3 days. On Monday, the polluted fog began to ease, and by Tuesday conditions were back to normal. Mortality records showed that deaths increased in a pattern very similar to that of the pollution measurements (Fig. 6-3). The maximum number of deaths occurred on the fourth day of the fog. It was estimated that 4000 extra deaths occurred (Martin, 1964).

Investigators at that time brought methods used in the evaluation of infectious disease outbreaks to bear on this air pollution event and convincingly demonstrated the hazard of this episode. Causality was accepted even though no specific hypotheses were tested statistically, no estimate of the exposure-response association was calculated, and no biologic mechanism was identified. As a result of this analysis, a Committee was formed, and ultimately controls were placed on coal combustion in London (Beaver, 1953).

Although the London 1952 episode identified the hazard of extreme air pollution episodes, it left open several important questions. It was not clear from this experience whether health effects were associated with lower concentrations. Moreover, the specific agent within the mix of pollutants that was responsible for the observed health effects could not be identified.

By the 1970s, a link had been well established between respiratory disease and particulate and/or sulfur oxide air pollution, but there remained disagreement as to the level of pollution that would significantly affect human health. In reviewing research published between 1968 and 1977, Holland and several other prominent British scientists (1979) concluded that particulate and related air pollution at high levels poses hazards to human health, but that health effects of particulate pollution at lower concentrations could not be "disentangled" from health effects of other factors. Other reviewers (Bates, 1980; Ellison and Waller, 1978; Shy, 1979; Ware et al., 1981) concluded that the epidemiologic evidence showed that human health may be adversely affected by particulate pollution even at relatively low concentrations.

Recent epidemiologic studies have provided additional quantification of the health effects associated with particulate pollution at levels common in contemporary urban areas of the developed world. More specific and precise measures of both pollution exposures and health end points plus advances in analytic techniques have permitted the evaluation of pollution associations in population and panel studies that would not have been possible in the 1970s.

Review Methods

This review presents a comparison of recent epidemiologic studies of the association of acute exposures to particulate air pollution with increased mortality and morbidity. The methods used to evaluate the associations of time-varying particulate air pollution exposures with daily measures of mortality and morbidity are discussed. The consistency and coherence of recent epidemiologic data regarding adverse health effects of particulate air pollution are assessed.

The epidemiologic studies included provide the following information: (1) exposure to particulates reported as PM_{10} concentrations, (2) health effects measured as change in mortality or indicators of respiratory disease with time scales of days up to weeks, and (3) measures of association and their standard errors. Epidemiologic studies are separated by comparable health end points (for example, mortality or exacerbation of asthma).

The estimated relative risks are usually small (1.1 or less). Therefore it is convenient to express these relative risks as the percentage increase in daily deaths associated with some specified increase in exposure. We have chosen to express these increases relative to an increase of $10 \mu g/m^3$ in PM_{10}, as a convenient unit of exposure well within the range of day-to-day fluctuations observed in these studies. For studies that have used logistic or Poisson regression and PM_{10}, this is a simple calculation based on reported regression coefficients and their standard errors. In some studies, particularly those with continuous health end points such as pulmonary function, associations are reported as linear rather than as proportional (or logarithmic) changes relative to particulate pollution. For these studies, the effect was reestimated as percentage change from the mean response associated with a $10 \mu g/m^3$ increase in PM_{10} above the mean exposure. This is a reasonable assumption for estimates close to the mean but will break down far from the mean.

For a few studies, particle concentrations had been transformed before being included in the analysis—for example, effects reported as a function of the logarithm of the particle mass concentrations. For these studies, the effect was estimated for a $10 \mu g/m^3$ increase in PM_{10} above the mean exposure. Again, this is appropriate close to the mean but will provide disparate estimated effects if extrapolated far from the mean.

Ninety-five percent confidence intervals were calculated for each exposure estimate. In most cases, reports included standard errors of the estimates or confidence intervals. In a few early studies, however, only P values were given. In these studies, standard errors were estimated assuming a normal distribution. When P values were reported as less than some arbitrary cutoff (e.g., $P < .05$), the standard errors were calculated on the basis of the upper limit of the cutoff probability (e.g., $z=1.96$ for $P < .05$).

To provide a combined estimate of the effect of a $10 \mu g/m^3$ increase in PM_{10} concentration for each health end point, a weighted-average effect estimate was calculated where the study-specific effect was weighted by its inverse variance (one over the standard error squared). The variance of the combined estimate was calculated as the inverse of the sum of the

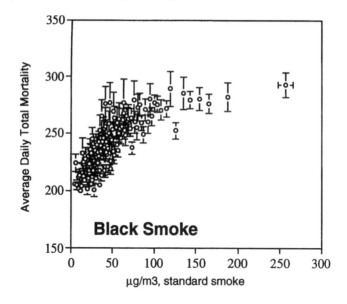

Figure 6-4. Average daily mortality in Greater London for period April 1, 1965, through December 31, 1972, versus British Smoke ($\mu g/m^3$). Each point represents average of 20 days sorted by smoke, with error bars of one standard deviation. (After Lippmann et al, 1995.)

study-specific inverse variances. Confidence intervals about the combined estimates were calculated assuming a normal variance.

Mortality studies

A series of recent epidemiologic studies have highlighted the association of particulate air pollution with increased daily mortality in a score of communities around the world. In 1990, Schwartz and Marcus (1990) published a reanalysis of daily mortality counts and daily BS and SO_2 measurements for the winters of 1959 to 1972 in London. This time series was originally compiled by MacFarlane (1977) and had been analyzed by several investigators (e.g. Mazumdar et al., 1982; Ostro, 1984). After sorting the data by particle (BS) concentrations and averaging each 20 consecutive observations, Schwartz and Marcus showed a striking nonlinear association between daily mortality and BS measurements. Lippmann and colleagues (1995) have recently presented an equivalent graphic analysis of these London data (Fig. 6-4). These analyses indicate that mortality increased with increasing BS down to the lowest measured concentrations. Schwartz and Marcus reported that positive, statistically significant associations remained after adjustment for possible confounding by temperature and season in multiple regression. In addition, multiple regression analyses showed that the estimated association with particulates (BS) was stable after adjustment for SO_2, whereas the estimated association with SO_2 was substantially reduced after adjustment for the BS measurements. This finding suggests that the association with SO_2 was due to confounding by the particulate air pollution measure (BS).

Analyses of the association of daily mortality in two cities in the United States—Steubenville, Ohio (Schwartz and Dockery, 1992) and Philadelphia (Schwartz and Dockery, 1992)—confirmed the London findings based on daily measurements of particles (measured as TSP) and of SO_2. Both of these analyses suggested that daily mortality was associated with the much lower particle concentrations observed currently in the United States and other developed countries, even after adjustment for SO_2 exposures.

Consistency of mortality associations

In addition to the analyses of daily mortality and suspended particulate measures in Philadelphia and Steubenville, increased daily mortality has been reported to be associated with measured suspended particulate air pollution concentrations in Detroit (Schwartz, 1991), Cincinnati (Schwartz 1994f), Erfurt, Germany (Spix et al., 1993), and Beijing, China (Xu et al., 1994). Positive associations with BS measures of particles have been reported in Athens, Greece (Touloumi et al., 1994) and Amsterdam, the Netherlands (Verhoeff et al., 1996). However, the lack of specific upper size cut for these particulate exposure measures makes it difficult to compare associations across studies. Therefore, the quantitative review is limited to the nine published studies that report associations between daily mortality and PM_{10} (Table 6-1).

There is good consistency in the estimated effect of PM_{10} across these studies. Effect estimates range between 0.5% and 1.6% increase in daily mortality for each 10 μg/m^3 increase in PM_{10} concentration, with a weighted mean of 0.75% (95% confidence interval, 0.59% to 0.91%).

Distributional characteristics and regression methods

Daily counts of deaths are classically modeled as generated by a Poisson process; that is, a process that generates independent and random occurrences across time or space. If time were divided into discrete periods such as days, daily death counts theoretically would be distributed as a Poisson distribution. Poissonian variation may account for most of the day-to-day variation in death counts, but the underlying mean of the process

Table 6-1. Studies of effects of PM_{10} on daily mortality

Location and Period	Reference	Particulate Measure	Mean PM_{10}	% Change in Daily Mortality for each 10 µg/m^3 Increase in PM_{10} (CI)
St. Louis, MO 1985–86	Dockery et al. (1992)	PM_{10} (prev. day)	28	1.5% (0.1%, 2.9%)
Kingston, TN 1985–86	Dockery et al. (1992)	PM_{10} (prev. day)	30	1.6% (−1.3%, 4.6%)
Birmingham, AL 1985–88	Schwartz (1993)	PM_{10} (3-day mean)	48	1.0% (0.2%, 1.9%)
Utah Valley, UT 1985–89	Pope et al. (1992)	PM_{10} (5-day mean)	47	1.5% (0.9%, 2.1%)
Los Angeles	Kinney et al. (1995)	PM_{10}	—	0.5% (0.0%, 1.0%
Chicago	Ito et al. (1995)	PM_{10}	—	0.5% (0.1%, 1.0%)
São Paulo, Brazil 1990–91	Saldiva et al. (1995)	PM_{10}	82.4	1.3% (0.7%, 1.9%)
Santiago, Chile 1989–91	Ostro et al. (1996)	PM_{10}	115	0.7% (0.4%, 0.9%)
Amsterdam 1986–92	Verhoeff et al. (1996)	PM_{10} (same day)	38	0.6% (−0.1%, 1.4%)
Combined		All PM_{10}		0.75% (0.59%, 0.91%)

PM_{10} = particulate matter smaller than 10µm aerodynamic diameter.

may be determined by pollution levels, season, weather, and other factors. For small cities (with low daily death counts) the distribution of counts is bounded on the left by zero and skewed toward large positive numbers. Therefore, Poisson regression techniques are often used to model mortality data and to estimate effects of pollution and other factors. For larger cities with larger mean daily death counts (more than 10 to 15), the Gaussian distribution is a close approximation of the Poisson distribution, and Gaussian (or normal) regression models are sometimes used. Poisson regression may still be preferred, even when the number of daily deaths is large, because the variance of the daily mortality data is not constant as assumed by normal least squares regression. Nevertheless, both Gaussian and Poisson regression approaches have been shown to produce comparable effect estimates and standard errors (Schwartz, 1994d; Kinney, 1995).

Confounding by time-varying covariates

Epidemiologic studies suffer from the weakness that observed associations with a specific exposure may result from an unmeasured association with an unknown or uncontrolled factor correlated with *both* exposure and disease—that is, from a confounder. Time-series studies have the advantage that many major causes of increased mortality (such as smoking, hypertension, or even age) cannot confound the observed associations with particulate air pollution because these factors do not vary with daily pollution exposures. This is not to say that response may not differ by these factors. Indeed, the mortality effects of particulate air pollution are most strongly seen in the elderly, which indicates that age is an effect modifier. Unfortunately data on smoking or preexisting chronic diseases are not available in the data sets of daily deaths used in these analyses, so the potential for stronger (or weaker) effect estimates among smoking or chronically debilitated subjects has not been evaluated.

Other time-varying factors such as season and weather conditions and changes in base population are potential confounders in these analyses. Indeed weather and seasonal factors are consistently found to be strong predictors of daily mortality. Thus it is important to control for these time-varying factors in the analysis.

A variety of methods and functional relations have been used to adjust for potential confounding by time-varying covariates. Of first concern has been control of seasonal patterns. Mortality tends to be highest in winter and lowest in summer. Historically, air pollution was also highest in winter. Early studies adjusted for long wave average (e.g., 15 days) of daily mortality. It was argued that such procedures would remove the seasonal and longer-term associations between air pollution and mortality, leaving only the acute day-to-day changes.

More recently, some analysts have used trigonometric functions of time to adjust for seasonal factors. Although any functional form can theoretically be fit by a sufficiently large number of trigonometric functions, these models intrinsically assume a level of long-term periodicity that is not necessarily found in real time series. A practical problem with these methods is that they require complete data. Although mortality or other count data are usually complete, exposure data are often missing. Application of these methods require estimation of missing values before the time-series analysis can be undertaken. These methods are designed for continuous Gaussian rather than count data and therefore also suffer from the weaknesses cited with the use of Gaussian regression methods.

Instead of or in addition to controlling for long-term trends and seasonal patterns by statistical modeling, time-varying factors can be modeled deterministically, that is, on the basis of hypothesized causal associations. For example, mortality rates are known to increase in extremes of both hot and cold temperature. Daily temperature—mean, maximum, or minimum—is usually considered as a predictor of mortality. It is often observed that daily mortality increases as temperature deviates substantially

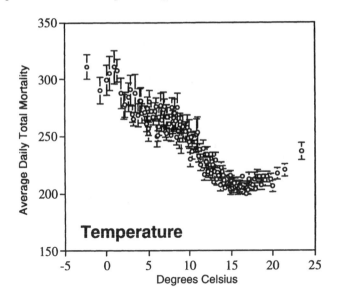

Figure 6-5. Average daily mortality in Greater London for period April 1, 1965, through December 31, 1972, versus temperature (°C). Each point represents average of 20 days sorted by temperature, with error bars of one standard deviation. (After Lippmann et al, 1995.)

above or below the average for a community. For example, daily mortality in London increased monotonically as temperature decreased below approximately 15°C and increased as temperature increased above approximately 17°C (see Fig. 6-5). Similar patterns are seen in most communities, although the temperature associated with minimum deaths and the slope of the temperature-mortality associations varies from city to city. Thus a simple linear function will not be sufficient to control the effects of temperature. Various measures of humidity, such as relative humidity and dew-point temperature, have likewise been shown to be predictive of daily mortality in a nonlinear fashion.

These weather factors are potential confounders because air pollution concentrations are in general associated with weather, and because these specific weather characteristics are independently associated with mortality, even in the absence of air pollution. Weather characteristics such as wind speed are strongly associated with air pollution levels because low wind speed implies less dilution of pollution emissions, but wind speed has not been shown to be associated with daily mortality independent of air pollution. It is easy to over-control for weather by the inclusion of multiple indicators of weather. For example, Mackenbach and colleagues (1993) showed that the strong univariate association between daily mor-

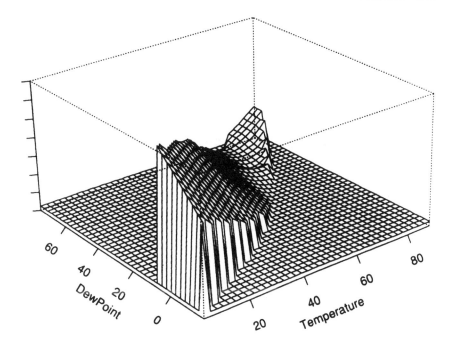

Figure 6-6. Smooth surface depicting relative effects of temperature (°F) and dew point temperature (°F) on total daily mortality (on vertical axis) for Philadelphia, 1973–1980. (From Samet et al., 1995.)

tality and air pollution (measured by SO_2) in the Netherlands could be adjusted away by including indicators of year, month, day of week, influenza epidemics, and 14 weather variables (nine measures of temperature lagged up to 15 days, four measures of precipitation and humidity lagged up to 5 days, and wind speed lagged up to 5 days).

Deterministic methods suffer because they depend on the model specified by the analyst. Thus the assumption of an inadequate functional form can lead to estimated effects biased by incomplete control of confounding.

An alternative modeling strategy makes no assumptions about the functional form of the association. Instead, the data are fit at each observation to the mean response for a neighborhood of data about that specific observation. These methods are called nonparametric smoothing techniques. They have the advantage of being able to fit very nonlinear relations that are not easily parameterized. For example, Fig. 6-6 shows the nonparametric smooth of the association among daily mortality, temperature, and dew point in Philadelphia (Samet et al., 1995). This plot shows the expected j-shape mortality for temperature association: mortality increases for temperatures above and below an optimal level. In addition, mortality increases with increasing dew point (i.e., humidity). Such smoothing methods allow simultaneous parametric and nonparametric fitting of multiple covariates, both for potential confounders and for posited risk factors. Thus, they provide a method for efficiently controlling potential confounders of unknown functional form. Moreover, nonparametric smoothing provides a method for determining the shape of the exposure–response association.

Ultimately the question is how sensitive the observed associations between daily mortality and particulate air pollution are to the analytic methods used. Several investigators have considered this issue (Schwartz, 1994b; Kinney et al., 1995; Samet et al., 1995) and found the results to be robust, that is, independent of the methods used.

How sensitive are the observed associations to confounding by season and weather? Although confounding is a potentially important issue in these studies, comparisons of effect estimates with and without control of weather have not shown these factors to be important confounders of the particulate air pollution associations once season effects are controlled. This is not to suggest that weather is not an important predictor of mortality, but rather that it does not confound the particulate air pollution associations. The reason for this apparent inconsistency is that the weather characteristics that are most strongly associated with mortality, such as temperature, are only weakly associated with particulate air pollution exposures. On the other hand, those weather factors most strongly associated with particulate air pollution, such as wind speed, are only weakly associated with daily mortality. Thus, although both air pollution and daily mortality are strongly associated with weather factors, the specific weather factors associated with each are different and largely independent.

Confounding by other pollutants

A more serious issue is control of confounding by co-pollutants. If the hypothesis is that particulate air pollution is associated with daily mortality, then correlated co-pollutants would act as confounders if they were themselves causally associated with mortality.

The degree of confounding is evaluated by comparing the magnitude of the estimated association with and without adjustment for the posited confounder. Possible confounding by various co-pollutants has been considered in many of the previously cited studies. Table 6-2 shows the results from these studies in which the particle–mortality association was evaluated for confounding by SO_2, O_3, and CO. There was some reduction in the effect estimates for particles; however, a positive association was found even after adjustment for each of the co-pollutants. On the other hand, it is generally found that the estimated effect of the posited confounder is substantially reduced after adjustment for particulate air pollution. Ostro et al. (1995) reported a similar lack of confounding of the particle–mortality association by SO_2, O_3, and CO in a study in Santiago, Chile, although quantitative comparisons of the effect estimates were not reported.

The alternative method for control of confounding is through restriction. If a covariate is not present or has little variation, it cannot confound the association. In most communities particulate air pollution is highly correlated with sulfur oxides and other pollutants, but a few communities have provided settings with exposure to particles in the presence of low exposures to other pollutants.

Fairley (1990) reported an analysis of daily mortality in Santa Clara Country, California, for the winters of 1980 to 1982 and 1984 to 1986. Daily mortality was positively associated with levels of particles measured as coefficient of haze, a measure of light transmission through a sample collected on a filter. When expressed in terms of equivalent PM_{10}, the estimated effect was 0.9% (95% CI 0.2% to 1.5%) increase in total daily mortality per $10\mu g/m^3$ PM_{10} (Dockery and Pope, 1994). Santa Clara has very limited emissions of SO_2 and, because this analysis was limited to winter, very low O_3 concentrations. Thus, it is unlikely that the observed particle associations were confounded by these pollutants.

A similar case of control of confounding by co-pollutants was reported in a study in Utah Valley, Utah (Pope et al., 1992). Utah Valley is approximately 1400 meters above sea level and is bordered on the east by the Wasatch Mountains and on the west by the Lake Mountains. During the winter, when snow covers the mountains and valley, shallow temperature inversions trap locally generated pollutants near the valley floor. During these inversions, concentrations of SO_2, O_3, and NO_2 are generally low, but PM_{10} concentrations are often above the NAAQS of 150 $\mu g/m^3$ (Pope, 1989). Despite a population of only about 200,000 in the valley, with an average of fewer than three deaths per day, a statistically significant increase in daily mortality was found associated with PM_{10} concentrations (see Table 6-3).

On the other hand, in communities with very high concentrations of O_3, such as Los Angeles (Kinney et al., 1995) or very high SO_2, such as eastern Europe (Spix et al., 1993), associations with particulate air pollution are still found that are comparable in magnitude to the estimates from other communities.

Thus, while these co-pollutants may be causally associated with mortality, they have not been found to substantially confound the observed particulate air pollution associations with mortality.

Table 6-2. Studies of effects of co-pollutants on particulate-mortality associations

Location and Period	Reference	Particulate Measure	Type of Analysis	% Change in Daily Mortality for each 10 $\mu g/m^3$ Increase in PM_{10} (CI)
SO_2 as a co-pollutant				
Philadelphia, 1973–80	Schwartz (1992)	TSP (2-Day mean)	Univariate Joint	1.2% (0.7%, 1.7%) 0.9% (0.3%, 1.6%)
Steubenville, OH 1974–84	Schwartz (1992)	TSP (prev. day)	Univariate Joint	0.7% (0.4%, 1.0%) 0.5% (0.1%, 1.0%)
Detroit, MI 1973–82	Schwartz (1991)	TSP	Univariate Joint	1.0% (0.5%, 1.6%) 0.9% (0.4%, 1.5%)
Athens, Greece 1984–1988	Touloumi et al. (1994)	Smoke	Univariate Joint	0.8% (0.6%, 1.0%) 0.4% (0.1%, 0.8%)
Erfurt, Germany 1988–89	Spix et al. 1993	SP (same day)	Univariate Joint	0.6% (0.1%, 1.1%) 0.5% (−0.1%, 1.1%)
São Paulo, Brazi 1990–91	Saldiva et al. (1995)	PM_{10} (2 day)	Univariate Joint	1.3% (0.7%, 1.9%) 1.4% (0.4%, 2.5%)
Amsterdam, Netherlands 1986–92	Verhoeff et al. (1996)	PM_{10} (same day)	Univariate Joint	0.6% (0.1%, 1.1%) 0.8% (0.2%, 1.3%)
Combined		PM_{10} Alone		0.8% (0.7%, 1.0%)
		Adjusted for SO_2		0.6% (0.4%, 0.8%)
CO as a co-pollutant				
Athens, Greece 1984–1988	Touloumi et al. (1994)	Smoke	Univariate Joint	0.8% (0.6%, 1.0%) 0.7% (0.3%, 1.1%)

Lagged associations

These studies consistently report lagged associations between particle exposure and increased mortality, usually with particle concentrations on the previous day. It would violate a basic tenet of causality if the observed effect were not either concurrent with or lagged behind the exposure. The pattern of daily mortality during the 1952 London fog episode showed that mortality peaked after the maximum air pollution exposures and remained high in the week after the episode compared to the week before. In the analysis of Utah Valley deaths, Pope et al. (1992) considered longer lag structures up to 7 days and found the strongest associations with the 5-day moving average—that is, with the mean PM_{10} of the current day and the four previous days.

It is not unreasonable to expect that an acute exposure may lead to death (or other adverse event) of some individuals on one day, but that

Table 6-2 (*continued*)

Location and Period	Reference	Particulate Measure	Type of Analysis	% Change in Daily Mortality for each 10 µg/m³ Increase in PM_{10} (CI)
São Paulo, Brazi 1990–91	Saldiva et al. (1995)	PM_{10} (2-day)	Univariate	1.3% (0.7%, 1.9%)
			Joint	1.4% (0.4%, 2.5%)
Los Angeles	Kinney et al. (1995)	PM_{10}	Univariate	0.5% (0.0%, 1.0%)
			Joint	0.4% (−0.1%, 0.9%)
Amsterdam, Netherlands 1986–92	Verhoeff et al. (1996)	PM_{10} (same day)	Univariate	0.6% (0.1%, 1.1%)
			Joint	0.6% (0.0%, 1.2%)
Combined		PM_{10} Alone		0.8% (0.6%, 1.0%)
		Adjusted for CO		0.7% (0.4%, 0.9%)
O_3 as a co-pollutant				
São Paulo, Brazi 1990–91	Saldiva et al. (1995)	PM_{10} (2 Day)	Univariate	1.3% (0.7%, 1.9%)
			Joint	1.4% (0.4%, 2.5%)
Los Angeles	Kinney et al. (1995)	PM_{10}	Univariate	0.5% (0.0%, 1.0%)
			Joint	0.5% (0.0%, 1.0%)
Chicago	Ito et al. (1995)	PM_{10}	Univariate	0.8% (0.4%, 1.1%)
			Joint	0.6% (0.2%, 1.0%)
Amsterdam, Netherlands 1986–92	Verhoeff et al. (1996)	PM_{10} (same day)	Univariate	0.6% (0.1%, 1.1%)
			Joint	0.5% (0.0%, 1.1%)
Combined		PM_{10} Alone		0.8% (0.5%, 1.0%)
		Adjusted for O_3		0.6% (0.3%, 0.9%)

PM_{10} = particulate matter smaller than 10 µm aerodynamic diameter;

TSP = total suspended particulates;

SP = suspended particulates

others may linger on before expiring the next or even the following day. Thus the response to an acute exposure could be distributed over a number of days. Methods for estimating distributed lag functions have been developed in econometrics, and their application to epidemiologic time-series data has been described by Pope and Schwartz (1996). In the simplest case, exposures at several days' lag are modeled simultaneously in a multiple regression. These simultaneous, day-specific effect estimates will give a sense of the distribution of the lag structure, but because of the high colinearity of pollution exposures day-to-day, the estimates for any given day will be very unstable. This simultaneous multi-day regression is called an unconstrained distributed lag model. The alternative is to place

Table 6-3. Studies of effects of particulates on cause-specific daily mortality

Location and Period	Reference	Particulate Measure	Mean PM_{10}	% Change in Daily Mortality for Each 10 μ/m^3 Increase in PM_{10} (CI)
Respiratory				
Santa Clara, CA 1980–82, 84–86	Fairley (1990)	Coefficient of haze	35	3.5% (1.5%, 5.6%)
Philadelphia, PA 1973–80	Schwartz (1992)	TSP (2-day Mean)	40	3.3% (0.1%, 6.6%)
Utah Valley, UT 1985–89	Pope (1992)	PM_{10} (5-day Mean)	47	3.7% (0.7%, 6.7%)
Birmingham, AL 1985–88	Schwartz (1992)	PM_{10} (3-day Mean)	48	1.5% (−5.8%, 9.4%)
Cincinnati, OH	Schwartz (1994)	TSP	76	2.8% (−0.9%, 6.6%)
Combined respiratory				3.4% (2.0%, 4.7%)
Cardiovascular				
Santa Clara, CA 1980–82, 84–86	Fairley (1990)	Coefficient of haze	35	0.8% (0.1%, 1.6%)
Philadelphia, PA 1973–80	Schwartz (1992)	TSP (2-day Mean)	40	1.7% (1.0%, 2.4%)
Utah Valley, UT 1985–89	Pope (1992)	PM_{10} (5-day Mean)	47	1.8% (0.4%, 3.3%)
Birmingham, AL 1985–88	Schwartz (1992)	PM_{10} (3-day Mean)	48	1.6% (−0.5%, 3.7%)
Cincinnati, OH	Schwartz (1994f)	TSP	76 (30.8)	1.5% (0.5%, 2.4%)
Combined cardiovascular				1.4% (1.0%, 1.8%)

PM_{10} = particulate matter smaller than 10 μm aerodynamic diameter;

TSP = total suspended particulates.

some constraint on the distribution of lagged effect estimates, possibly based on results of an unconstrained analysis. Conceptually, in a constrained distributed lag model an overall effect is estimated for the particulates over a defined period of lagged days, with weights assigned to the contribution from each individual day. A model estimating the effect of pollution on the same day is a constrained model with a weight of 1 for the same day and 0 for all other days. Similarly, estimating the effects at various prior days univariately is also a constrained model, with weights of 1 on the day of interest and 0 for all other days. A moving-average model gives equal weight to all lagged days for a specified period. A geometric distributed lag model gives weights that decrease geometrically with lag time. This model has the intuitive appeal that the influence of a given day's pollution diminishes with time. However, there may be a finite lag between exposure and response. An alternative lag model is the polynomial distributed lag, which assigns weights constrained to fit a polynomial function. The polynomial weighting function permits a more flexible weighting scheme for individual days, such that the maximum effect could be lagged by a day or more.

The use of constrained distributed lag models has been important in understanding the associations in time-series analyses of mortality and morbidity end points. Effects of particulate pollution episodes on mortality have been observed on the same or previous day, but have also been observed to persist for several days. Ignoring these lag structures can lead to errors in the estimates of the associations. Estimates based on single-day effects will overestimate the effect for that specific day. The cumulative effects over several days will be underestimated if lag structures are not considered.

Autocorrelation

Daily counts of deaths are correlated day-to-day. This correlation arises from the day-to-day correlation of the determinants of deaths, and not because deaths on any given day are causally linked to deaths of previous or succeeding days. There is a high day-to-day correlation of weather parameters and air pollution concentrations, due in part to the fact that weather patterns are largely determined by the movement of air masses. Air masses are large enough that any given area is usually under the influence of a specific air mass for 2 or 3 days before there is a change of air mass and therefore a change in the weather.

A complete model of daily mortality should be free of autocorrelation in the model residuals. Day-to-day correlation of model residuals is not an indication of an underlying autoregressive process, but rather an indication that the determinants of daily mortality have not been completely specified or adequately modeled. Nevertheless, it has become common practice to include adjustment autoregressive structure in the residuals as a means of ensuring that associations are conservatively estimated. Although this autoregressive adjustment is appropriate, it should be recognized that it is a statistical correction for an inadequate model, and the preferred solution would be to improve the underlying mortality model.

Harvesting

A weakness of time-series studies is that those individuals who die as a result of pollution exposure cannot be identified. Reports show that the associations of mortality with particle air pollution are stronger in the elderly (Schwartz and Dockery, 1992) and that deaths are associated with chronic respiratory or cardiovascular problems. But it is not clear who is dying. Are they people who would have died within the next couple of days anyway? Is air pollution "harvesting" those who were on the verge of mortality? If so, the few days' loss of life expectancy may not have major public health significance.

If harvesting is occurring, then there should be fewer deaths than expected following an air pollution or other episode that produces excess deaths. Following the London 1952 episode, there was no indication of lower-than-expected mortality. In fact, the observed number of deaths per day in the week following the episode was substantially higher than the number of deaths per day before the episode. Spix et al. (1993) looked for a negative correlation between the number of deaths in the preceding period (up to 2 weeks) and the level of air pollution. There was an indication of weak harvesting, but the effect was small compared with the estimated air pollution effect.

If harvesting were operating in the mortality time-series, then each increase in mortality should be balanced by a subsequent decrease in mortality. Thus the change in the annual mortality rate should be less than expected on the basis of the change in mean particle concentrations. Between August 1, 1986, and September 1, 1987, the major source of particulate air pollution in Utah Valley, a steel mill, was closed by a labor dispute. During the 13 months that the mill was not operating, average particulate air pollution concentrations dropped from 50 to 35 $\mu g/m^3$ PM_{10} (Pope et al., 1992). Based on the 1.5% increase in mortality for each 10 $\mu g/m^3$ PM_{10} observed in the valley, a 2.3% reduction in mortality would be expected. There was actually a 3.2% reduction in overall mortality during this period. Comparable associations between city-specific mortality rates and mean particulate pollution rates have been observed in cross-sectional studies. For example, Pope et al. (1995) show that age-, sex-, and race-adjusted mortality rates increased with particle concentrations in 50 communities with fine particle measures in 1980 (Fig. 6-7). These observed differences in mortality rates suggest that the increased deaths associated with short-term particulate air pollution exposures were not balanced by decreased mortality in the following days.

Coherence of observed health effects

Bates (1992) has argued that the observation of increased mortality associated with air pollution exposures implies that measures of morbidity

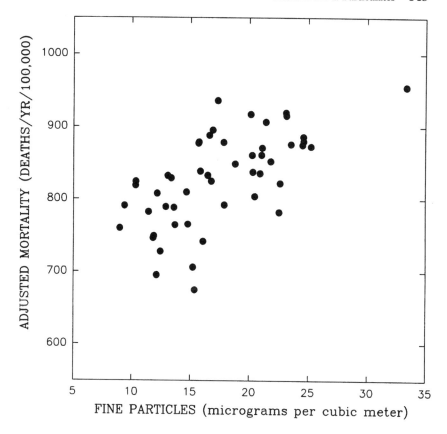

Figure 6-7. City-specific age-, sex-, and race-adjusted population-based mortality rates for 1980 plotted against mean fine particulate air pollution concentrations for 1979 to 1983. (From Pope *et al*, 1995.)

also must necessarily be increased—for example, hospital admissions, hospital emergency room visits, and outpatient or doctor's visits. Among potentially responsive subjects (such as asthma patients), we expect to observe increased symptoms, lower lung function, increased medication use, and, ultimately, higher use of hospital services. A similar cascade of associations also may be detected among less sensitive individuals, that is, among members of the general population. Bates (1992) has described this as *coherence* of effects—that is, the adverse effects of air pollution should be observable across a range of related health outcomes. Adverse effects of air pollution also should be reproducibly observed by different investigators in different settings—that is, there should be *consistency* of effects across independent analytic studies.

Cause-specific mortality

If total daily mortality is associated with particulate air pollution, then there should be marked differences in the magnitude of this effect by cause of death. Six of the mortality studies (Fairley, 1990; Pope et al., 1992; Schwartz, 1993; Schwartz and Dockery, 1992; Schwartz, 1994; Ostro et al., 1996) have provided a breakdown of mortality by broad cause-of-death categories (Table 6-3). Cardiovascular deaths accounted for about 45% of all deaths in these studies. Effect estimates for cardiovascular deaths ranged between 0.7% and 1.8% (weighted mean, 1.4%; 95% confidence interval [CI], 1.0% to 1.8%) increase for each 10 $\mu g/m^3$ PM_{10}. Respiratory deaths, which were 2% to 8% of the total, had effect estimates between 1.5% and 3.7% (weighted mean, 3.5%; 95% CI, 2.0% to 4.7%) increase for each 10 $\mu g/m^3$ PM_{10}. No associations with cancer or with other causes of death were reported in any of these studies. Thus the strongest associations consistently are observed with respiratory and cardiovascular mortality.

Hospital usage

If daily particulate pollution levels are associated with daily mortality, then associations should also be expected with increased hospital admissions and emergency department visits, which, like mortality, are counts of events in specified time intervals. Thus the analyses of these data use the same methods applied to the daily mortality time-series. The principal difference is that mortality records are readily available, but hospital usage records are not. Daily counts must be collected from review of discharge records or other data files, usually collected for billing purposes. Thus, although the methods for analyzing these data are well developed, the application has been limited by the lack of readily available hospital usage data.

In a unique natural experiment, Pope (1989, 1991) observed that hospital admissions of children for respiratory disease in Utah Valley dropped by over 50% during the winter of 1986–87 compared with adjacent years. During this winter, the strike by workers at the local steel mill led to much lower PM_{10} concentrations—a mean of 51 $\mu g/m^3$ and maximum of 113 $\mu g/m^3$ compared with a mean of 90$\mu g/m^3$ and a maximum of 365 $\mu g/m^3$ in the previous year. Regression analyses estimated a 4.2% decrease in asthma and bronchitis admissions and a 7.1% decrease in all respiratory admissions of children associated with a 10 $\mu g/m^3$ decrease in the 2-month mean PM_{10} concentration. No associations were found with all other, i.e. nonrespiratory, hospital admissions.

Burnett and colleagues (1995) reported increased respiratory hospital admissions in southern Ontario for the summers of 1983 to 1988 associated with increased sulfate concentrations. Sulfate particles make up more than half of the fine particle mass in Southern Ontario. These sulfate particle associations were independent of associations with ozone exposures. Thurston and colleagues have reported associations of respiratory hospital admissions with $PM_{2.5}$ concentrations in Toronto, Ontario (1994) and sulfate particles in New York City and Buffalo, New York (1992). For comparison with other studies, the effect estimates were converted to equivalent effects of PM_{10} assuming a $PM_{2.5}$ to PM_{10} ratio of 0.55 and a SO_4^{2-} to PM_{10} ratio of 0.25 (Dockery and Pope, 1994). The combined estimate for the effect of each 10 $\mu g/m^3$ increase in PM_{10} in these studies was 1.1% (95% CI, 0.8% to 1.5%).

Emergency department visits for all respiratory complaints were associated with daily TSP concentrations in Steubenville, Ohio (Samet et al., 1981). Expressed as the equivalent effect of a 10 $\mu g/m^3$ increase in PM_{10} (Dockery and Pope, 1994), respiratory emergency room visits increased by 0.5% (95% CI, 0.0% to 1.0%)

Hospital admissions for asthma were reported to increase in association with particles in both the Ontario and New York studies (Table 6-4). Schwartz (1994a) has reported associations between daily PM_{10} concentrations and daily hospital admissions for asthma among the elderly (65+ yr) in Detroit, Michigan. Taken together, these studies indicate that asthma hospital admissions increase by about 1% for each 10 $\mu g/m^3$ increase in PM_{10} (95% CI, 0.4% to 1.6%). An analysis of asthma emergency department visits in Seattle (Schwartz et al., 1993) found an increase of 3.4% (95% CI, 0.9% to 6.0%) associated with each 10 $\mu g/m^3$ increase in PM_{10}.

Schwartz estimated the association between daily PM_{10} exposures and hospital admissions for pneumonia among the elderly in Birmingham, Alabama (1994d), Detroit, Michigan (1994a), and Minneapolis–St. Paul, Minnesota (1994b). Together these studies give an estimated increase of 1.4% (95% CI, 0.7% to 2.0%) in pneumonia admissions for each 10 $\mu g/ m^3$ increase in PM_{10} (Table 6-4). These associations do not imply that particulate air pollution is producing new cases of pneumonia, but rather that particulate pollution is aggravating existing pneumonia cases sufficiently to send patients to the hospital.

Schwartz also reported increased admissions for aggravation of chronic obstructive pulmonary disease in these same cities (Table 6-4). Burnett et al. (1995) found increased hospital admissions for COPD associated with sulfate particles in southern Ontario. The combined effect estimate from these studies is a 2.4% (95% CI, 1.5% to 3.4%) increase in hospital ad-

Table 6-4. Studies of acute effects of particles on hospital usage

	Location and Period	Reference	Particulate Measure	Patient Age Group	% Change in Hospital Usage for Each 10 μg/m³ Increase in PM_{10} (CI)
Admissions					
Respiratory Asthma	New York City Buffalo, NY Summer 1988, 1989	Thurston (1992)	Daily mean SO_4		1.9% (0.4%, 3.4%)
					2.1% (−0.6%, 5.0%)
	Toronto, Ont Summer 1986–88	Thurston (1994)	Daily mean $PM_{2.5}$		2.1% (−0.8%, 5.1%)
	Detroit, MI 1986–89	Schwartz (1994)	Daily mean PM_{10}	>65 yr	0.5% (−3.3%, 4.4%)
	Southern Ontario 1983–88	Burnett et al. (1995)	Daily mean SO_4	All ages	1.0% (0.4%, 1.6%)
	Combined Asthma				1.0% (0.8%, 1.6%)
Pneumonia	Birmingham, AL 1986–89	Schwartz 1994d	Daily mean PM_{10}	>65 yr	1.8% (0.7%, 2.8%)
	Detroit, MI 1986–89	Schwartz (1994)	Daily mean PM_{10}	>65 yr	1.2% (0.4%, 1.9%)
	Minneapolis–St. Paul, MN 1986–89	Schwartz (1994)	Previous Day PM_{10}	>65 yr	1.6% (0.3%, 2.9%)
	Combined Pneumonia				1.4% (0.7%, 2.0%)
COPD	Birmingham, AL 1986–89	Schwartz (1994d)	Daily mean PM_{10}	>65 yr	2.5% (0.3%, 4.7%)

Detroit, MI 1986–89	Schwartz (1994a)	Daily mean PM_{10}	>65 yr	2.0% (0.9%, 3.2%)
Minneapolis–St. Paul, MN 1986–89	Schwartz (1994e)	Previous 2-Day PM_{10}	>65 yr	4.6% (1.8%, 7.5%)
Southern Ontario 1983–88	Burnett et al. (1995)	Daily mean SO_4	All ages	1.5% (0.8%, 2.2%)
Combined COPD				2.4% (1.5%, 3.4%)
All Respiratory				
New York City Buffalo, NY	Thurston	Daily mean SO_4		1.0% (0.2%, 1.8%)
Summer 1988, 1989	(1992)			2.2% (0.6%, 3.8%)
Toronto, ONT Summer 1986–88	(1994)	Daily mean $PM_{2.5}$		3.4% (0.4%, 6.4%)
Southern Ontario Summer 1983–88	Burnett (1995)	Daily mean SO_4	All ages	0.8% (0.4%, 1.1%)
Southern Ontario 1983–88	Burnett et al. (1995)	Daily mean SO_4	All ages	1.1% (0.7%, 1.4%)
Combined All Respiratory				1.1% (0.8%, 1.5%)
Coronary Artery Disease				
Detroit, MI 1986–89	Schwartz (1994a)	Daily mean PM_{10}	>65 yr	0.6% (0.2%, 0.0%)
Southern Ontario 1983–88	Burnett et al. (1995)	Daily mean SO_4	All ages	0.7% (0.2%, 1.2%)
Combined Coronary Artery Disease				0.6% (0.3%, 0.9%)

(continued)

Table 6-4. Studies of acute effects of particles on hospital usage (*continued*)

	Location and Period	Reference	Particulate Measure	Patient Age Gruop	% Change in Hospital Usage for Each 10 μg/m³ Increase in PM₁₀ (CI)
Dysrhythmias	Southern Ontario (1983–88	Burnett et al. (1995)	Daily mean SO_4	All ages	0.4% (−0.6%, 1.4%)
	Detroit, MI 1986–89	Schwartz (1995)	Daily mean PM_{10}	>65 yr	0.6% (−0.1%, 1.3%)
	Combined Dysrhythmias				0.5% (−0.1%, 1.1%)
Congestive Heart Failure	Southern Ontario 1983–88	Burnett et al. (1995).	Daily mean SO_4	All ages	0.9% (0.2%, 1.7%)
	Detroit, MI 1986–89	Schartz (1994a)	Daily mean PM_{10}	>65 yr	1.0% (0.4%, 1.6%)
	Combined Congestive Heart Failure				1.0% (−0.5%, 1.4%)
Emergency Department Visits					
Asthma (<65 yr)	Seattle, WA 1989–90	Schwartz et al. 1993b	Daily mean PM_{10}		3.4% (0.9%, 6.0%)
Respiratory disease	Steubenville, OH Fall 1974–77	Samet et al (1981)	Daily Mean TSP		0.5% (0.0%, 1.0%)
COPD	Barcelona, Spain Winter 1985–89	Sunyer et al. (1993)	British smoke		2.3% (1.4%, 3.2%)
	Combined COPD				1.0%

PM₂.₅ = particulate matter smaller than 2.5 μm aerodynamic diameter

PM₁₀ = particulate matter smaller than 10 μm aerodynamic diameter;

TSP = total suspended particulates.

missions for COPD associated with each 10 $\mu g/m^3$ increase in PM_{10} (Table 6-4). Emergency department visits for chronic obstructive pulmonary disease were associated with black smoke concentrations in Barcelona (Sunyer et al., 1993. The estimated effect corresponded to a 2.3% (95% CI, 1.4% + 3.2%) increase in emergency visits for COPD associated with a 10 $\mu g/m^3$ increase in PM_{10} (Dockery and Pope, 1994).

The evidence of increased cardiovascular mortality suggests that associations should also be observed for cardiovascular hospital admissions. Indeed Schwartz (1994a) and Burnett et al. (1995) have reported increased cardiovascular admissions associated with increased particle concentrations in Detroit and southern Ontario (Table 6-4). For each 10 $\mu g/m^3$ increase in PM_{10}, these two analyses combined estimated a 1.0% (95% CI, 0.5% to 14%) increase in congestive heart failure (ischemia), a 0.6% (95% CI, 0.3% to 0.9%) increase in coronary artery disease, and a 0.5% (95% CI, -0.1% to 1.1%) increase in dysrhythmias.

Asthma attacks

Hospital admission and emergency department visit data suggest that particle exposures may be directly associated with asthma attacks. Records of daily asthma attacks or other clinical or subclinical measures of asthma status are not routinely collected. To assess the association of air pollution and other time-varying factors with exacerbation of asthma, daily reports have been collected in defined cohorts (i.e., panels) of asthmatics. The measure of health status is typically a dichotomous or binary indicator of an asthma attack. Binary data are produced by a binomial process and therefore require different regression methods than apply to count data. Logistic regression is commonly applied to these data, although a probit regression is also appropriate. The analytic issues in analyzing these time-series data are the same as in daily mortality studies. One major difference is the role of autocorrelation. In mortality studies there was no reason to believe that deaths on one day were causally related to deaths on succeeding days. On the other hand, asthma attacks might represent a heightened state of responsiveness, such that an asthma attack one day might induce a higher risk of attack on subsequent days. How much of the day-to-day correlation in exacerbation of asthma is due to autocorrelation of risk factors and how much is due to intrinsic autocorrelation of asthma is not clear. Whittemore and Korn (1980) analyzed the association of asthma attacks and air pollution in 16 panels of asthmatics in the Los Angeles area. They found a strong association with asthma status on the previous day and with particle exposures (measured as TSP) independent of the association with ozone. This study demonstrated methods for the analysis of panel data. Subject-specific regression coefficients of asthma attacks versus air pollution were calculated with adjustment for asthma attacks on the previous day. The subject-specific effect estimates were pooled to produce a common effect estimate. While this analysis was important in providing a methodology to consider random effects between subjects, the effect estimates may have been overcontrolled by inclusion of the previous day's asthma status in the model. Associations attributed to asthma status on the previous day would have included any lagged effects of particulate air pollution exposures. Given the evidence for such lagged effects of particles that has developed, the failure to consider particle exposures on the previous days may have underestimated the cumulative effects of these air pollution exposures.

Winter studies of asthmatic children with chronic respiratory symptoms in the Netherlands (Roemer et al., 1993) and of asthmatic adults in Denver (Ostro et al., 1991) both found substantial increases in reported asthmatic attacks associated with particle exposures. Ostro et al. (1995) also found that children in an asthma summer camp in Los Angeles had increased attacks of shortness of breath associated with increased PM_{10} concentrations. These studies (Table 6-5) give a combined effect estimate of 8.8% (95% CI, 6.9% to 11.4%) increase in asthmatic attacks associated with 10 $\mu g/m^3$ PM_{10}.

The use of bronchodilators has been evaluated as a measure of exacerbation in a panel of asthmatics in the Netherlands (Roemer et al., 1993) and panels of symptomatic children and asthmatic patients in the Utah Valley (Pope et al., 1991) (Table 6-5). The weighted mean of these studies gives an estimated effect of a 2.9% (95% CI, 1.5% to 4.5%) increase in bronchodilator use associated with each 10 $\mu g/m^3$ increase in PM_{10}.

Respiratory symptoms

Daily diaries of respiratory symptoms are an inexpensive method of evaluating acute changes in respiratory health status that have been widely used in evaluating acute effects of particulate air pollution. In a commonly applied study design, panels of subjects (e.g., schoolchildren,) record the presence of specific respiratory symptoms daily on weekly or monthly calendars. These symptom reports are often aggregated into *upper respiratory symptoms* (runny or stuffy nose, sinusitis, sore throat, wet cough, head cold, hayfever, and burning or red eyes) and *lower respiratory symptoms* (wheezing, dry cough, phlegm, shortness of breath, and chest discomfort or pain). In addition, *cough*, the most frequently reported symptom, is often analyzed separately.

The frequency of reported respiratory symptoms is generally taken as

Table 6-5. Studies of acute effects of particles on exacerbation of asthma

Location and Period	Reference	Particulate Measure	Subjects	% Change in Daily Asthma Response for Each 10 μg/m³ Increase in PM_{10} (CI)
Bronchodilator use				
Utah Valley, UT Winter 1989–90	Pope et al. (1991)	Daily mean PM_{10}	School panel Asthma panel	11.2% (2.4%, 20.7%) 12.0% (4.7%, 19.7%)
2 Dutch cities Winter 1990–91	Roemer et al. (1993)	Daily mean PM_{10}	School panel	2.3% (0.7%, 3.8%)
Combined Bronchodilator Use				2.9% (1.5%, 4.5%)
Asthmatic Attacks				
2 Dutch cities Winter 1990–91	Roemer et al. (1993)	Daily mean PM_{10}	School panel	1.1% (−3.5%, 5.9%)
Denver, CO Winter 1987–88	Ostro (1991)	$PM_{2.5}$	Asthma panel	11.5% (8.9%, 14.3%)
Combined Asthma Attacks				8.8% (6.9%, 11.4%)

PM_{10} = particulate matter smaller than 10μm aerodynamic diameter;
$PM_{2.5}$ = particulate matter smaller than 2.5μm aerodynamic diameter.

the prevalence of specific symptoms, that is, the fraction of participating children reporting a symptom complex on each day. In some cases (Schwartz et al., 1994), however, incident cases were reported, where "incidence" requires that the child be symptom-free for 2 days prior to the incident symptom report. Other studies have focused on the duration of symptoms related to air pollution exposure. These three measures of respiratory symptoms—prevalence, incidence, and duration—are related. The analysis of each measure addresses separate, but related questions.

Studies of lower respiratory symptoms have been conducted in Utah Valley (Pope et al., 1991; Pope and Dockery, 1992), the Netherlands (Hoek and Brunekreef, 1993; Hoek and Brunekreef, 1994), in six U.S. cities (Schwartz et al., 1994) and Pennsylvania (Neas et al., 1995) (Table 6-6).

The combined weighted average from these studies gives an estimated effect of 3.0% (95% CI, 1.5% to 4.5%) increase in lower respiratory symptoms with each 10 μg/m³ increase in daily mean PM_{10} concentrations. For upper respiratory symptom reports, the weighted average effect estimate was only a 0.7% (95% CI, −0.1% to 1.5%) increase in upper respiratory symptoms with each 10 μg/m³ increase in daily mean PM_{10} (see Table 6-6).

Cough reports were analyzed in three of these studies as well as in a winter diary study in the Netherlands (Roemer et al., 1993), a study of two Swiss cities (Braun-Fahrlander et al., 1992), and the summer diary

Table 6-6. Studies of acute effects of particles on respiratory symptom reports

Location and Period	Reference	Particulate Measure	Sample	% Change in Daily Symptom Reporting for Each 10μg/m³ Increase in PM_{10}
Lower respiratory symptoms				
Utah Valley, UT Winter 1989–90	Pope et al. (1991)	Daily mean PM_{10}	Children Asthmatics	5.1% (1.1%, 9.3.%) 0.2% (−4.2%, 4.8%)
Utah Valley, UT Winter 1990–91	Pope et al. (1992)	Daily mean PM_{10}	Symptomatic children Asymptomatic children	4.8% (1.5%, 8.3%) 2.4% (−1.8%, 6.8%)
6 U.S. cities Summer 1984–88	Schwartz et al. (1994)	Daily mean PM_{15}	Schoolchildren	15.2% (6.3%, 24.9%)
Wageningen, Netherlands Winter 1990–91	Hoek (1993)	Daily mean PM_{10}	Schoolchildren	1.2% (−3.1%, 5.7%)
4 Dutch cities Winter 1987–90	Hoek (1994)	Prev. day PM_{10}	Schoolchildren	1.5% (−1.1%, 4.32%)
Combined Lower Respiratory Symptoms				3.0% (1.5%, 4.5%)
Upper respiratory symptoms				
Utah Valley, UT Winter 1989–90	Pope et al. (1991)	Daily mean PM_{10}	Children Asthmatics	3.7% (0.7%, 6.8%) −0.2% (−4.2%, 4.0%)
Utah Valley, UT Winter 1990–91	Pope et al. (1992)	Daily mean PM_{10}	Symptomatic children Asymptomatic children	3.7% (0.6%, 6.9%) −0.2% (−4.9%, 4.7%)

Location / Period	Study	Exposure	Population	Effect (95% CI)
6 U.S. cities Summer 1984–88	Schwartz (1993)	Daily mean PM$_{15}$	Schoolchildren	6.9% (0.7%, 15.0%)
Wageningen, Netherlands Winter 1990–91	Hoek (1993)	Daily mean PM$_{10}$	Schoolchildren	2.6% (0.1%, 5.3%)
4 Dutch cities Winter 1987–90	Hoek (1994)	Previous Day PM$_{10}$	Schoolchildren	−0.2% (1.2%, 0.8%)
Combined Upper Respiratory Symptoms				0.7% (−0.1%, 1.5%)

Cough symptoms

Location / Period	Study	Exposure	Population	Effect (95% CI)
Utah Valley, UT Winter 1990–91	Pope et al. (1992)	Daily mean PM$_{10}$	Symptomatic children / Asymptomatic children	5.2% (2.3%, 8.2%) / 3.4% (−0.1%, 7.0%)
6 US Cities Summer 1984–88	Schwartz (1993)	Daily mean PM$_{15}$	Schoolchildren	6.9% (0.9%, 13.1%)
2 Dutch Cities Winter 1990–91	Roemer et al. (1993)	Previous Day PM$_{10}$	Symptomatic children	0.1% (−0.8%, 1.1%)
4 Dutch Cities Winter 1987–90	Hoek (1994)	Previous Day PM$_{2.5}$	Schoolchildren	1.3 (−0.1, 2.7%)
Uniontown, PA Summer 1990	Neas et al. (1995)	Daily mean PM$_{2.5}$	Children	18.6% (3.1%, 36.4%)
Combined Cough				1.3% (0.5%, 2.0%)

study in Uniontown, Pennsylvania (Neas et al., 1995) (see Table 6-6). The weighted mean effect estimate from these studies was a 1.3% (95% CI, 0.5% to 2.0%) increase in cough associated with each 10 $\mu g/m^3$ increase in daily mean PM_{10}.

Lung function

Lung function has been shown to be a sensitive indicator of acute response to ozone in controlled exposure and chamber studies (Lippmann, 1989). Repeated measures of lung function in panels of subjects also have been used to evaluate the effect of particulate air pollution episodes. Lung function is a continuous measure and can be analyzed by Gaussian regression. The same modeling issues described previously need to be considered.

Panels of elementary school children in Steubenville, Ohio had their lung function measured weekly before, during, and after particulate and sulfur dioxide episodes during four periods in 1978 through 1980 (Dockery et al., 1982). Forced expired volume in three-quarters of a second ($FEV_{.75}$) was reported to decline following these episodes. There was a suggestion that $FEV_{.75}$ remained depressed for up to 2 weeks following the episode. A study of weekly lung function measurement of schoolchildren in the Netherlands following a sulfur dioxide and particulate episode in January 1985 reported decreases in forced expired volume in one second (FEV_1) that were similar in magnitude and in lag structure to those observed in Steubenville. Subsequent studies of panels of schoolchildren with weekly lung function measurements (Hoek and Brunekreef, 1993a,b) have also shown decreased FEV_1 associated with increased daily PM_{10} concentrations.

Pope and Kanner (1993) analyzed repeated FEV_1 measurements in a panel of chronic obstructive pulmonary disease patients participating in the Lung Health Study. Measurements were taken 10 to 90 days apart. A 0.2% decrease in FEV_1 for each 10 $\mu g/m^3$ increase in daily PM_{10} was reported.

Analysis of longer lags in the Netherlands panel (Hoek and Brunekreef, 1993b) found a significant association between decreased FEV_1 and increased mean PM_{10} over the previous 7 days. Similarly, in a reanalysis of the Steubenville data, Brunekreef et al. (1991) found the strongest association with increased mean TSP over the previous 5 days.

Taken together, these studies found a decrease of between 0.05% and 0.35% or a weighted average of 0.15% decrease in FEV_1 associated with each 10 $\mu g/m^3$ increase in daily mean PM_{10} (see Table 6-7). For longer averaging times, the weighted mean decrease in FEV_1 was 0.2% for each 10 $\mu g/m^3$ increase in mean PM_{10} over the previous 5 to 7 days.

Peak flow measurements have been widely used as a simple, inexpensive indicator of acute changes in lung function among asthmatic patients. Peak flow measurements were made in the weekly panel studies of schoolchildren in the Netherlands (Hoek and Brunekreef, 1993a,b). In these two studies, peak flow declined approximately 0.16% for each 10 $\mu g/m^3$ increase in PM_{10}.

In two studies in the winters of 1989–90 and 1990–91 in Utah Valley, (Pope et al., 1991; Pope and Dockery, 1992), panels of schoolchildren measured their peak flow daily before going to bed. In both cases, small but significant reductions in peak flow were found associated with increased mean PM_{10} concentrations that day. In both studies, there appeared to be associations between lower peak flow and higher PM_{10} concentrations for up to 5 preceding days, and stronger associations were found when these lag structures were included in the models. In the second study (Pope and Dockery, 1992), the estimated effect was about twice as large with the 5-day lagged mean as with the 1-day mean PM_{10}.

Similar winter panel studies of schoolchildren have been conducted in the Netherlands (Roemer et al., 1993). Effects were observed between evening peak flow and daily mean PM_{10} concentrations, and 7-day mean PM_{10} concentration, which were similar to those observed in Utah.

A panel study of children was conducted in the summer of 1992 in Uniontown, Pennsylvania (Neas et al. 1995) to evaluate peak flow changes in an area of high aerosol acidity. Although the strongest associations were found with aerosol acidity, there also was an association between evening peak flow and daily mean PM_{10} that was consistent with the estimates from other studies.

Comparing the results from these studies with repeated peak flow measurements, there was a decrease of between 0.04% and 0.25% in peak flow (weighted mean of 0.08%) associated with each 10 $\mu g/m^3$ increase in daily mean PM_{10} concentration (see Table 6-7).

In summary, studies of repeated measure of lung function consistently show a small decrement in FEV_1 (weighted mean, 0.15%; 95% CI, 0.09% to 0.21%) and peak flow (weighted mean, 0.08%; 95% CI, 0.05% to 0.11%) associated with each 10 $\mu g/m^3$ in PM_{10} daily mean concentration. There is a strong suggestion in these data that changes in lung function may reflect the cumulative exposure of several (5 to 7) days preceding the measurement.

Summary

Evidence from the selected epidemiologic studies presented in this chapter suggests a *coherence* of effects across a range of related health outcomes

Table 6-7. Studies of acute effects of particles on lung function

Location and Period	Reference	Particulate Measure	Sample (Mean PFT)	% Decrease in Daily Lung Function for Each 10μg/m^3 Increase in PM$_{10}$
Forced Expired Volume				
FEV$_{.75}$				
Steubenville, OH 1978–80	Dockery (1982)	Daily mean TSP	School children (1.57 L)	0.05% (0.00%, 0.10%)
FEV$_1$				
4 Cities, NL Winter 1987–90	Hoek and Brunekreef 1991 (1994)	Daily mean PM$_{10}$	Lacks mean (Assume 1.57 L)	0.06% (−0.01%, 0.14%)
Wageningen, NL Winter 1990–91	Hoek and Brunekreef 1991 (1993)	Daily mean PM$_{10}$	Lacks mean (Assume 1.57 L)	0.35% (0.23%, 0.48%)
Salt Lake City, UT 1987–89	Pope and Kanner (1993)	Daily mean PM$_{10}$	COPD patients (2.72 L)	0.21% (0.05%, 0.37%)
Combined				0.15% (0.21%, 0.09%)
Peak Expiratory Flow				
Daily (evening)				
Utah Valley, UT 1989–90	Pope et al. (1991)	Daily mean PM$_{10}$	Symptomatic children (260 L/min)	0.25% (0.10%, 0.39%)

Location and Period	Reference	Particulate Measure	Sample (Mean PFT)	% Decrease in Daily Lung Function for Each $10\mu g/m^3$ Increase in PM_{10}
Utah Valley, UT 1990–91	Pope and Dockery (1992)	Daily mean PM_{10}	Symptomatic children (297 L/min)	0.06% (0.00%, 0.12%)
			Symptomatic children (308 L/min)	0.04% (−0.02%, 0.09%)
Wageningen, NL 1990–91	Roemer et al. (1993)	Daily mean PM_{10}	Symptomatic children (297 L/min)	0.09% (−0.01%, 0.20%)
Uniontown, PA Summer 1990	Neas et al. (1995)	Daily mean PM_{10}	Children (330 L/min)	0.19% (0.01%, 0.37%)
≥ Weekly				
4 Cities, NL Winter 1987–90	Hoek and Brunekreef (1994)	Daily mean PM_{10}	Lacks mean (Assume 300L/min)	0.16% (0.05%, 0.28%)
Wageningen, NL Winter 1990–91	Hoek and Brunekreef (1993)	Daily mean PM_{10}	Lacks mean (Assume 300L/min)	0.16% (−0.03%, 0.36%)
Combined				0.08% (0.05%, 0.11%)

$FEV_{.75}$ = forced expiratory volume in three quarters of a second; FEV_1 = forced expiratory volume in 1 sec.

PFT = pulmonary function test

PM_{10} = particulate matter smaller than 2.5µm aerodynamic diameter.

TSP = total suspended particulates.

COPD = chronic obstructive pulmonary disease.

Table 6-8. Estimated effects of each 10 µg/m³ increase in PM_{10}

Health Indicator	% Change in Health Indicator Reporting for each 10µg/m³ Increase in PM_{10} (95% CI)
Mortality	
All causes	0.7% (0.6%, 0.9%)
Cardiovascular	1.4% (1.0%, 1.8%)
Respiratory	3.4% (2.0%, 4.7%)
Hospital Admissions	
All respiratory	1.1% (0.8%, 1.5%)
Asthma	1.0% (0.4%, 1.6%)
Pneumonia	1.4% (0.7%, 2.0%)
COPD	2.4% (1.5%, 3.4%)
Congestive heart failure	1.0% (0.5%, 1.4%)
Coronary artery disease	0.6% (0.3%, 0.9%)
Dysrythmias	0.5% (−0.1%, 1.1%)
Exacerbation of Asthma	
Bronchodilator use	2.9% (1.5%, 4.5%)
Asthma attacks	8.8% (6.9%, 11.4%)
Respiratory Symptoms	
Upper respiratory	0.7% (−0.1%, 1.5%)
Lower respiratory	3.0% (1.5%, 4.5%)
Cough	1.3% (0.5%, 2.0%)
Decreased Pulmonary Function	
FEV_1	0.15% (0.09%, 0.21%)
PEF	0.08% (0.05%, 0.11%)

and a *consistency* of effects across independent analytic studies with different investigators in different settings. This review also provides insights into the relative magnitude of effects observed in various studies (see Table 6-8).

Total mortality is observed to increase by approximately 0.7% per 10 µg/m³ increase in PM_{10}, with somewhat stronger associations for cardiovascular mortality (approximately 1.4% per 10 µg/m³ PM_{10}), and considerably stronger associations for respiratory mortality (approximately 3.4% per 10 µg/m³ PM_{10}). No acute effects are detected with cancer and other nonpulmonary and noncardiovascular causes of mortality. These relative differences in cause-specific mortality are plausible, given the respiratory route of particle exposures.

If respiratory mortality is associated with particulate pollution, then health care visits for respiratory illness would also be expected to be associated with particulate pollution. Respiratory hospital admissions increase by approximately 1.1% per 10 µg/m³ PM_{10}. Particle exposures are most strongly associated with COPD admissions (2.4% increase per 10 µg/m³ PM_{10}), and pneumonia admissions (1.4% increase per 10 µg/m³ PM_{10}). Cardiovascular hospital admissions are associated with particle exposures: 1.0%, 0.6%, and 0.5% increase per 10 µg/m³ PM_{10} for congestive heart failure, coronary artery disease, and dysrhythmias, respectively.

Asthma admissions to hospital are associated with particle exposures (1.0% increase per 10 µg/m³ PM_{10}). Asthmatic subjects report substantial increases in asthma attacks (an approximate 11% increase per 10 µg/m³ PM_{10}) and in bronchodilator use (an approximate 12% increase per 10 µg/m³ PM_{10}).

Less severe measures of respiratory health also are associated with particle exposures. Lower respiratory symptom reporting increases by approximately 3.0% and cough by 1.3% per 10 µg/m³ PM_{10}. Weaker effects are observed with upper respiratory symptoms (approximately 0.7% per 10 µg/m³ PM_{10}). While lung function provides accurate objective measures, the observed effects are fairly modest: approximately 0.15% decrease for FEV_1 or $FEV_{.75}$ and 0.08% decrease for peak flow per 10 µg/m³ PM_{10}. Despite the relatively small size of these lung-function effect estimates, they consistently achieve statistical significance.

Limitations

Mass concentration of inhalable particles is only one measure of a complex mixture of gaseous and particulate air pollution to which people are exposed. PM_{10} includes a wide array of potentially toxic chemical species. In this review the possible contribution of gaseous co-pollutants has been ignored. It is, therefore, presumptuous to assign these observed health effects solely to the mass concentration of particulates. On the other hand, the consistency of these observed effects across so many communities suggests that, lacking an explicit hypothesis, these associations are assigned to a nonspecific definition of inhalable or fine particle concentrations common to urban areas.

The physical and chemical characteristics of ambient particles are generally not known and so are impossible to duplicate in controlled animal- or human-exposure studies. Many of the health effects of particles are thought to reflect the combined action of the diverse components in the pollutant mix. Until controlled animal-and human-exposure studies identify the active component(s) of these complex mixtures and can characterize their underlying mechanisms of toxicity, it is prudent to ascribe health effects observed by epidemiologists to the undifferentiated particle mass rather than to any specific component.

The results of epidemiologic studies of acute effects of particulate air pollution, particularly those describing associations with cardiovascular mortality, have been called into question because of the lack of a biologically plausible mechanism (Utell and Samet, 1993; Waller and Swan, 1992). While the specific biologic mechanism for these acute increases in mortality is not clear, the internal consistency of the mortality studies and the external consistency with evidence of acute increases in morbidity measures suggest that these results are not artifacts.

Recommendations

Mortality has always been a key health end point in epidemiologic studies; that is, it serves as a leading indicator for hypothesis generation. It is a well-defined health outcome, and mortality data are routinely collected and readily available for epidemiologic analysis. When the numerous time-series studies of the association of mortality with particulate air pollution are compiled, using measures of effect (% increase) and exposure (PM_{10}) as in Table 6-1, the quantitative consistency of estimated effects becomes clear. When estimated effects of particulate air pollution are similarly combined for other health indicators, the consistency of results also becomes apparent. These findings highlight the importance of using equivalent exposure metrics and health end points in air pollution studies.

Thus, we recommend that researchers report results such that they can be readily compared with previous (and future) investigations. The groupings of health end points considered here present some guidance. Likewise, the reporting of associations with PM_{10} concentrations is important. This recommendation should not be interpreted as a request for regimentation or an attempt to limit innovation. Rather, it is recommended that the associations with common end points and PM_{10} exposures be reported in addition to other, potentially more sensitive or specific, indicators of health effect or exposure.

A quantitative effect estimate and its estimated standard error should be reported in all cases. Reports of statistical significance without explicit effect estimates are not very informative. Likewise, correlation coefficients and other unscaled measures of association fail to provide useful information.

Epidemiologic research regarding the health effects of particulate air pollution has been impeded by the lack of daily (or more frequent) particle measurements (Dockery et al., 1992). In communities that are not likely to violate (or that clearly exceed) the NAAQS for particles, PM_{10} measurements are made only once every 6 days, as required by the EPA (1987). Fortunately for epidemiologists, the EPA has required daily monitoring in communities likely to violate the NAAQS for particles. These regulations have had the unanticipated (but beneficial) effect of making feasible new epidemiologic studies of the acute effects of particles. Inasmuch as associations are being observed between daily particle exposures and adverse health effects down to the lowest measurable concentrations, it is recommended that daily PM_{10} concentrations be measured whenever possible. When alternative measures of particle concentrations are used, then a description of the relationship to PM_{10} concentrations should be provided.

Research into mechanisms of the adverse health effects of PM_{10} mass concentrations observed in recent epidemiologic studies needs to be undertaken in controlled exposure studies of humans and animals. It is only through integration of the complementary evidence from laboratory animal and controlled human exposure studies with the results from epidemiologic studies that the risk of particle exposures can be fully evaluated. Nevertheless, these recent epidemiologic studies implicate particulate air pollution as contributing to respiratory morbidity and mortality even at exposure levels below the current NAAQS in the United States.

Acknowledgments

This review updates a previous review by the same authors (Dockery and Pope, 1994) and was supported in part by National Institute of Environmental Health Sciences grant ES-00002.

References

Bates DV. 1980. The health effects of air pollution. J Respir Dis 1:29–37.

Bates DV, Sizto R. 1987. Air pollution and hospital admissions in Southern Ontario: the acid summer haze effect. Environ Res 43:317–331.

Bates DV. 1989. Respiratory Function in Disease, 3rd ed. W. B. Saunders, Philadelphia, PA.

Bates DV. 1992. Health indices of the adverse effects of air pollution: the question of coherence. Environ Res 59:336–349.

Beaver H. 1953. Committee on air pollution: Interim report. Her Majesty's Stationery Office. London. Cmd 9011.

Braun-Fahrlander C, Ackermann-Liebrich U, Schwartz J, Gnehm HP, Rutishauser M, Wanner, HU. 1992. Air pollution and respiratory symptoms in preschool children. Am Rev Respir Dis 145:42–47.

Brimblecombe P. 1987. The Big Smoke: A History of Air Pollution in London Since Medieval Times. Methuen & Co., London, p 161.

Brunekreef B, Kinney PL, Ware JH, Dockery DW, Speizer FE, Spengler JD, Ferris BG Jr. 1991. Sensitive subgroups and normal variation in pulmonary function response to air pollution episodes. Environ Health Perspect 90:189–193.

Burnett RT, Krewski D, Vincent R, et al. Associations between ambient particulate sulfate and Admissions to Ontario Hospitals for Cardiac and Respiratory Disease. Am J Epidemiol 142:15–22 1995.

Cohen D, Arai SF, Brain JD. 1979. Smoking impairs long-term clearance from the lung. Science 204:514–517.

Dockery DW, Schwartz J, Spengler JD. 1992. Air pollution and daily mortality: associations with particulates and acid aerosols. Environ Res. 59: 362–373.

Dockery DW, Pope CA III. 1994. Acute respiratory effects of particulate air pollution. Ann Rev Public Health 15:107–132.

Dockery DW, Ware JH, Ferris BG Jr., Speizer FE, Cook NR, Herman SM. Change in pulmonary function in children associated with air pollution episodes. APCA Journal 1982; 32:937–942.

Dzubay TG, Stevens RK. 1975. Ambient air analysis with dichotomous sampler and x-ray fluorescence spectrometer. Environ Sci Tech 9:663–668.

Ellison JM, Waller RE. 1978. A review of sulphur oxides and particulate matter as air pollutants with particular reference to effects on health in the United Kingdom. Environ Res 16:302–325.

Environmental Protection Agency. 1987. 40 CFR Part 50. Revisions to the National Ambient Air Quality Standards for Particulate Matter: Final Rules. Federal Register 52(126):24634–24669.

Fairley D. 1990. The relationship of daily mortality to suspended particulates in Santa Clara County, 1980–1986. Environ Health Perspect 89:159–168.

Firket J. 1936. Fog along the Meuse Valley. Trans Faraday Soc 32:1192–1197.

Friedlander SK. 1978. Smoke, Dust and Haze: Fundamentals of Aerosol Behavior. John Wiley and Sons, New York.

Hatch GE, Boykin E, Graham JA, Lewtas J, Pott F, Loud K, Mumford JL. 1985. Inhalable particles and pulmonary host defenses: *in vivo* and *in vitro* effects of ambient air and combustion particles. Environ Res 36:67–80.

Hoek G, Brunekreef B. 1993. Acute effects of a winter air pollution episode on pulmonary function and respiratory symptoms of children. Arch Environ Health 48:328–335.

Hoek G, Brunekreef B. 1994. Effects of low level winter air pollution concentrations on respiratory health of Dutch children. Environ Res 64:136–150.

Holland WW, Bennett AE, Cameron IR, Florey CduV, Leeder SR, Schilling RSF, et al. 1979. Health effects of particulate pollution: reappraising the evidence. Am J Epidemiol 110:525–659.

Ito K, Kinney RK, Thurston GD. 1995. Variations in PM-10 concentrations within two metropolitan areas and their implications for health effects analyses. Inhalation Toxicol 7:735–745.

Kinney PL, Ito K, Thurston GD. 1995. A sensitivity analysis of mortality/PM_{10} association in Los Angeles. Inhalation Toxicol 7:59–70.

Lippmann M, Lioy PJ. 1985. Critical issues in air pollution epidemiology. Environ Health Perspect 62: 243–258.

Lippmann M. 1989. Health effects of ozone—a critical review. J Air Pollut Control Assoc 39:672–695.

Lippmann M, Ito K. 1995. Separating the effects of temperature and season on daily mortality from those of air pollution in London: 1965–1972. Inhalation Toxicol 7:85–97.

MacFarlane A. 1977. Daily mortality and environment in English conurbanations. 1: air pollution, low temperature, and influenza in greater London. Br J Prev Med 31: 54–61.

Mackenbach JP, Looman CWN, Kunst AE. 1993. Air pollution, lagged effects of temperature, and mortality: the Netherlands 1979–1987. J Epidemiol Comm Health 47:121–126.

Martin AE. 1964. Mortality and morbidity statistics and air pollution. Proc Roy Soc Med 57:969.

Ministry of Health. 1954. Mortality and morbidity during the London fog of 1952. London, HMSO (Reports on Public Health and Medical Subjects, No. 95).

Mazumdar S, Schimmel H, Higgins ITT. 1982. Relation of daily mortality to air pollution: an analysis of 14 London winters, 1958/59–1971/72. Arch Environ Health 37:213–220.

Miller FJ, Gardner DE, Graham JA, Lee RE Jr, Wilson WE, Bachmann JD. 1979. Size considerations for establishing a standard for inhalable particles. J Air Pollut Control Assoc 29:610–615.

Neas LM, Dockery DW, Koutrakis P, Tollerud DJ, Speizer FE. 1995. The association of ambient air pollution with twice daily peak expiratory flow rate measurements in children. Am J Epidemiol 141:111–122.

Neas LM, Dockery DW, Burge H, Koutrakis P, Speizer FE. 1996. Fungus spores, air pollutants and other determinants of peak expiratory flow rate in children. Am J Epidemiol 143:797–807.

Ostro B. 1984. A search for a threshold in the relationship of air pollution to mortality: a reanalysis of data on London winters. Environ Health Perspect 58:397–399.

Ostro BD, Lipsett MJ, Wiener MB, Selner JC. 1991 Asthmatic response to airborne acid aerosols. Am J Pub Health 81:694–702

Ostro BD, Lipsett MJ, Mann JK, Braxton-Owens H, White MC. 1995. Air pollution and asthma exacerbations among African-American children in Los Angeles. Inhalation Toxicol 7:711–722.

Ostro BD, Sanchez JM, Aranda C, Eskeland GS. 1996. Air pollution and mortality: results from a study of Santiago, Chile. J Expo Assess Environ Epid 6:97–114.

Pavia D, Bateman JRM, Sheahan NF, Agnew JE, Newman SP, Clarke SW. 1980. Techniques for measuring lung mucociliary clearance. In: Berglund E, Nilsson BS, Mossberg B, Bake B, eds. Cough and Expectoration. Eur J Respir Dis 61(107):157–168.

Phalen RF, Cuddihy RG, Fisher GL, Moss OR, Schlessinger RB, Swift DL, Yeh HC. 1991. Main features of the proposed NCRP respiratory tract model. Radiat Protect Dosim 38:179–184.

Pope CA III. 1989. Respiratory disease associated with community air pollution and a steel mill, Utah valley. Am J Public Health 79:623–628.

Pope CA III, Dockery DW, Spengler JD, Raizenne ME. 1991. Respiratory health and PM_{10} pollution: a daily time series analysis. Am Rev Respir Dis 144:668–674.

Pope CA III, Dockery DW. 1992. Acute health effects of PM_{10} pollution on symptomatic and asymptomatic children. Am Rev Respir Dis 145:1123–1128.

Pope CA III, Schwartz J, Ransom MR. 1992. Daily mortality and PM_{10} pollution in Utah Valley. Arch Environ Health 47:211–217.

Pope III CA, Kanner RE. 1993. Acute effects of PM_{10} pollution on pulmonary function of smokers with mild to moderate chronic obstructive pulmonary disease. Am Rev Respir Dis 147:1336–1340.

Pope CA III, Dockery DW, Schwartz J. 1995. Review of epidemiological evidence of health effects of particulate air pollution. Inhal Tox 7:1–18.

Pope CA III, Thun MJ, Namboodiri MN, Dockery DW, Evans JS, Speizer FE, Heath CW Jr. 1995. Particulate air pollution as a predictor of mortality in a prospective cohort study of US adults. Am J Respir Crit Care Med 151:669–674.

Pope CA III. 1996. Particulate pollution and health: a review of the Utah Valley experience. J Exp Anal Environ Epid 6:23–34.

Pope CA III, Schwartz J. 1996. Time series for the analysis of pulmonary health data. Presented at the joint ATS/ERS Workshop on the Analysis of Longitudinal Respiratory Data, Barcelona, September 21–22, 1995.

Roemer W, Hoek G, Brunekreef B. 1993. Effect of ambient winter air pollution on respiratory health of children with chronic respiratory symptoms. Am Rev Respir Dis 147:118–124.

Saldiva PHN, Pope CA, Schwartz J, Dockery DW, Lichtenfels AJ, Salge JM, Barone I, Bohm GM. 1995. Air Pollution and mortality in elderly people: a time series study in Sao Paulo, Brazil. Arch Environ Health 50:159–163.

Samet JM, Speizer FE, Bishop Y, Spengler JD, Ferris BG Jr. 1981. The relationship between air pollution and emergency room visits in an industrial community. J Air Pollut Control Assoc 31:236–240.

Samet JM, Zeger SL, Berhane K. 1995. The association of mortality and particulate air pollution. In: Particulate Air Pollution and Daily Mortality: Replication and Validation of Selected Studies. Health Effects Institute, Cambridge, MA: pp. 1–104.

Schwartz J, Marcus A. 1990. Mortality and air pollution in London: a time series analysis. Am J Epidemiol; 131:185–794.

Schwartz J. 1991 Particulate air pollution and daily mortality in Detroit. Environ Res 56:204–213.

Schwartz J, Spix C, Wichmann HE, Malin E. 1991. Air pollution and acute respiratory illness in five German communities. Environ Res 56:1–14.

Schwartz J, Dockery DW. 1992. Increased mortality in Philadelphia associated with daily air pollution concentrations. Am Rev Respir Dis 145:600–604

Schwartz J. 1993a. Air pollution and daily mortality in Birmingham Al. Am J Epidemiol 137:1136–1147.

Schwartz J, Slater D, Larson TV, Pierson WE, Koenig JQ. 1993b. Particulate air pollution and hospital emergency room visits for asthma in Seattle. Am Rev Respir Dis 147:826–831.

Schwartz J. 1994a. Air pollution and hospital admissions for the elderly in Detroit, Michigan. Am J Respir Crit Care Med 150:648–655.

Schwartz J. 1994b. Air pollution and daily mortality: a review and meta analysis. Environ Res 64:36–52.

Schwartz J. 1994c. What are people dying of on high air pollution days? Environ Res 64:26–35.

Schwartz J. 1994d. Air pollution and hospital admissions for the elderly in Birmingham, Al. Am J Epidemiol 139:589–598.

Schwartz J. 1994e. PM_{10}, ozone, and hospital admissions for the elderly in Minneapolis–St. Paul, Minnesota. Arch Environ Health 49:366–374.

Schwartz J. 1994f. Particulate air pollution and daily mortality in Cincinnati, Ohio. Environ Health Perspect 102:186–189.

Schwartz J. 1994g. Nonparametric smoothing in the analysis of air pollution and respiratory illness. Canadian Journal of Statistics 22:471–487.

Schwartz J. 1994h. The use of generalized additive models in epidemiology. In: International Biometric Society XVII International Conference: Proceedings. Invited Papers, pp. 55–80. Hamilton Ontario, 1994.

Schwartz J, Dockery DW, Neas LM, Wypij D, Ware JH, Spengler JD, Koutrakis P, Speizer FE, Ferris BG Jr. 1994. Acute effects of summer air pollution on respiratory symptom reporting in children. Am J Respir Crit Care Med 150:1234–1242.

Schwartz J. 1996. Short term fluctuations in air pollution and hospital admissions for respiratory disease. Thorax 50:531–538.

Seaton A, MacNee W, Donaldson K, Godden D. 1995. Particulate air pollution and acute health effects. Lancet 345:176–178.

Shrenk HH, Heimann H, Clayton GD, Gafafer WM, Wexler H. 1949. Air pollution in Donora, PA: epidemiology of the unusual smog episode of October 1948, Preliminary Report. Public Health Bulletin No. 306. Public Health Service, Washington, DC.

Spix C, Heinrich J, Dockery DW, Schwartz J, Volksch G, Schwinkowski K, Collen C, Wichmann, HE. 1993. Air pollution and daily mortality in Erfut, East Germany, 1980–1989. Environ Health Perspect 101(6):518–525.

Shy CM. 1979. Epidemiologic evidence and the United States air quality standards. Am J Epidemiol 110:661–671.

Sunyer J, Saez M, Murillo C, Castelsaque J, Martinez F, Anto JM. 1993. Air pollution and emergency room admissions for chronic obstructive pulmonary disease: a 5-year study. Am J Epidemiol 137:701–705.

Taubes G. 1995. Epidemiology faces its limits. Science 269(5221):164–169.

Thurston GD, Ito K, Kinney PL, Lippmann M. 1992. A multi-year study of air pollution and respiratory hospital admissions in three New York state metropolitan areas: results for 1988 and 1989 summers. J Expos Anal Environ Epidem 2:429–450.

Thurston GD, Ito K, Hayes CG, Bates DV, Lippmann M. 1994. Respiratory hospital admissions and summertime haze air pollution in Toronto, Ontario: Consideration of the role of acid aerosols. Environ Res 1994; 65:270–290.

Touloumi G, Pocock SJ, Katsouyanni K, Trichopoulos D. 1994. Short term effect of air pollution on daily mortality in Athens: a time series analysis. Int J Epidemiol 23:957–967.

Utell MJ, Samet JM. 1993. Particulate air pollution and health: new evidence on an old problem (editorial). Am Rev Respir Dis 147: 1334–1335.

Verhoeff AP, Hoek G, Schwartz J, van Wijuen JH. 1996. Air pollution and daily mortality in Amsterdam, the Netherlands. Epidemiology 7:225–230.

Ware JH, Thibodeau LA, Speizer FE, Colome S, Ferris BG Jr. 1981. Assessment of the health effects of atmospheric sulfur oxides and particulate matter: evidence from observational studies. Environ Health Perspect 41:255–276.

Waller RE, Swan AV. 1992. Invited commentary: Particulate air pollution and daily mortality. Am J Epidemiol 135:20–22.

Whittemore AS, Korn EL. 1980. Asthma and air pollution in the Los Angeles area. Am J Public Health 70:687–696.

Wilson WE, Suh HH. 1996. Fine and coarse particles: concentration relationships relevant to epidemiological studies. J Air Waste Management Association. (in press).

World Health Organization, Regional Office for Europe. 1987. Air quality guidelines for Europe. WHO Regional Publications, European Series No. 23, pp. 426.

Xu X, Gao J, Dockery DW, Chen Y. 1994. Air pollution and daily mortality in residential areas of Beijing, China. Arch Environ Health 49:216–222.

Outdoor Air II: 7

Nitrogen Dioxide

JORDI SUNYER

NITROGEN dioxide (NO_2) is an air pollutant generated by combustion. It occurs both in homes, primarily from gas stoves or heaters, and in the outdoor air, primarily from cars. Indoor levels have been more of a concern because they can exceed outdoor levels. The main focus of epidemiologic studies has been on respiratory effects in children; children in homes with gas stoves have often been compared to children in homes without them.

One reason for concern about NO_2 is that there is evidence that it increases respiratory infection in rodents; it is also known to reduce lung clearance in humans at high doses. A variety of human experimental studies under controlled conditions have shown that NO_2 increases airway responsiveness in normal adults at high levels and in asthmatics at low levels. The clinical implications of these effects for the general population, however, are unknown. In addition, there are limited data indicating that NO_2 may heighten the response to allergens.

These experimental data illustrate a common theme in environmental epidemiology. Experimental data are often summarized as negative to weakly positive. Those who prefer to rely on experimental rather than epidemiologic data as the basis for assessing hazards are usually unimpressed with the evidence at the exposure levels of regulatory interest. While experimental studies of human volunteers can provide markedly refined understanding of mechanisms, however, the fundamental question of whether there are adverse effects in free-living human populations is ultimately better addressed by epidemiologic studies. Experimental studies are conducted on a limited number of select subjects (e.g., healthy adults). They are therefore incapable of incorporating the variation in susceptibility based on genetics or preexisting disease, and the variation in lifestyle factors, that occur in the general population. They also are unable to mimic real exposures, which are characterized by a complex mixture of pollutants.

Notwithstanding the above caveats, the epidemiology of NO_2 to date is generally consistent with experimental studies in not showing consistent or strong health effects. Although some studies of children have revealed an increase in respiratory infections, the better-designed studies of children with actual exposure measurements have not. In adults studies of outdoor NO_2 have also shown no consistent effects on respiratory function on disease, for either healthy individuals or asthmatics.

In contrast to other pollutants such as particulates or sulfates, levels of NO_2 in the environment have been increasing over time. The data so far do not generally indicate health effects at the low levels commonly encountered in the environment, but there is some suggestion that NO_2 may exacerbate the effect of allergens. Asthmatics with allergic asthma may prove to be a uniquely susceptible population.

Nitrogen dioxide is a common air pollutant both in homes (indoor air) and in the urban outdoor atmosphere. NO_2 is an oxidant gas generated directly from any combustion appliance. The pollution of indoor environments is produced by indoor combustion sources (gas stoves, water and space heaters) in addition to outdoor air entry. Indoor air pollution is an important determinant of human exposure to NO_2 (Spengler et al., 1983) because people usually spend more of their time in indoor environments. Indoor NO_2 air levels may reach average concentrations of 0.2 to 0.4 parts per million (ppm), and even higher transient peaks while cooking with gas stoves (Spengler et al., 83).

In outdoor air the combustion of fossil fuels by cars is the main source of NO_2, by direct release or by the secondary oxidation of nitric oxide, a primary generated gas. NO_2 outdoor concentration in the urban atmosphere is increasing with traffic density (Broughton 1993). Hence, the decline in sulfur dioxide and particles that occurred in all the western industrialized cities during recent decades was not paralleled by a decline in NO_2 and ozone (EPA 1991). In outdoor air, 1-hour values of NO_2 range from around 0.025 ppm in non-polluted cities to around 0.1 ppm in cities with high traffic density (Katsouyanis et al., 1995). Occasionally, outdoor levels may reach higher hourly levels, i.e., 0.4 ppm during a pollution episode in London (Broughton 1993). There is little seasonal variation for NO_2, unlike the classic outdoor pollutants, SO_2 and particles, which show a higher winter concentration in most of the settings.

NO_2 is not highly soluble; most inhaled NO_2 is retained in the large and small airways of the lungs (Goldstein et al., 1980). At high concentrations in animals and in humans accidentally exposed, NO_2 damages the lung by oxidant injury, adversely affects lung defense mechanisms, and reduces the clearance of infecting organisms, particularly bacteria (the modification of viral effects being less clear) (NRC 1976, Pennington, 1988). This toxicological evidence suggests that NO_2—at the low concentrations found in life—may play a role in increasing the incidence and severity of respiratory infections and contributing to airways injury and obstruction in persons with previous bronchial diseases (Samet and Utell, 1990).

Since the 1970s, a large body of research has been developed on the respiratory effects of real-life concentrations of NO_2, based on both clinical studies with controlled exposures to volunteers and epidemiologic studies. Experimental studies show on average an increase in airways reactivity with NO_2 exposure in comparison with clean air, although the approach of exposing persons to individual pollutants has little relevance to the real world. Recent experiments reflected the complexity of human exposures, challenging volunteers with allergens and NO_2 alone or in combination with other pollutants. Epidemiologic studies are more relevant to populations but face the difficulty of measuring the personal exposure to one contaminant among the complex mixture of pollutants.

Laboratory Studies

Controlled exposures to air pollutants undergone by volunteers in a chamber have been broadly used to assess acute respiratory functional responses. These chamber studies (also called clinical studies) have been a rich tool to understand air pollution health effects. The major advantage of these studies is the precise control of the air pollutant exposure. In addition, some of the atmosphere characteristics such as humidity and temperature may also be controlled, as well as other cofactors such as exercise or other pollutants.

Some chamber studies with volunteers have shown a small effect on bronchial responsiveness in asthmatics exposed at NO_2 concentrations similar to those found during the high urban peaks or near home combustion appliances (between 0.1 and 0.3 ppm per hour) (Oherek et al., 1976; Kleinman et al., 1983; Mohensin, 1987; Bauer et al., 1986), but other studies have fail to find such increase in bronchial responsiveness (Linn et al., 1985; Hazucha et al., 1983). A recent comprehensive review (Folinsbee, 1992) of the experiments carried out between 1971 and 1991, including 20 studies of asthmatics with a total of 355 subjects (201 of them challenged with exercise), and five studies including healthy subjects, shows that there is a statistically significant bronchial responsiveness effect in asthmatics at rest (70% responded at NO_2 concentrations between 0.05 and 0.3 ppm), whereas the response during exercise was not statistically significant (51% of the subjects responded). Bronchial responsiveness is merely a functional disorder, used as an operative marker of the tendency of the airways to bronchoconstrict when challenged by environmental stimuli. It has been associated with the progress of chronic obstructive pulmonary disease, and it has been used to measure asthma, but it is an indirect measure of the actual impact of air pollutants on respiratory disease. Healthy subjects showed a significant response at NO_2 concentrations above 1 ppm (a very high concentration rarely observed in real life). The effect of NO_2 exposure on lung function was less clear than on bronchial responsiveness, the majority of studies failing to demonstrate any effect (Bylin, 1993), even in severe asthmatics (Avol et al., 1988).

Real urban atmospheres are complex chemical mixtures that are continuously reacting. Laboratory studies with a unique air pollutant permit an analysis of the separate effects of each particular component of the atmosphere, but such results are not easily transferred to real life. Experiments may become more complex with the addition of different pollutants, but chamber studies with gas mixtures can provoke a response caused by discomfort and limitation of the inspiration rather than bronchoconstriction (Hazucha et al., 1989). Such reactions have to be controlled by restricting the volumes of gas breathed relative to the remaining volumes (Tunnicliffe et al., 1994).

Recent controlled studies using allergens (*Dermatophagoides* Pt.) have shown an increase of bronchial responsiveness (Tunnicliffe et al., 1994; Devalia et al., 1994). These findings have to be considered preliminary because they found a weak effect in very small populations (eight subjects) that were highly selected (mild asthmatics, nonsmokers without steroid medication). However, the finding could explain the discrepancies of previous experiments that only involved challenges with NO_2 and did not take into account the likely modification of the effect due to the presence of allergens in subjects with allergic asthma. Thus, it is possible that NO_2 may modify the immune response, resulting in sensitization or increased allergic responses in the airway; or it may be that subclinical airways in-

Table 7-1. Differences between clinical and epidemiological studies

	Clinical	Epidemiological
Design	Experiment	Observational
Subjects	Volunteers	General population
Sample size	Small	Large
Outcome	Bronchial responsiveness	Respiratory symptoms, Respiratory illnesses, Pulmonary function
Time-pattern	Acute	Acute and chronic
Exposure	Controlled, unique	Environment mixture
Confounders	Volume inhaled	Meteorology smoking social class
Effect modifiers	Exercise, allergy, medication, virus infection	Allergy infections, smoking
Internal validity	Strong	Weak underestimate
External validity	Low: selection Artificial air	High: no selection Real air

flammation produced by other agents, such as allergens, is a prerequisite for any detrimental effects of the NO_2. Most of the clinical studies have measured bronchial responsiveness or pulmonary function as the marker of the NO_2 health effects. However, inflammation may be another important end point (Aris et al., 1993). A recent study showed induced inflammatory changes in the bronchi with NO_2 controlled exposure (Devalia et al., 1993). These inflammatory changes may have a clinical impact in sensitive subjects such as those suffering from asthma. The approach of exposing persons to pollutants individually may have little relevance to the real world (Table 7-1).

NO_2 has been found to increase the frequency of respiratory tract infectious in animal studies (NRC 1976). To test this hypothesis in humans, Goings et al. (1989) simultaneously exposed healthy volunteers intranasally to an attenuated influenza virus and NO_2. The amount of recovery virus or the antibody levels did not differ by NO_2 concentrations, signaling a lack of differences in respiratory infection. However, the negative results might be the result of the use of attenuated virus (Samet and Utell, 1990).

Epidemiologic Studies

Epidemiological studies, unlike laboratory studies, measure the effect of the actual air on large populations, often representative of the overall population (Table 7-1). Epidemiologic studies are natural experiments in which the study design allows inference about the relationship between exposure and disease. Epidemiologic studies of NO_2 have focused on respiratory effects, both short term (exacerbation of preexisting diseases or transient illnesses or pulmonary function decrement in healthy subjects), and long term (the cumulative exposure to NO_2 may contribute to the development of disease incidence, for example, asthma).

The main limitation in epidemiologic studies is the measure of the actual exposure to air pollution. NO_2 in the outdoor air is a component of a complex pollutant mixture and the relationships often cannot be attributed to NO_2 alone. Selecting places for studies where NO_2 is the major outdoor air pollutant has helped to reduce this limitation. Studies conducted in the indoor air also solve, in part, the problem of measuring the effects of NO_2, because NO_2 is often the principal pollutant in indoor air, and in many places NO_2 indoor concentrations exceeded outdoor concentrations (NRC 1976).

Effects of NO₂ in indoor air

Although the setting of these studies was the home, their conclusions may also be valid for the effects of the outdoor environment. On the other hand, NO_2 is always present in a complex mixture with other components that may also have adverse respiratory effects, such as nitrous acid, and the indoor and outdoor mixtures are different; thus, the validity of the extrapolation from indoor NO_2 findings to outdoor NO_2 is limited (Samet et al., 1993). One theoretical advantage of studying the effects of NO_2 in the indoor environment is that epidemiologic studies may measure more easily the actual exposure to NO_2, reducing the potential bias produced in the studies with outdoor air caused by the error in the measurement of the exposure. However, most of the indoor studies have been based on comparisons between children from homes with and without gas appliances, and have lacked actual NO_2 measurements. The assumption was made that homes with gas had higher levels of NO_2, because in general NO_2 levels in homes with gas stoves are markedly higher than in homes with electric stoves. This is true on average (Spengler et al., 1983), but the distribution of NO_2 levels in homes with gas and electric stoves overlap, and NO$_2$ concentration in homes with gas stoves showed a broad range (Samet and Utell, 90).

Studies of indoor air and NO$_2$ are shown in Table 7-2. Results have not been consistent. The most recent studies have improved the measurement of personal exposure to NO$_2$ (Koo et al., 1990; Rutihauser et al., 1990). Among these, the prospective cohort study of New Mexico newborns during 18 months was noteworthy for the quality of both exposure and the disease measurements (Samet et al., 1993). One thousand two hundred and five newborns from homes without smokers were enrolled. Every 2 weeks, mothers reported daily occurrence of symptoms and illnesses, and a nurse practitioner validated the reports, doing home visits in addition to the revision of the outpatient clinical records. Two-week NO$_2$ measurements in the bedroom were done each season, in addition to 2-week measurement in the kitchen and living room during the cool season. The bedroom measurement were used as a valid indicator of the personal exposure and time-activity weighted patterns in the house did not improve such measurement. The authors found that neither lower respiratory tract illness incidence (defined as wheezing and wet cough) nor illness duration during the first 18 months were associated with NO$_2$ exposure. The authors concluded that their findings may be extended to homes of the United States where outdoor air pollution for NO$_2$ is not high, like in New Mexico, and to healthy children not exposed to tobacco smoke and not in full-time day care. These remarks lead to two considerations: exposure characteristics are place-specific and concomitant exposures and other factors such as viral infection may modify the effect of NO$_2$.

One of the important findings in the report of Samet (Samet et al., 1993) is that children in the United States are not highly exposed to NO$_2$ from gas cooking (70% of the children spent no time in the kitchen during cooking, and only 22% of the time children were exposed to levels higher than 0.02 ppm in the bedroom). However, other populations may have higher exposures. Furthermore, the presence of other indoor air pollution sources such as smoking may modify the role of NO$_2$ on the lower respiratory tract diseases, as may frequent exposure to viruses as the result of day-care attendance.

Formal meta-analysis of indoor NO$_2$ studies have been conducted (e.g., Hasselblad et al., 1992), but have had to combine studies with different ages and different respiratory outcomes. Bronchial illness during the first 2 years of life is a different medical entity than the same illness at older ages (Martinez et al., 1995). In addition, the authors combined respiratory symptoms and respiratory diseases. Furthermore, the authors had to as-

Table 7-2. List of the principal studies on NO_2 and indoor air and the association with respiratory symptoms, diseases, and function

Study (Main Author)	Design	Population	Exposure to NO_2	Association with[a] Symptoms	Association with[a] Diseases	Association with[a] Function	Comments
Melia, 1977, 1979	Survey, national	Children, 6–11 years	Type of stove	+	+		
Speizer, 1980	Survey	8000 schoolchildren	Type of stove		+	+	
Melia, 1983	Cohort, first year	390 infants	Type of stove	NS	+		Symptoms in first year using medical records
Ware, 1984	Survey	10,000 schoolchildren	Type of stove	−/+	−/+		After adjusting for parental education association decreases
Ogston, 1985	Follow-up, first year	1565 newborns	Type of stove		−/+		Periodic collection of information
Koo, 1990	Survey	362 schoolchildren	Personal samplers	NS			NO_2 related with outdoor rather than indoor levels
Rutishauser, 1990	Panel, 6 weeks	1225 children, 0–5 years	Personal samplers	NS			Outdoor NO_2 related with symptoms
Neas, 1991	Follow-up, 5 years	1567 schoolchildren	Weekly samplers indoor	+		NS	In girls but not in boys
Samet, 1993	Follow-up, 18 months	1205 newborns	2-week samplers in bedroom	NS	NS		Low indoor exposure

[a]significant association; NS, nonsignificant association; −/+, association at the limit of the significance.

sume a certain amount of exposure for all the studies that reported only qualitative information exposure. The confounding variables from one study to another also varied broadly. These problems limit the validity of the meta-analysis carried out.

Samet and Utell (1990) have reviewed the common limitation of the indoor NO_2 studies signaling three main drawbacks: errors in the exposure measurement, errors in the disease measurement and sample size. As Samet has pointed out (Samet and Utell, 1990), the misclassification errors in the disease and in the exposure are multiplicative, and consequently studies having both problems may be severely biased toward showing no effect. The question remains if the lack of consistent evidence for NO_2 indoor health effects is due to the limits of the studies available or due to true lack of effect.

Acute effects of outdoor NO₂

PANEL STUDIES

Most of the studies with outdoor air measured the short-term effects of NO_2 using a panel design, which assesses the temporal variation in NO_2 in relation to acute temporal variation in the outcome in a given set of individuals. Outcomes have included both (1) subjective symptoms measured by diaries and (2) changes in pulmonary function. These longitudinal studies are characterized by repeated cross-sectional measures of the exposure and the outcome in populations of a relative moderate size (hundreds of subjects), measured in a large number of occasions during a short time period (months). Such studies require methods for the analysis of longitudinal data that incorporate the intrinsic correlation of the repeated measurements within the same individual.

Table 7-3 presents the panel studies. Two such studies have followed groups of subjects defined by a baseline health condition using the daily environmental urban city-average NO_2 to assess the individual NO_2 exposure (Pershagen et al., 1984; Vedal et al., 1987). In a different panel, NO_2 exposure was estimated based on the outdoor measures and the individual time-activity pattern of each individual (Clench-Aas et al., 1991). A model attributed to each subject a different value of NO_2 exposure for each hour. The author found a significant relation with symptoms but not with peak expiratory flow measurements, a rather more objective measurement of effects. Studies conducted in places polluted mainly by vehicle exhausts showed a positive association between outdoor NO_2 and symptoms in young adults (Schwartz et al., 1991), duration of the lower respiratory tract symptoms in children (Braun-Farhrlander et al., 1992), and pulmonary function (peak-flow) in asthmatics (Moseholm et al.,

1993). By contrast, a panel study of schoolchildren suffering current respiratory symptoms carried out during winter episodes of air pollution did not find any effect (Roemer et al., 1993). The authors suggested that the lack of association for NO_2 may be due to the high correlation with the other pollutants assessed. An alternative explanation could be that at the low levels of NO_2 observed in this study the association was too small to be detected with this type of study, or even that a threshold level exists below which no effects appeared. Limitations in measuring exposure often preclude the assessment of a possible threshold with epidemiologic studies.

TEMPORO-ECOLOGIC STUDIES

Temporo-ecologic studies of acute responses to air pollutants are studies of populations rather than individuals. For example, the population may be a city and the outcome variable the daily number of recorded hospital visits or deaths, which is to be related with daily air pollution. These studies may be considered longitudinal studies of one unit, where the exposure and the output are measured cross-sectionally in a repeated series of days during a large period. These types of studies are also called time-series studies. They have become popular in the assessment of the relation between particulate pollution and mortality. Methods to account for the autocorrelation of repeated outcomes, as well as the control of the possible confounding effects played by the temperature and season are very well developed. These studies do not have problems of subject selection, because all the subjects of a given population are inherently included in the study population, but they have to face the limits of the so-called ecological fallacy, in which findings pertaining to populations may not accurately reflect what would have been found if individuals had been studied.

Daily counts of hospital visits for croup in German cities polluted by cars were related with daily NO_2 outdoor levels in children (Schwartz et al., 1991). Similarly, daily counts in asthma visits were related with NO_2 in Finland, where particulate levels were very low (Ponka 1991; Rossi and Kimula, 1993). Other studies of hospital admissions for chronic respiratory disease, however, have failed to find an association with NO_2—but they have shown a relation with particulates or SO_2 (Sunyer et al., 1991), which may be explained by the specificity of the NO_2 effects for asthma or croup. The degree of severity of the outcome measured in this type of study differs from the previous studies, because hospital visits are measuring a more extreme potential effect, compared with symptoms or functional changes. A common problem in time-series studies of this type is the inability to separate out the effects of different pollutants. For exam-

Table 7-3. Summary of panel studies of outdoor NO_2 and respiratory symptoms, diseases, and function.

Study (Main Author)	Population	Exposure to NO_2	Association with[a]			Comments
			Symptoms	Diseases	Function	
Pershagen, 1984	COPD[b] patients	City-average		NS	NS	Near a coal-power plant
Vedal, 1987	Children with respiratory symptoms	City-average	NS		NS	Near a coal-power plant
Cleen-Ass, 1991	General	City-average with individual weight	+		NS	
Schwartz, 1991	Nurses	Sampler near the school	+			
Braun-Fahrlander, 1992	Children	Passive sampler outside each house and city-average		+		
Roemer, 1993	Children with respiratory symptoms	City-average	NS		NS	Air pollution episodes
Moseholm, 1993	Asthmatics	City-average			+	

[a] + significant association; NS, nonsignificant association.
[b] Chronic obstructive pulmonary disease.

ple, in a study of the relation between mortality and air pollution in Los Angeles using data for a large period (1970–1979), the authors observed a relationship between total or cardiovascular mortality and NO_2, but they were not able to disentangle the effects caused by NO_2 from those caused by the rest of pollutants generated by motor vehicles (Kinney and Özkaynak, 1991).

In conclusion, studies of outdoor exposures have failed to show a consistent short-term effect of outdoor NO_2 on respiratory disease.

Chronic effects of outdoor air

Differences between acute and chronic effects are not clearly defined. The link between measures of acute transient end points (e.g., symptoms, short-term changes in lung function) and the chronic effects (e.g., permanent changes in lung function) has not been established. Acute changes in pulmonary function may signal chronic underlying damage in the small airways. Similarly, the relative importance of acute exposures (peaks) and cumulative exposures (averages) has not been established for air pollutants. It has been suggested that subjects repeatedly exposed may adapt to the exposure and attenuate the responses (Ostro, 1993). Nevertheless, it is useful to consider separately studies on the long-term effects of cumulative exposure.

Chronic effects of cumulative exposures are inherently difficult to measure because they need long-term studies. However, most studies have been cross-sectional ecologic studies comparing disease rates in subjects from geographical areas with different levels of exposures, assuming that the current exposure reflects differences in the cumulative exposure. Therefore, this type of study uses an imprecise estimate of past exposure (Shy et al., 1970; Pearlman et al., 1971; Cohen et al., 1972; Euler et al., 1988).

A study of nonsmokers by Detels and colleagues (Detels et al., 1981), is an exception because of its longitudinal design. During 5 to 6 years of follow-up, these authors found a higher reduction of pulmonary function among those living in the high-pollution area (Detels 91). The follow-up design allowed data on past exposure and control for migration. However, the number of subjects lost during the follow-up was very high, and as in the other studies the air pollution effects could not be attributed to a single pollutant.

Overall, studies of the chronic effects of living in areas with higher NO_2 pollution suggest a respiratory effect; however the inability to single out the responsible agent precludes a direct link with NO_2.

Conclusions

Epidemiologic studies of indoor NO_2 suggest some increase in respiratory diseases in normal children, but results of these studies are not consistent, and exposure has not been well defined in many. Similarly, outdoor studies did not find consistent effects on respiratory diseases or pulmonary function of normal people or asthmatics. Positive studies of outdoor air have often been unable to separate the effects of NO_2 from those of other pollutants. Furthermore, clinical studies have provided conflicting results when only NO_2 was used, although in general bronchial responsiveness in asthmatics was produced at low levels and in normal population at high levels. Recent laboratory studies on the effects of combined exposures to allergens and NO_2 suggests that NO_2 may act as an effect modifier, particularly in subjects with allergic asthma. This complex casual role should be considered in the forthcoming epidemiologic studies.

References

Aris RM, Christian D, Hearne PQ, Finkbeiner WE, Balmes JR. 1993 Ozone-induced airway inflammation in human subjects as determined by airway lavage and biopsy. Am Rev Respir Dis 148:1363–1372.

Avol EL, Linn Ws, Peng RC, Valencia G, Little D, Hackney JD. 1988. Laboratory study in asthmatic volunteers exposed to nitrogen dioxide and to ambient air pollution. Am Ind Hyg Assoc J; 49:143–149.

Bauer MA, Utell MJ, Morrow PE, Speers DM, Gibb FR. 1986. Inhalation of 0.3 ppm nitrogen dioxide potentiates exercise-induced bronchospasm in asthmatics. Am Rev Respir Dis 134:1203–1208.

Braun-Fahrlander C, Ackerman-Lievrich U, Scwartz J, Gnehm HP, Rutishauser M, Wanner HU. 1992. Air pollution and respiratory symptoms in preschool children. Am Rev Respir Dis 145:42–47.

Brought on GFJ. 1993. Air quality in the UK: a summary of results from instrumental monitoring networks in 1991–92. Warren Springs laboratory, report LR 941. Stevenage: WSL.

Bylin G. 1993. Controlled studies on humans. Scand J Environ Health 19, 2:37–43.

Clench Aas J, Larssen S, Bartonova A, Aarnes MJ, Myhre K, Christensen CC, et al. 1991. The health effects of traffic pollution as measured in the Vˆalerenga Area of Oslo. Lilleström: Norwegian Institute for Air Research (NILU 7/91).

Cohen CA, Hudson AR, Clausen JL, Kuelson JH. 1972. Respiratory symptoms, spirometry, and oxidant air pollution in non-smoking adults. Am Rev Respir Dis 105:251–261.

Detels R, Tashkin DP, Sayre JW, Rokaw SN, Massey FJ Jr, Coulson AH, et al. 1991. The UCLA population studies of CORD: X. A cohort study of changes in respiratory function associated with chronic exposure to SO_x, NO_x and hydrocarbons. Am J Public Health 81:350–359.

Detels R, Sayre JW, Coulson AH, Rokaw SN, Massey FJ Jr, Tashkin DP, et al. 1981. The UCLA population studies of chronic obstructive respiratory disease: IV. Respiratory effect of long-term exposure to photochemical oxidants, nitrogen dioxide, and sulfates on current and never smokers. Am Rev Respir Dis 124:673–680.

Devalia JL, Sapsford RJ, Cundell DR, Rusznak C, Campbell AM, Davies RJ. 1993. Human bronchial epithelial cell dysfunction following in vitro exposure to nitrogen dioxide. Eur Respir J 6:1308–1316.

Devalia JL, Rusznack C, Herdman MJ, Trigg CJ, Tarraf H, Davies RJ. 1994. Effect of nitrogen dioxide and sulphur dioxide on airway response of mild asthmatic patients to allergen inhalation. Lancet 334:1688–1671.

Environmental Protection Agency. 1991. National air quality and emissions trends report, 1990. Research Triangle Park, N.C.: Environmental Protection Agency. (Publication no. EPA-450/4-91-023).

Euler GL, Abbey DE, Hodgkin JE, Magie AR. 1988. Chronic obstructive pulmonary disease symptom effects of long-term cumulative exposure to ambient levels of total oxidants and nitrogen dioxide in California Seventh-Day Adventist residents. Arch Environ Health 43:279–285.

Folinsbee LJ. 1992. Does nitrogen dioxide exposure increase airways responsiveness? Toxicol Ind Health 8:273–283.

Goings SAJ, Kulle TJ, Bascom R, Sauder LR, Green DJ, Hebel JR, Clements ML. 1989. Effect of nitrogen dioxide exposure on susceptibility to influenza A virus infection in healthy adults. Am Rev Respir Dis 139:1075–1081.

Goldstein E, Goldstein F, Peek NF, Parks NJ. 1980. Absorption and transport of nitrogen oxides. In: Lee SD ed. Nitrogen Oxides and Their Effects on Health. Ann Arbor Science, Ann Arbor, MI; pp. 143–160.

Harlos DP, Marbury M, Samet J, Spengler JD. 1987. Relating indoor NO_2 levels to infant personal exposures. Atmos Environ 21:369–376.

Hasselblad V, Eddy DM, Kotchmar DJ. 1992. Synthesis of environmental evidence: nitrogen dioxide epidemiology studies. J Air Waste Manag Assoc 42:662–671.

Hazucha MJ, Ginsberg JF, McDonnel WF, Haak ED, Pimmel RL, Salaam SA, et al. 1983. Effects of 0.1 ppm nitrogen dioxide on airways of normal and asthmatic subjects. J Appl Physiol Respir 54: 730–739.

Hazucha MJ, Bates DV, Bromberg PA. 1989. Mechanisms of action of ozone on the human lung. J Appl Physiol 67:1535–1541.

Katsouyanni K, Zmirou D, Spix C, Sunyer J, Shoutten JP, Ponka A, et al. 1995. Short-term effects of air pollution on health: a european approach using epidemiologic time series data. The aphea project: background, objectives, design. Eur Respi J 8:1030–1038.

Kleinman MT, Bailey RM, Linn WS, Anderson KR, Whynot JD, Shamoo DA, et al.

1983. Effects of 0.2 ppm nitrogen dioxide on pulmonary function and response to bronchoprovocation in asthmatics. Am Rev Respir Dis 12:815–826.

Kinney PL, Özkaynak H. 1991. Associations of daily mortality and air pollution in Los Angeles county. Environ Res 54:99–120.

Koo LC, Ho JH-C, Ho C-Y, Matsuki H, Shimizu H, Mori T, et al. 1990. Personal exposure to nitrogen dioxide and its association with respiratory illness in Hong Kong. Am Rev Respir Dis 141:1119–1126.

Linn WS, Solomon JC, Trim SC, Spier CE, Shamoo DA, Venet TG, Avol EL, Hackney JD. 1985. Effects of exposure to 4 ppm nitrogen dioxide in healthy and asthmatic volunteers. Arch Environ Health 40:234–238.

Love GJ, Lan S-P, Shy CM, Riggan WB. 1930. Acute respiratory illness in families exposed to nitrogen dioxide ambient air pollution in Chattanooga, Tennessee. Arch Environ Health; 37:75–80.

Martinez FD, Wright AL, Taussing LM, et al. 1995. Asthma and wheezing in the first six years of life. N Engl J Med 332:133–138.

Melia RJW, Florey C du V, Altman DG, Swan AV. 1977. Association between gas cooking and respiratory disease in children. BMJ 2:149–152.

Melia RJW, Florey C du V, Chinn S. 1979. The relation between respiratory illness in primary schoolchildren and the use of gas for cooking: I. Results from a national survey. Int J Epidemiol 8:333–338.

Melia RJW, Florey C du V, Morris RW, Goldstein BD, John HH, Clark D, Craighead IB, Mackinlay JC. 1982. Childhood respiratory illness and the home environment: II. Association between respiratory illness and nitrogen dioxide, temperature and relative humidity. Int J Epidemiol 11:164–169.

Melia RJW, Florey C du V, Sittampalam Y, Watkins C. 1983. The relation between respiratory illness in infants and gas cooking in the US: a preliminary report. In: Proceedings of the 6th Congress in Air Quality. Paris: International Union of Air Pollution Prevention Associations.

Mohensin V. 1987. Airway responses to nitrogen dioxide in asthmatic subjects. J Toxicol and Environ Health 22:371–380.

Molfino NA, Wright SC, Katz I, et al. 1991. Effect of low concentrations of ozone on inhaled allergen responses in asthmatic subjects. Lancet 338:199–203.

Moseholm L, Taudorf E, Frosing A. 1993. Pulmonary function changes in asthmatics associated with low-level SO_2 and NO_2 air pollution, weather, and medicine intake. Allergy 48:334–344.

National Research Council. 1976. Subcommittee on Nitrogen Oxides, Committee on Medical and Biological Effects of Environmental Pollutants. Nitrogen Oxides. National Academy Press, Washington, DC.

Neas LM, Dockery DW, Ware JH, Spengler JD, Speizer FE, Ferris BG Jr. 1991. Association of indoor nitrogen dioxide with respiratory symptoms and pulmonary function in children. Am J Epidemiol 134:204–219.

Ogston SA, Florey C du V, Walker CHM. 1985. The Tayside infant morbidity and mortality study: effect on health of using gas for cooking. BMJ 290:957–960.

Orehek J, Massari JP, Gayrard P, Grimaud C, Charpin J. 1976. Effect of short-term, low-level nitrogen exposure on bronchial sensitivity of asthmatic patients. J Clin Invest 57:301–307.

Ostro B. 1993. Examining acute health outcomes due to ozone exposure and their subsequent relationship to chronic disease outcomes. Environ Health Perspect 101:213–216.

Ozkaynak H, Ryan PB, Spengler JD, Letz R. 1984. Presented at the Air Pollution Control Association and American Society for Quality Control Speciality Conference on: Quality Assurance in Air Pollution Measurements, Boulder, Colorado.

Pearlman ME, Finklea JF, Creason JP, Shy CP, Young MM, Horton RJM. 1971. Nitrogen dioxide and lower respiratory illness. Pediatrics 47:391–398.

Pennington JE. 1988 Effects of automotive emissions on susceptibility to respiratory infections. In: Watson AY, Bates PR, Kennedy D, eds. Air Pollution, and Public Health. Washington, National Academy Press; 499–518.

Pershagen G, Hrubec Z, Lorich U, Ronnqvist P. 1984. Acute respiratory symptoms in patients with chronic obstructive pulmonary disease and in other subjects living near a coal-fired plant. Arch Environ Health 39:27–33.

Pershagen G, Norberg S. 1993. Epidemiological studies. Scand J Environ Health 19, 2:57–69.

Ponka A. 1991. Asthma and low level air pollution in Helsinki. Arch Environ Health 46:262–270.

Rossi OV, Kimula VL. 1993. Association of severe asthma attacks with weather, pollen and air pollution. Thorax 48:244–248.

Roemer W, Hoek G, Brunekreef B. 1993. Effect of ambient winter air pollution on respiratory health of children with chronic respiratory symptoms. Am Rev Respir Dis 147:118–124.

Rutishauser M, Ackerman U, Braun CH, Gnehm HP, Wanner HU. 1990. Significant association between outdoor NO_2 and respiratory symptoms in preschool children. Lung 168 (suppl): 347–352.

Samet JM, Tager IB, Speizer FE. 1983. The relationship between respiratory illness in childhood and chronic airflow obstruction in adulthood. Am Rev Respir Dis 127:508–523.

Samet JM, Utell MJ. 1990. The risk of nitrogen dioxide: What have we learned from epidemiological and clinical studies? Toxicol Ind Health 6:247–262.

Samet JM, Cushing AH, Lambert WE, Hunt WC, McLarten LC, You SA, et al. 1993. Comparability of parent-reported respiratory illnesses to clinical diagnoses. Am Rev Respir Dis 148:441–446.

Schwartz J, Spix C, Wichman HE, Malin E. 1991. Air pollution and acute respiratory illness in five German communities. Environ Res 56:1–4.

Schwarz J, Zeger S. 1990. Passive smoking, air pollution, and acute respiratory symptoms in a diary study of student nurses. Am Rev Respir Dis 141:62–67.

Shy CM, Creason JP, Pearlman ME, McClain KE, Benson FB, Young MM. 1970. The Chattanooga school children study: effects of community exposure to nitrogen dioxide. J Air Pollut Control Assoc 20:539–545.

Speizer FE, Ferris B Jr, Bishop YMM, Spengler J. 1980. Respiratory disease rates and pulmonary function in children associated with NO_2 exposure. Am Rev Respir Dis 121:3–10.

Spengler JD, Duffy CP, Letz R, Tibbitts TW, Ferris BG Jr. 1983. Nitrogen dioxide inside and outside 137 homes and implications for ambient air quality standards and health effects research. Environ Sci Technol 17:164–168.

Sunyer J, Anto JM, Murillo C, Saez M. 1991. Air pollution and emergency room admissions from chronic obstructive pulmonary diseases. Am J Epidemiol 134:277–286.

Tunnicliffe WS, Burge PS, Ayres JG. 1994. Effect of domestic concentrations of nitrogen dioxide on airway responses to inhaled allergen in asthmatic patients. Lancet 344:1733–1736.

Vedal S, Schenker MB, Muñoz A, Samet JM, Batterman S, Speizer FE. 1987. Daily air pollution effects on children's respiratory symptoms and peak expiratory flow. Am J Public Health 77:694–698.

Walker AM, Blettner M. 1985. Comparing imperfect measures of exposure. Am J Epidemiol 121:783–790.

Ware JH, Dockery DW, Spiro A III, Speizer FE, Ferris BG Jr. 1984. Passive smoking, gas, cooking and respiratory health of children living in six cities. Am Rev Respir Dis 129:366–374.

Outdoor Air III: 8

Ozone

VICTOR HUGO BORJA-ABURTO

DANA LOOMIS

OZONE (O_3) in the stratosphere protects human health, but at low levels in the troposphere it is a cause for concern. Tropospheric ozone, the subject of this chapter, is the main component of urban smog. Ozone is produced largely through the combination of exhaust from automobiles and sunlight. Levels have been steady or increasing over time. The number of cars has increased but pollution controls on cars have also been adopted. Levels are higher in the summer when visible smog can cause respiratory irritation.

Both experimental and epidemiologic studies have shown short-term reversible decreases in lung function resulting from ozone in normal subjects. These decreases last from hours to days. Several studies have also shown an increase in hospital admissions for respiratory disease when ozone levels are high. Furthermore, some time-series studies of mortality demonstrate increases in death rates that correlate with ozone levels—although these increases are usually also correlated with other pollutants, and in some cases disappear when other pollutants are taken into account.

Despite this evidence of acute effects, it is unknown whether ozone has any long-term effect on chronic respiratory disease. This remains the major epidemiologic question about ozone. There have been few studies of chronic exposure and chronic respiratory health effects. A prospective study of populations with different levels of ozone exposure, controlled for major confounders and including good measurement of other air pollutants, will be required. The inclusion of areas in which levels of other pollutants are low, if possible, would be an advantage.

Asthmatics are a susceptible population. However, experimental stud-

184

ies have not shown short-term effects of ozone on asthmatics. On the other hand, a number of epidemiologic studies have documented exacerbation of symptoms in asthmatics exposed to ozone, and increases in hospital admissions for asthma in urban populations when ozone levels are high. It is possible that this discrepancy between experimental data and epidemiologic data is due to a synergistic effect of ozone and other air pollutants. Again, an issue to be resolved is whether chronic exposure to ozone might increase the incidence of asthma.

Ozone is an important outdoor air pollutant to which large numbers of people are exposed worldwide. Resolution of its effect on respiratory disease should be a high priority.

In the earth's stratosphere, a naturally occurring layer of ozone protects us against the harmful effects of ultraviolet light. In contrast, ambient ozone in the troposphere is a widespread artificial pollutant that has been hard to control. As an air pollutant, ozone is one member of a family of secondary oxidants produced from primary air contaminants by photochemical reactions in the atmosphere.

Tropospheric ozone pollution comes from a complex series of chemical reactions involving sunlight and volatile organic compounds derived largely from incomplete combustion of fuel in motor vehicles. The initial reaction is the photolysis (via sunlight) of nitrogen dioxide, resulting in the production of nitric oxide (NO) and atomic oxygen (O). The latter combines with O_2 to yield ozone, O_3. Concurrent photodissociation of organic compounds results in the production of various free radicals, which in turn can combine with O_3. The levels of ozone and oxidized hydrocarbons resulting from these reactions depend on the mix of primary pollutants, their chemical characteristics, and on meteorologic conditions. The visible components of this oxidant mix are the principal components of urban smog.

Because of the key role of sunlight in its formation, the level of ozone is highly variable over the course of a day, peaking in the afternoon and falling close to zero at night. In addition, ozone is highly reactive, and levels indoors are typically much lower than outdoors, with the ratio depending upon ventilation. Despite the introduction of the catalytic converter, which reduced hydrocarbon emissions per vehicle-mile traveled, ozone levels have remained fairly stable since the mid-seventies. This may be because of increasing numbers of automobiles and driving distances worldwide. High levels of ozone are especially characteristic of areas with sunny, dry, warm climates and large numbers of automobiles, such as Los Angeles and Mexico City. As with other secondary pollutants formed in atmospheric reactions, the highest concentrations of ozone often occur away from the sources of their precursors, depending on speed and wind direction.

The initial National Ambient Air Quality Standard (NAAQS) for the United States was set in 1971 at 0.80 parts per million (ppm) of total oxidants, which include ozone and other oxidation products such as peroxyacyl nitrate and aldehydes. Based on clinical studies, the standard was revised in 1979 to a 1-hour maximum of 0.12 ppm of O_3, not to be exceeded more than one day per year. In 1988, a year with a particularly hot summer, 112 million people in the United States lived in areas where the standard was not attained (Koenig, 1995). Ambient ozone in urban areas is a surrogate for total photochemical smog, so any health effects of ambient ozone could also be the result of exposures to other photochemical oxidants.

Health Effects of Ozone

In discussing the health effects of air pollution, it is useful to distinguish long-term exposures and chronic health outcomes from short-term exposures and acute health effects. These distinctions are particularly important for ozone because most of the available information pertains to short-term exposures and acute effects, but the major uncertainties and the most challenging questions for research and public health center on the significance of these observations over longer periods of time. Nevertheless, it is equally important to remember that there are generally no clear, natural boundaries between acute and chronic or long and short term. As a result, such attempts at classification are always somewhat arbitrary and may not be equally useful in all cases.

This chapter emphasizes findings from observational epidemiologic studies. However, knowledge of the diverse health effects of ozone is based on toxicologic experiments with animals and controlled experimental studies of humans, in addition to epidemiologic research. Each type of research offers advantages and disadvantages.

Epidemiologic studies are based on real exposures and record health effects in natural human populations. They can be used to study the full range of exposures and health outcomes over short or long intervals of time. However, they are often limited by the ability to control for confounding factors, such as socioeconomic conditions, occupational exposures, and tobacco smoke. Epidemiologic studies can also entail considerable challenges in characterizing the complex mixture of human exposures in urban environments, often a serious problem because of limitations in the quality and quantity of the data that can be obtained at reasonable cost.

In contrast, experiments with animals, typically rodents, allow precise quantification of exposure duration and concentration. They also facilitate accurate identification of a wide variety of end points, as well as the study of extreme exposures, even at lethal levels. However, the interpretation of these studies is hampered by the difficulty of extrapolating results from animal models to humans. Animal experiments are amenable to the study of both acute and chronic effects of pollutants. However, because the lifespan of most experimental species is short in comparison to that of humans, there are additional uncertainties concerning the comparability of exposures and health outcomes over the long term.

Human clinical studies in laboratory settings combine some advantages of the other two types of investigation. They can be used to characterize dose-response relationships in small groups of subjects under controlled conditions in exposure chambers for relatively short periods of time. Some susceptible populations, such as people with asthma, can be studied. However, high concentrations and irreversible effects cannot be studied. In addition, the experimental conditions may be rigorously controlled but unrealistic. The experimental subjects are often volunteers, who may not be representative of the exposed population. Finally, the complex conditions of real exposures can be very difficult to reproduce in the laboratory.

Thus, observational epidemiology provides an appropriate approach to determining the health effects of exposure to ozone air pollution, but leaves important uncertainties that are not easily resolved by other types of research.

Acute Effects and Short-term Exposures
Respiratory changes

Ozone exposure has been associated with an array of transient adverse respiratory effects in healthy people, as well as in people with preexisting respiratory disease such as asthma, and with increased frequency of hospital and emergency room visits. Thorough reviews have been conducted by Lippman (1993) and Lipfert and Hammerstrom (1992). We will provide only a brief overview of the extensive literature concerning these effects.

Assessments of lung function among people exposed to ozone in chamber experiments have demonstrated transient, apparently reversible effects after short-term exposure of normal subjects during exercise lasting from minutes to a few hours (Fouke et al., 1988; Folisbee et al., 1988;

McDonnell, et al., 1991). The inhalation of ozone causes concentration-dependent decreases in average lung volume and flow resistance (Hazucha, 1987; Higgins et al., 1990), epithelial permeability, and reactivity to bronchoactive challenges (Becket, 1988; Seltzer, 1986). Such effects can be observed within the first hours after the start of the exposure and may persist for many hours or days after the exposure ceases (Lipmann, 1989b).

Changes in lung function appear to be caused by involuntary inhibition of inspiration (Hazucha et al., 1989) mediated by the activation of C fibers in the large airways, rather than to changes in respiratory mechanical properties. Vagal afferent stimulation may be responsible for the pattern of decreased tidal volume and increased respiratory rate. Because of its physical properties and high reactivity and relative insolubility, ozone when inhaled irritates the respiratory tract, from the nose to the alveoli. Nasal inflammation in response to ozone exposure has been assessed by nasal lavage, with quantification of inflammatory cells in the fluid returned (Calderón-Garcidueñas et al., 1994). Acute ozone exposure also induces inflammatory responses in the upper and lower airway. Bronchoalveolar lavage studies have shown an eightfold increase in polymorphonuclear leukocytes (PMN) accompanied by increased recovery of inflammatory mediators (Horstman et al., 1990; Devlin, et al., 1991). This inflammatory response to single exposures occurs approximately 6 hours after exposure and does not correlate closely with symptoms or changes in spirometric response. However, the clinical and long-term importance of these transient effects remains uncertain.

Given the findings of the responses of healthy subjects to controlled exposures to ozone, one would expect asthmatics to be particularly sensitive to ozone. One on hand, most controlled-exposure studies have failed to document greater response for asthmatics (Kagawa, 1984; Shepard et al., 1983; Balmes, 1993; Koening et al., 1987; Balmes et al., 1995). On the other hand, several epidemiologic studies have demonstrated exacerbation of asthma in panel studies (Whittemore and Korn, 1980; Holguin et al., 1985) and in time series of hospital admissions or emergency room visits for asthma (Cody et al., 1992; Romieu et al., 1995). This discrepancy in identifying asthmatics as a sensitive population could be the result of the exclusion of severe asthmatics in the controlled exposure studies, or the failure to simulate the complex mix of air pollutants to which such individuals may be exposed. However, it could also be argued that the effects in the epidemiologic studies are due to another pollutant in smog rather than ozone. Another reason for discrepancy is the study of different end points. Most controlled studies assess functional responsiveness; epidemiologic studies evaluate the frequency of asthma attacks following ozone exposure. Probably lung function is not the most relevant end point to monitor. In a controlled exposure study, Balmes et al. (1995) compared pulmonary functional responses of asthmatic subjects to those of healthy subjects. Although both groups showed significant ozone-induced changes in airway resistance and forced expiratory volume in 1 second (FEV_1), there were no significant differences between asthmatics and non-asthmatics. In contrast, the inflammatory response, as measured by the increase in percent neutrophils in bronchoalvealar lavage, was more intense for people with asthma.

Acute exposure to ozone results in specific changes in lung function that are very reproducible over time in an individual. However, there is high inter-individual variability in response to ozone exposure. There is also inconclusive evidence of greater functional responsiveness in older adults (Drechsler-Parks et al., 1987; Reisenau et al., 1988; Koenig et al., 1987; Linn et al., 1983) and patients with chronic obstructive pulmonary disease (Linn et al., 1983; Solic et al., 1982).

Transient decrements in lung function of exercising schoolchildren have been observed under ambient natural conditions (Braun-Fahrlander et al., 1994; Castillejos et al., 1992; Higgins et al., 1990) and in panel studies of camp settings during summer vacations (Krzyanowski et al., 1993). Mean decrements in lung function associated with outdoor exercise among children are larger than those reported for adults exposed to ozone in purified air chambers. A recent meta-analysis by Kinney et al. (1960) found a decline of FEV_1 of 0.5 mL/ppb O_3. Other constituents of the ambient mixture could be potentiating the effect of ozone.

Symptoms

Epidemiologic studies have also provided evidence of respiratory and other symptoms of ozone and related photochemical oxidants at exposures as low as 0.10 ppm/hour. The symptoms that have been observed include eye, nose, and throat irritation; cough; increased mucus production; chest tightness; substernal pain; lassitude; malaise; and nausea (Hammer et al., 1974). Lower respiratory tract symptoms have been observed at low levels of ozone in adults (Ostro et al., 1993), and in a nonsmoking population (Abbey et al., 1993). Associations were observed not only with the occurrence of respiratory symptoms, but also with the duration of coughing, phlegm, and sore throat (Shwartz, 1992). The threshold for symptoms is lowered by exercise and heat, which increases the inspired dose (Folinsbee et al., 1984; McDonnell et al., 1983).

Infections

Both in vivo and in vitro studies in animals have demonstrated that ozone can affect the ability of the immune system to defend against infection (Miller et al., 1978; Goldstein, 1971; Ehrlich, 1980). The major limitation of these data is that they require uncertain interspecies extrapolation in order to estimate the possible effects of ozone on infectivity in humans.

Hospital admissions

The frequency of admissions to hospital has been used as a measure of morbidity in a number of epidemiologic studies of air pollution. Elevated levels of ambient ozone have been associated with increased frequency of hospital and emergency department visits in analysis of time series in Ontario, Canada (Bates and Sizto, 1987; Bates and Sizto, 1983; Lipfert et al., 1992; Burnett et al., 1994; Thurston et al., 1994), hospital visits for asthma in New Jersey and Mexico City (Cody et al., 1992; Romieu et al., 1995) hospital admissions for respiratory causes in New York (Thurston et al., 1992). Admissions for pneumonia in St. Paul, Minnesota (Schwartz, 1994a) and Birmingham, Alabama (Schwartz, 1994b) also suggest that high levels of atmospheric ozone lead people to seek medical attention with greater frequency. Additionally, high levels of ozone have been associated with school absenteeism because of respiratory disease among children in Mexico (Romieu et al., 1992).

Chronic Health Outcomes and Long-term Exposures

While much is known about some of the transient health effects following short-term exposures to ozone, there has been controversy regarding their ultimate significance for health. In addition, knowledge about the effects of long-term exposures and health end points with a chronic time course is much less complete.

The chronic effects of exposure to ozone may include alterations in lung function or structure (Schwartz, 1989). Such effects may result from cumulative damage due to chronic or repeated, intermittent exposure. Epidemiologic studies are essentially the only method available for studying exposures and health outcomes over extended time periods. However, such research is particularly challenging. Limitations in the assessment of long-term exposures to ozone are notably important in this area of investigation. Short term exposure can be readily evaluated from fixed stations and recently developed personal monitors, but long-term and intermittent exposure databases are limited.

Mortality is the most serious outcome that has been associated with ozone in epidemiologic studies. However, the study of mortality is one situation in which the distinction between acute and chronic health end points is somewhat less useful. We have rather arbitrarily placed mortality studies under the heading of research into chronic effects because death is irreversible, but the relationship to air pollution and mortality can be considered on either a chronic or an acute time scale.

Existing epidemiologic studies focus on short-term relationships between mortality and ozone exposures. Two reports have indicated positive associations between daily changes in mortality and ozone levels in different cities. In a 10-year study of records from Los Angeles County, California, total non-injury mortality and cardiovascular mortality were associated on a daily basis with ozone lagged by one day, controlling for temperature and nitrogen dioxide; annual regressions demonstrated the consistency of the results over time (Kinney and Ozkaynak, 1991). The analysis was later extended to New York City, where the ozone–mortality association was stronger than in Los Angeles, perhaps reflecting an influence of other unmeasured pollutants (Kinney and Ozkaynak, 1992). However, another study by Dockery and others (1992) did not find an effect on mortality at low levels of ozone (mean ozone concentration=22 ppb) in St. Louis and Tennessee. A study of daily mortality in Mexico City in 1990–1992 suggested a positive relationship with ambient ozone concentration when other air pollutants were not considered (Loomis et al., 1996). Ozone concentrations were above the U.S. NAAQS on most days in this study, and the association with mortality was strongest for lags of 0–2 days and among the elderly. However, the association was eliminated by controlling for particulate pollutants. In São Paolo, daily respiratory mortality among infants was not associated with ozone, but it was associated with nitrogen oxides when all pollutants were simultaneously included in a model (Saldiva et al., 1994).

The suggestive but inconsistent results of these mortality studies suggest that there may be interdependence between ozone and other pollutants in both the occurrence of exposure and the health effects they produce.

Case Study: Epidemiologic Study of Children in Summer Camp

The study of acute effects of ambient ozone exposures on respiratory function can be exemplified by a field study of healthy children undertaken by Spektor et al. (1991) at the Fairview Lake YMCA summer camp in northwestern New Jersey. This is part of a series of studies that have been performed in areas of the United States periodically exposed to hazy summer air masses enriched in secondary pollutants (Lioy et al., 1985; Lippmann et al., 1983; Spektor et al., 1988a; Spektor et al., 1988b). Typically, daily measurements of lung function for each child are regressed on ozone levels measured by fixed monitors outdoors. These studies exploit a "natural experiment" of sorts, the rationale being that children attending summer camp are involved in outdoor exercise and therefore have elevated potential to experience ambient pollution and its effects.

Forty-six children (13 girls and 33 boys) 8 to 14 years of age with no history of lung disease or atopy participated in the 1991 study by Spektor and colleagues. The investigators improved on previous studies by measuring the lung function of each child twice each day. This allowed examination of the change in function in relation to acute ozone exposure, as well as the use of morning measurements to examine whether baseline shifts were occurring in relation to cumulative exposure. Children were followed for the entire time they spent in the summer camp, with follow-up time ranging from 7 days to 4 weeks. Lung function measurements were performed during breaks between programmed activities, once before 11:00 A.M, and a second time between 4 and 7:30 P.M, with a portable spirometer inside a mobile laboratory.

Measurements of ambient atmospheric conditions included temperature, humidity, concentrations of ozone, and aerosol acidity. Of the 30 days of ozone measurements, only 5 exceeded the current NAAQS of 120 ppb. On 7 days, the acid aerosols concentrations were higher than 10 $\mu g/m^3$.

Table 8-1 shows selected results of regression analyses of lung function measures on different indices of ozone exposure. These are average slopes for all 46 children after separate linear regressions were calculated for each child. Regressions of morning baseline function on the prior day's exposure provide evidence that ambient ozone at relatively low levels is associated with a statistically significant decrement in lung function, which persists into the following day. The regression of changes in lung function parameters, including ΔFVC, ΔFEV_1, $\Delta PEFR$, ΔFEF_{25-75}, and $\Delta FEV_1/FVC$, between morning and afternoon measurements allowed evaluation of the acute effect controlling for daily fluctuations in baseline function. The regression of afternoon lung function on average ozone exposures on the same day or on the ozone concentration in the hour preceding generally had mean values more strongly negative than those based on the daily change in function.

The magnitude of these functional changes observed in natural set-

Table 8-1. Average regression slopes (± standard error) for respiratory function indices vs ambient ozone concentration, field study by Spektor et al. (1991) at Fairview Lake, NJ, YMCA camp, summer of 1988

Time of Day for Measurement	Ozone Average Period	Children (n)	FVC (mL/ ppb O₃)	FEV (mL/ ppb)	PEFR (mL/ sec/ppb)	FEF 25%-75% (mL/sec/ppb)	FEV₁/FVC (%/ ppb)
PM	Previous hour	46	−1.53 ± 0.38	−1.60 ± 0.30	−5.38 ± 0.92	−2.13 ± 0.59	−0.019 ± 0.004
PM	Average for day	46	−1.27 ± 0.86	−1.65 ± 0.73	−1.90 ± 1.07	−2.30 ± 0.85	−0.010 ± 0.010
PM	1 hour maximum	46	−2.38 ± 0.32	−2.29 ± 0.26	−3.00 ± 0.62	−2.56 ± 0.26	−0.018 ± 0.004
PM-AM	Previous hour	46	−1.56 ± 0.27	−1.18 ± 0.27	−5.89 ± 1.12	−1.18 ± 0.57	−0.034 ± 0.006
PM-AM	Between AM and PM	46	−0.80 ± 0.10	−0.63 ± 0.09	−3.24 ± 0.48	−1.17 ± 0.17	−0.015 ± 0.002
PM-AM	1 hour maximum	46	−0.93 ± 0.15	−0.82 ± 0.12	−3.22 ± 0.49	−1.07 ± 0.28	−0.18 ± 0.003
AM	Previous day average	35	−0.38 ± 0.11	−0.43 ± 0.08	−1.20 ± 0.28	−0.61 ± 0.11	−0.023 ± 0.003
AM	Previous day 1 hour maximum	35	−0.49 ± 0.14	−0.50 ± 0.12	−1.32 ± 0.35	−0.76 ± 0.17	−0.025 ± 0.007

FVC = forced vital capacity; FEV = forced expiratory volume; PEFR = peak expiratory flow rate.
FEF 25%-75% = forced expiratory flow, mid-expiratory

tings is larger than that observed among people receiving controlled exposures in chambers. The authors attribute these discrepancies to three factors: (1) longer exposures; (2) potentiation by other aspects of ambient exposure; (3) persistence of effects from prior day's exposures; and (4) persistence of a transient response associated with the daily peak exposure.

These interpretations highlight the principal challenges that attend epidemiologic research concerning the effects of ambient ozone. Although much is known about the transient, non-serious effects of ozone from experimental studies, the complex environments in which real human populations live can be difficult to reconcile with the simpler, controlled conditions of the laboratory. Effects observed in natural settings may be due to exposures that are present but unmeasured, as well as to combined effects that are not easily disentangled with existing methodology.

In addition, the results of this epidemiologic study suggest persistent effects from ozone exposure in the recent past. Although no direct link has been demonstrated with more serious health outcomes, the observation of persistent, mild effects after several days' exposure does make the notion that long-term exposures may produce chronic or irreversible effects more plausible.

Conclusions

Ozone is a widespread air pollutant whose concentration has been increasing in much of the world. In this respect, it contrasts with other historically important pollutants, such as particulates, which have declined. Short-term exposures to ozone are known from experimental and epidemiologic studies to have a variety of acute, reversible health effects, including respiratory irritation, symptoms of respiratory ill health, and reduced lung function. Some epidemiologic studies also indicate that short-term increases in ozone concentration lead to higher rates of hospital admission for respiratory and other diseases.

Whether ozone exposures in the short or long term also have irreversible or serious health effects has been more difficult to determine. The investigation of protracted exposures and serious outcomes requires epidemiologic, rather than laboratory, methods. Epidemiologic studies in the United States and Latin America have been inconclusive as to whether day-to-day changes in ambient ozone level and mortality are related. However, these studies do suggest that exposures to ozone, their health effects, or both may be intertwined with other agents. Interdependence between exposures to ozone and other pollutants was also suggested in the study of lung function among children in summer camp that we considered as an example.

The complexity and variability of the mixtures in which pollutants co-exist in urban environments makes isolating the specific, biologically active agents responsible for empirical associations between health end points and measured pollutant levels a challenging task. Ozone indexes exposure to photochemical oxidants, a mixture whose components share common sources, and it may also be a marker for exposure to acid aerosols, which have been hypothesized as the causal agent in the association of ozone with increments in hospitalization and mortality (Thurston et al., 1994). Further challenges attend the interpretation of the relative importance of different pollutants based on empirical exposure–disease relationships. Comparing risk coefficients for different pollution indices is problematic when they differ in scale and quality of measurement (Ito, 1993).

The summer camp study and several others also suggest reversible health effects persisting for several days. Studies of chronic health conditions, such as the development of chronic respiratory conditions, would help to resolve key uncertainties about the importance of ozone exposures by defining the "middle ground" between the known transient effects of ozone and the suggestive results of a few studies of ozone and more serious health outcomes, including mortality. Likewise, follow-up studies of serious health outcomes in relation to long-term exposures may help to define the consequences of living in environments with chronically elevated ozone levels, like those that exist in numerous cities. Neither type of study has not been conducted to date, however.

The significant uncertainties concerning the health effects of ozone are reason for concern. With large populations already exposed throughout the world and ambient levels stable or increasing, even a modest increase in the occurrence of adverse health effects could have a large impact in terms of the overall burden of illness. Further epidemiologic research is clearly needed, particularly on the long-term, serious consequences of exposure to ozone. The extent to which such effects derive from ozone alone is also a question of some interest, but the scientific validity of attempting to isolate the effect of a single pollutant among people chronically exposed to complex mixtures requires careful consideration.

References

Abbey DE, Peterson F, Mills PK, Beeson WL. 1993. Long-term ambient concentrations of total suspended particulates, ozone, and sulfur dioxide and respiratory symptoms in a nonsmoking population. Arch Environ Health 48:33–46.

Balmes JR. 1993. The role of ozone exposure in the epidemiology of asthma. Environ Health Perspect 101 (suppl 4): 219–224.

Balmes JR, Scannel CH, Chen LL, Tager Y, Christian D, Welch B, Ferrando R, Boylen K, Kelly TJ. 1995. Effects of a multi-hour exposure to 0.2 ppm ozone on proximal airways and distal lung in subjects with asthma. Health Effects Institute Annual Conference Abstracts: 22.

Bates DV, Sizto R. 1983. Relationship between air pollutant levels and hospital admissions in Southern Ontario. Can J Public Health 74:117–122.

Bates DV, Sizto R. 1987. Air pollution and hospital admissions in Southern Ontario: the acid summer haze effect. Environ Res 43:317–331.

Beckett WS, Freed AN, Turner C, Menkes HA. 1988. Prolonged increased responsiveness of canine peripheral airways after exposure to ozone. J Appl Physiol 64:605–610.

Braun-Fahrlander C, Kunzli N, Domenighetti G, Carell CF, Ackermann-Liebrich U. 1994. Acute effects of ambient ozone on respiratory function of Swiss schoolchildren after a 10-minute heavy exercise. Pediatr Pulmunol 17:169–177.

Burnett RT, Dales RE, Raizenne ME, Krewski D, Summers PW, Roberts GR, Raad-Young M, Dann T, Brook J. 1994. Effects of low ambient levels of ozone and sulfates on the frequency of respiratory admissions to Ontario hospitals. Environ Res 65:172–194.

Calderon Garciadueñas L, Rodriguez-Alcaraz A, Garcia R, Sanchez G, Barragan G, Camacho R, Ramirez L. 1994. Human nasal mucosal changes after exposure to urban pollution. Environ Health Perspect 102:1074–1080.

Castillejos M, Gold DR, Dockery D, Tosteson T, Baum T, Speizer FE. 1992. Effects of ambient ozone on respiratory function and symptoms in Mexico City schoolchildren. Am Rev Respir Dis 145:276–282.

Cody RP, Weisel CP, Birnbaum G, Lioy PJ. 1992. The effect of ozone associated with summertime photochemical smog on the frequency of asthma visits to hospital emergency departments. Environ Res 58:184–194.

Devlin RB et al. 1991. Exposure of humans to ambient levels of ozone for 6.6 hours causes cellular and biochemical changes in the lung. Am Rev Respir Cell Mol Biol 4:72–81.

Dockery DW, Schwartz J, Spengler JD. 1992. Air pollution and daily mortality: associations with particulates and acid aerosols. Environ Res 59:362–373.

Drechsler-Parks DM, Bedi JF, Horvath SM. 1987. Pulmonary function responses of older men and women to ozone exposure. Exp Geront 22:91.

Ehrlich R. 1980. Interaction between environmental pollutants and respiratory infections. Environ Health Perspect 35:89.

Folinsbee LJ et al. 1984. Pulmonary function changes after 1 h of continuous heavy exercise in 0.21 ppm ozone. J Appl Physiol 5.

Folinsbee LJ, McDonnel WF, Horstman DH. 1988. Pulmonary function and symptoms responses after 6.6 hour exposure to 0.12 ppm ozone with moderate exercise. JAPCA 38:28.

Fouke JM, Delemos ER, McFadden ER. 1988. Airway response to ultra short term exposure to ozone. Am Rev Respir Dis 137:326.

Golstein BD, Hamburger SJ, Falk GW, Amoruso MA. 1977. Effect of ozone and nitrogen dioxide on the agglutination of rat alveolar macrophages by concanavalin A. Life Sci 21:1637.

Goldstein IF, Rausch LE. 1978. Time Series Analysis of Morbidity Data for Assessment of Acute Environmental Health Effects. Environ Res 17:266–275.

Hammer DI, Hasselblad V, et al. 1974. Los Angeles student nurse study: daily symptoms reporting and photochemical oxidants. Arch Environ Health 28:255.

Hazucha MJ. 1987. Relationship between ozone exposure and pulmonary function changes. J Appl Physiol 62:1671.

Hazucha MJ, Bates DV, Bromberg PA. 1989. Mechanism of action of ozone on the human lung. J Appl Physiol 67:1535–1541.

Higgins IT, D'Arcy JB, Gibbons DI, Avol EL, Gross KB. 1990. Effect of exposures to ambient ozone on ventilatory lung function in children. Am Rev Respir Dis 141:1136–1146.

Holguin AH. Buffler PA, Contant CF, Stock TH, Kotchmar D, Hsi BP, Jenkins DE, Gehan BM, Noel LM, Mei M. 1985. The effects of ozone on asthmatics in the Houston area. Trans APCA, TR-4, 262–280.

Horstman DH et al. 1990. Ozone concentration and pulmonary response relationshipps for 6.6-hour exposures with five hours of moderate exercise to 0.08, 0.10 ans 0.12 ppm. Am Rev Respir Dis 142:1158–1163.

Ito K, Thurston GD, Hayes C, Lippman M. 1993. Association of London, England, daily mortality with particulate matter, sulfur dioxide, and acidic aerosol pollution. Arch Environ Health 48 (4):213–220.

Kagawa J. 1984. Exposure effect relationship of selected pulmonary function measurements in subjects exposed to ozone. Int Arch Occup Environ Health 54(3): 345–358.

Kinney P, Ozkaynak H. 1991. Association of daily mortality and air pollution in Los Angeles County. Environ Res 54:99–120.

Kinney P, Ozkaynak H. 1992. Associations between ozone and daily mortality in Los Angeles and New York City. Am Rev Respir Dis 145:A95.

Kinney P, Thurston G, Raizenne M. 1996. The effects of ambient ozone on lung function in children: a reanalysis of six summer camp studies. Environ Health Perspect 104:170–174.

Koenig JQ, Covert DS et al. 1987. The effects of ozone and nitrogen dioxide on pulmonary function in healthy and asthmatic adolescents. Am Rev Res Dis 136:1152.

Koenig J, 1995. Efect of ozone on respiratory responses in subjects with asthma. Environ Health Perspect 103 (suppl 2):103–105.

Krzyzanowski M, Quackenboss JJ, Lebowitz M. 1993. Relation of peak expiratory flow rates and symptoms to ambient ozone. Arch Environ Health 47:107–115.

Linn WS, Shamoo DA et al. 1983. Response to ozone in volunteers with chronic obstructive pulmonary disease. Arch Environ Health 38:278.

Lioy PJ, Vollumuth TA, Lippmann M. 1985. Persistence of peak flow decrement in children following ozone exposure exceeding the national ambient air quality standard. J Air Pollut Control Assoc 35: 1068–1071.

Lipfert FW, Hammerstrom T. 1992. Temporal patterns in air pollution and hospital admissions. Environ Res 59:374–399.

Lippmann M., Lioy PJ, Leikuaf G, Green KB, Baxter D, Morandi M, Pasternack B, Fife D, Speizer FE. 1983. Effects of ozone on the pulmonary function of children. Adv Mod Environ Toxicol 5:423–466.

Lippmann M. 1989. Health effects of ozone: a critical review. JAPCA 39:672–695.

Lippmann M. 1993. Health effects of tropospheric ozone: review of recent research findings and their implications to ambient air quality standards. J Exp Anal Environ Epidemiol 3:103–129.

Loomis D, Borja-Aburto V, Bangdiwala S, Shy C. 1996. Ozone exposure and daily mortality in Mexico City: a time-series analysis, Health Effects Institute, Boston, Mass, in press

McDonnell WF, et al. 1983. Pulmonary effects of ozone during exercise, dose-response characteristics. J Appl Physiol 54:1345.

McDonnell W, Horstman D, Hazucha M et al. 1991. Respiratory response of humans exposed to low levels of ozone for 6.6 hours. Arch Environ Health 46:145–150.

Miller FJ, et al. 1978. Effect of urban ozone levels on laboratory induced infections. Toxicol Lett 2:163.

Ostro B, Lipsett MJ, Mann JK, Krupnick A, Harrington W. 1993. Air pollution and respiratory morbidity among adults in Southern California. Am J Epidemiol 137:691–700.

Reisenauer CS, Koening JQ, et al. 1988. Pulmonary response to ozone in healthy individuals aged 55 years or greater. JAPCA 38:51–55.

Romieu Isabelle, et al. 1995. Effects of urban air pollutants on emergency visits for childhood asthma in Mexico City. Am J Epidemiol 141:546–553.

Romieu Isabelle, et al. 1992. Air pollution and school absenteeism among children in Mexico City. Am J Epidemiol 136: 1524–1531.

Saldiva PH, et al. 1994. Association between air pollution and mortality due to respiratory diseases in children in Sao Paulo Brazil: A preliminary report. Environ Res 65:218–225.

Schwartz J. 1989. Lung function and chronic exposure to air pollution: a cross-sectional analysis of NHANES II. Environ Res 50:309–321.

Schwartz J. 1992. Air pollution and the duration of acute respiratory symptoms. Arch Environ Health 47(2):116–122.

Schwartz J. 1994a. PM10, ozone, and hospital admissions for the elderly in Minneapolis–St. Paul, Minnesota. Arch Environ Health 49:366–374.

Schwartz J. 1994b. Air pollution and hospital admissions for the elderly in Birmingham, Alabama. Am J Epidemiol 139:589–598.

Seltzer J, Bigby BG, Stulbarg M. Holtzman MJ, Nadel JA. 1986. 03 induced change in bronchial reactivity to metacholine and airway inflammation in humans. J Appl Physiol 60:1321–1326.

Shepard RJ, Silverman UF, Corey PN. 1983. Interaction of ozone and cigarette smoke exposure. Environ Res 31:125.

Solic JJ, Hazucha MJ, et al. 1982. The acute effects of 0.2 ppm ozone in patients with chronic obstructive pulmonary disease. Am Rev Respir Dis 38:664.

Spektor DM, Lippmann M, Lioy PJ, Thurston GD, Citak K, James DJ, Bock N, Speizer FE, Hayes C. 1988a. Effects of ambient ozone on respiratory function in active normal children Am Rev Respir Dis 137:313–320.

Spektor DM, Lippmann M, Thurston GD, Lioy PJ, Stecko J, O'Connor G, Garshick E, Speizer FE, Hayes C. 1988b. Effects of ambient ozone on respiratory function in healthy adults exercising outdoors. Am Rev Respir Dis 138.821–828.

Specktor DM, Thurston GD, Mao J, He D, Heyes C, Lippmann M. 1991. Effects of single-and multiday ozone exposures on respiratory function in active normal children. Environ Res 55:107–122.

Thurston GD, Ito K, Hayes CG, Bates DV, Lipmann M. 1994. Respiratory hospital admissions and summertime haze air pollution in Toronto, Ontario: consideration of the role of acid aerosols. Environ Res 65:271–290.

Thurston GD, Ito K, Kinney PL, Lipmann M. 1992. A multiple-year study of air pollution and respiratory hospital admissions in three New York State metropolitan areas: results from 1988 and 1989 summers. J Exposure Analysis and Environmental Epidemiology 4:429–450.

Whittemore A, Korn E. 1980. Asthma and air pollution in the Los Angeles area. Am J Public Health 70:687–696.

Environmental Tobacco Smoke I: Childhood Diseases

9

RUTH A. ETZEL

ENVIRONMENTAL tobacco smoke (ETS) is ubiquitous. The Third National Health and Nutrition Examination Survey (NHANES III) provided data on levels of serum cotinine, a metabolite of nicotine, in a representative sample of approximately 12,000 nonsmokers from the U.S. population in the late 1980s. Using a more sensitive assay than previous studies, the investigators found that 88% of U.S. nonsmokers had detectable levels of serum cotinine. Forty-three percent of children under age 12 lived in a home with at least one smoker.

There is a large body of epidemiologic evidence associating ETS with childhood respiratory disease. Young children live primarily indoors in a single residence. If smokers live in the same residence, children may have particularly high and prolonged exposures to ETS. They may also be particularly susceptible to respiratory disease.

This chapter covers childhood illness associated with ETS exposure. Although it is not possible to directly compare the public health burden of mortality from chronic disease (i.e., lung cancer and heart disease) with morbidity among children, it seems clear that a major public health burden from childhood respiratory illnesses is caused by ETS. The strongest evidence of an ETS association relates to lower respiratory tract illness in the first year of life, middle ear disease during childhood, and severe asthma attacks among asthmatic children. There is also suggestive evidence linking ETS exposure to sudden infant death syndrome and to decreased pulmonary function.

The typical study design for most of these outcomes, which are common and occur with a short induction period, is a cohort design. The fact that children are not smokers facilitates the study of ETS, as does the fact that the home is often the principal if not the only site where exposure occurs.

This chapter will review the evidence that passive smoking is associated in children with higher rates of lower respiratory tract illness in the first year of life, decrements in pulmonary function, higher rates of middle ear effusion, sudden infant death syndrome, and more severe asthma attacks. It will also review some of the biochemical markers such as cotinine that are used to measure exposure to environmental tobacco smoke, and the relative advantages and disadvantages of using markers and questionnaires.

In 1992, 48 million American adults (26.5%) were current cigarette smokers (CDC, 1994). A recent national survey indicated that 43% of children aged 2 months to 11 years live in a home with at least one smoker (Pirkle et al., 1996). An estimated 8.7 to 12.4 million U.S. children under age 5 are exposed to cigarette smoke at home (American Academy of Pediatrics, 1986). Because many young children spend a large proportion of their time indoors, they may have significant exposures to environmental tobacco smoke.

Environmental tobacco smoke is composed of more than 3800 different chemical compounds (National Research Council, 1986). Concentrations of respirable suspended particulate matter (particulates < 2.5 micrometers) can be 2 to 3 times higher in homes with smokers than in homes with no smokers (Spengler et al., 1981). Cigarette smoking is the most important factor determining the level of suspended particulate matter and respirable sulfates and particles in the indoor air (Dockery and Spengler 1981; Lefcoe et al., 1971).

Passive Smoking and Lower Respiratory Tract Illness Among Children

The first effect of passive smoking to be documented in children was an increased rate of illnesses affecting the lower respiratory tract. Cameron reported a positive correlation between the presence of a smoker in the home and the incidence of perceived disease in children (Cameron, 1967).

Since that first report, numerous other investigators have demonstrated a consistent association between lower respiratory tract illness and parental smoking. The association appears to be strongest for infants during the first year of life, and for maternal smoking rather than paternal smoking. Infants with two smoking parents were more than twice as likely to have had pneumonia and bronchitis as were infants with nonsmoking parents. (Harlap and Davies, 1974; Rantakallio, 1978; Colley et al., 1974; Fergusson et al., 1980)

More recent studies of childhood lower respiratory tract illness in relation to ETS can be found in Table 9-1.

Passive Smoking and Serious Infectious Illnesses Among Children

Berg and her colleagues (1991) determined that among children aged 3 months to 59 months passive smoking increased the risk of serious infectious illnesses requiring hospitalization almost fourfold.

Passive Smoking and Lung Growth Among Children

Children have slower rates of lung development if they are exposed to environmental tobacco smoke (Tager et al., 1983; Ware et al., 1984). Estimates indicate that current maternal smoking reduces forced expiratory volume in 1 second (FEV_1) by approximately 0.5% per year for each pack of cigarettes smoked per day.

Passive Smoking and Middle Ear Effusions in Children

Children who lived in households where cigarettes are smoked are more likely to be admitted to the hospital for tympanostomy tube placement than children whose parents do not smoke (Kraemer et al., 1983, Black, 1985; Hinton, 1989). Children in day-care centers whose parents smoke are more likely to develop middle ear effusion as measured by tympanometry (Iversen et al., 1985; Etzel et al., 1992; Owen et al., 1993). Passive smoking has also been associated with type B tympanograms (suggesting middle ear effusion) (Strachan et al., 1989).

Table 9-2 summarizes recent epidemiologic studies of the effects of passive smoking on acute and chronic middle ear diseases.

The mechanism by which tobacco smoke exposure leads to middle ear effusions is likely to be related to ciliostasis, goblet cell hyperplasia, and mucus hypersecretion, which could cause accumulation of mucus and bacteria in the inner ear. Also, exposure to environmental tobacco smoke

Table 9-1. Recent epidemiological studies of effects of passive smoking on acute lower respiratory tract illnesses (LRIs) [a]

Authors	Population Studied	ETS exposure Assessment	Outcome Variable	Results [b]	Observations
Breese-Hall et al. (1984)	Cases: 29 infants hospitalized with bronchiolitis due to respiratory syncytial virus (RSV) Controls: 58 infants hospitalized for nonrespiratory conditions; 58 infants hospitalized due to LRIs not due to RSV	Parental questionnaire	See population studied	Cases vs. controls Odds ratio (OR) = 4.8 (1.8, 13.0) (>5 cig./day vs. none) LRI controls vs. non-LRI controls OR = 2.7 (1.3, 5.7)	Cases matched to controls for age, sex, race, month of admission, form of payment; selection bias not ruled out
Chen et al. (1986)	1058 infants born in Shanghai, China	Parental self-administered questionnaire; number of cigarettes smoked by household members	Admissions to hospital for respiratory illnesses as reported by parents	Cig./day OR 1–9 1.2 (0.6,2.3) >9 1.9 (1.1,3.4)	Controlling for crowding, paternal education, feeding practices, birthweight, family history of chronic respiratory illness
Chen et al. (1988)	2227 infants born in Shanghai, China	Household self-administered questionnaire	Incidence of hospitalization for respiratory illness, incidence of bronchitis or pneumonia first 18 mo. of life	First 6 mo. of life: OR = 3.0 (1.6, 5.7); 7–18 mo. of life: OR = 1.8 (1.0, 3.2)	No smoking mothers; controlling for sex, birthweight, feeding practices, nursery care, paternal education, use of coal for cooking, family history of chronic respiratory illness

(continued)

Table 9-1. Recent epidemiological studies of effects of passive smoking on acute lower respiratory tract illnesses (LRIs) [a] (*continued*)

Authors	Population Studied	Outcome Variable	ETS exposure Assessment Results[b]	Observations	
Chen (1989)	Same as above	Same as above	Same as above	First 18 mo. of life incidence density ratio (IDR) 1.6 for breast-fed babies; IDR 3.4 for non-breast-fed babies; confidence intervals not calculable	
McConnochie and Roghmann (1986)	53 infants with bronchiolitis; 106 controls	Parental questionnaire at mean age 8 yr.	See population studied	Cases *vs.* controls OR = 2.4 (1.2, 4.8) smoking mother vs. nonsmoking mother	Cases matched to controls for sex and age; controlling for family history of asthma, social status, older siblings, crowding; selection bias not ruled out
Ogston et al. (1987)	1565 infants in New Zealand	Maternal and paternal smoking habits during pregnancy by questionnaire	Upper and lower respiratory illnesses during first year of life	Paternal smoking OR = 1.43 (1.05, 1.96); maternal smoking OR 1.82 (1.25, 3.64)	Upper and lower respiratory illnesses not distinguished; controlling for maternal age, feeding practices, heating type, social class

Reference	Population	Exposure measure	Outcome	Results[b]	Comments
Anderson et al. (1988)	102 children hospitalized in Atlanta, Georgia, <2 yr.; 199 controls	Self-reported smoking habits of family members	LRI	No effect of parental smoking after controlling for other risk factors	Selection bias possible
Woodward et al. (1990)	2125 children aged 18 mo. to 3 yr.	Self-administered mailed questionnaire	Respiratory score regarding 13 different symptoms; top 20% compared with low 20%	OR = 2.0 (1.3, 3.4) of having a smoking mother for high scores compared with low scores; no effect of paternal smoking	Controlling for parental history of respiratory illness, child care, parental occupation, maternal stress
Wright et al. (1991)	847 white children born in Tucson, Arizona	Self-administered questionnaire and cotinine levels in a subsample	LRIs as assessed by the infants' pediatricians	OR = 1.5 (1.1, 2.2) of having smoking mother; no effect of paternal smoking	Effects significant only for LRIs occurring in the first 6 mo. of life; controlling for day care, room sharing, parental history of respiratory illnesses, feeding practices, sex, and maternal education
Reese et al. (1992)	491 children aged 1 mo. to 17 yr.	Cotinine levels in urine of children; questionnaire of parents' current smoking	Hospitalization for bronchiolitis	Higher levels in children hospitalized for bronchiolitis than in controls (p < 0.02)	No effects of ETS on hospitalization for asthma

[a] Adapted from: U.S. Environmental Protection Agency, 1992.

[b] 95% confidence intervals in parentheses.

Table 9-2. Recent epidemiologic studies of effects of passive smoking on acute and chronic middle ear diseases[a]

Authors	Population Studied	ETS Exposure Assessment	Outcome Variable	Results[b]	Observations
Willatt (1986)	93 children aged 2–15 yr. admitted to hospital for tonsillectomy; 61 age- and sex-matched controls	Questionnaire answered by parents	Tonsillectomy for middle ear infection	OR = 2.1 (1.1, 4.0) of having smoking mothers	Controlling for birthweight, sex, age, feeding practices, social class, crowding, sore throats in other household members
Fleming et al. (1987)	575 children <5 yr.	Questionnaire answered by child's guardian	Upper respiratory illnesses (URI) and infections in previous 2 weeks	OR = 1.7 for URI when mother smoked; no effect on ear infection	Controlling for feeding practices, income, crowding, day care, siblings, sex, race
Tainio et al. (1988)	198 Finnish newborns followed from birth to age 2.3 yr.	Questionnaire to parents	Recurrent otitis media as diagnosed by pediatricians	No effects	No distinction between maternal and paternal smoking; small sample
Reed and Lutz (1988)	24 cases of acute otitis media; 25 controls	Questionnaire to parents	Abnormal tympanometry	OR = 4.9 (1.4, 17.2) of having smokers at home	Small sample; selection bias cannot be ruled out
Hinton (1989)	115 children aged 1–12 yr. admitted for grommet insertion; 36 controls aged 2–11 yr. in Great Britain	Questionnaire to parents	Being admitted for grommet insertion	OR = 2.1 (1.0, 4.5) of having smoking parents	No control for confounders; selection bias not ruled out
Teele et al. (1989)	877 children observed for 1 yr.; 698 observed for 3 yr.; 498 observed for 7 yr. in Boston, Massachusetts	Questionnaire to parents	Acute otitis media; number of days with middle ear effusion	13% more acute otitis during first yr. of life; more days with middle ear effusion ($p < .009$) only during first year; no effects after controlling for confounders	No distinction between paternal and maternal smoking; parents smoking 1 cig./day included among smokers

Reference	Population	Exposure measure	Outcome	Results[b]	Comments
Corbo et al. (1989)	1615 children aged 6–13 yr. in Abruzzo, Italy	Questionnaire to parents	Child's snoring as reported by parents	OR = 1.8 (1.1, 3.0) for moderate smokers (1–19 cig./day); OR = 1.9 (1.2, 3.1) for heavy smokers (≥20 cig./day)	No distinction between maternal and paternal smoking
Strachan et al. (1989)	736 children in third elementary class in Edinburgh, Scotland	Salivary cotinine level	Prevalence of middle ear effusion as assessed by tympanogram	OR for doubling salivary cotinine = 1.4 (1.03, 1.27)	One-third of cases of middle ear effusion attributable to passive smoking; controlling for sex, housing tenure, social class, crowding, gas cooking, damp walls
Takasaka (1990)	77 children aged 4–8 yr. with otitis media with effusion; 134 controls matched for age and sex in Sendai, Japan	Questionnaire to parents	See population studied	No effect	Low power
Etzel et al. (1992)	132 children aged < 3 yr. from day-care facility	Serum cotinine levels	Otitis media with effusion	Incidence density ratio 1.4 (1.2, 1.6) for exposed children; increases significant for ages ≤ 2 years only	8% of cases attributable to ETS exposure
Owen et al. (1993)	435 healthy infants followed until age 2 yrs	Parental questionnaire	Otitis media with effusion (OME)	11% increase in amount of OME for each additional pack of cigarettes smoked in the home between age 12–18 mos.	No effect seen during 1st yr. of life
Ey et al. (1995)	1013 infants in a large health maintenance organization followed for 1st year of life	Questionnaire to parents	At least 3 episodes of acute otitis media in 6 mo. or 4 episodes in 12 mo.	OR = 1.78 (1.01, 3.11) for maternal smoking (≥20 cigs/day)	Paternal smoking showed no effect

[a] Adapted from U.S. Environmental Protection Agency, 1992.
[b] 95% confidence intervals in parentheses.

and viral infections may reduce phagocyte antibacterial defenses, with re-sulting bacterial colonization of the middle ear (Etzel et al., 1992).

Passive Smoking and Asthma

Children with asthma whose parents smoke may have more frequent ex-acerbations and more severe symptoms (Burchfiel et al., 1986; Chilmon-czyk et al., 1993; Ehrlich et al., 1992; Evans et al., 1987; Krzyzanowski et al., 1990; Murray and Morrison, 1989; O'Connor et al., 1987; Oldigs et al., 1991; Sherman et al., 1990; Weitzman et al., 1990). Table 9-3 sum-marizes recent epidemiologic studies of the effects of passive smoking on asthma in childhood. In one of the few interventions reported in the literature, Murray and Morrison demonstrated that if parents expose their asthmatic children to less cigarette smoke, their asthmatic symptoms will be less severe (Murray and Morrison, 1993).

Passive Smoking and Sudden Infant Death Syndrome

There is a growing body of evidence linking exposure to environmental tobacco smoke to sudden infant death syndrome (SIDS) (Bergman and Weisner, 1976; Haglund and Cnattingius, 1990; Hoffman et al., 1988; Le-wak et al., Malloy et al., 1988; Mitchell et al., 1991; Naeye et al., 1976; Steele and Longworth, 1966). Table 9-4 summarizes epidemiologic studies of the effects of passive smoking on the incidence of sudden infant death syndrome. This relationship appears to be independent of socioeconomic status, birthweight, and gestational age. Investigators have not determined the mechanism for the effect of passive exposure to tobacco smoke on SIDS. Future research will be needed to determine whether exposure to tobacco smoke and infant positioning act synergistically.

Measurement of Exposure to ETS

In most of the studies that have been mentioned in this chapter, the estimate of a child's passive exposure to environmental tobacco smoke was based on parents' self-reports on questionnaires asking about their usual cigarette consumption.

Questionnaires have the advantage of being noninvasive and inexpen-sive; in addition, from a questionnaire one can determine exposure history for any time period. However, questionnaires have several disadvantages as measuring tools for passive smoking. They may give the investigator an imprecise estimate of the child's exposure, because the amount of tobacco smoke products actually absorbed by a child could vary considerably depending on the amount of smoke present in the environment, the child's proximity to the source of the smoke, and the room's ventilation characteristics. Furthermore, as smoking becomes increasingly socially unacceptable, a child's parents may underreport their actual cigarette consumption, or report that they smoke only outdoors, away from the child.

To overcome the problems of recall bias and misclassification, investigators have tried to identify objective, biochemical measures of tobacco smoke exposure to evaluate the health risks of passive smoking. In epidemiologic studies of tobacco-related diseases, measurement of such biological markers is an essential adjunct to questionnaire responses about smoking and passive tobacco smoke exposure.

Five different biochemical markers have been evaluated among active smokers to measure compliance with smoking cessation programs and thus offer some potential as biochemical markers. They are carboxyhemoglobin, expired air carbon monoxide, thiocyanate, nicotine, and cotinine.

Carboxyhemoglobin

This test has the advantage of being rapid and relatively inexpensive. However, it requires a blood sample and thus may be ill-suited for large epidemiologic studies. Furthermore, carboxyhemoglobin has a short half-life (about 4 hours) and thus reflects only very recent exposure. Moreover, there is the possibility of a false-positive result when the individual has been exposed to the products of incomplete combusion (such as from a wood stove). Also, the carboxyhemoglobin concentration must be measured promptly (within a few hours of blood drawing) and cannot be stored for future analysis.

Expired air carbon monoxide

Expired air carbon monoxide is another measure of smoke exposure that has advantages over carboxyhemoglobin. The test is noninvasive, requiring only that the person produce a blood sample, which can be analyzed on the spot, providing immediate feedback. Furthermore, expired air carbon monoxide is an inexpensive test. However, measuring expired air carbon monoxide has many of the same disadvantages as measuring carboxyhemoglobin concentrations; it has a short half-life, identifying only

Table 9-3. Recent epidemiologic studies of effects of passive smoking on asthma in childhood [a]

Authors	Population Studied	ETS Exposure Assessment	Outcome Variable	Results[b]	Observations
Burchfiel et al. (1986)	3482 nonsmoking children 0 to 19 yr., in Tecumseh, Michigan	Questionnaire answered by subjects or parents	Prevalence of asthma	OR = 1.7 (1.2, 2.5) for boys; OR = 1.2 (0.8, 1.9) for girls	Independent of parental respiratory illness, age, parental education, family size, and allergies
Evans et al. (1987)	191 children aged 4 to 17 yr. in New York, New York	Parental questionnaire	Emergency room visits and hospitalizations for asthma (from medical records)	3.1 ± 0.4 vs. 1.8 ± 0.3 ($p = .008$) emergency room visits in children of smoking and nonsmoking parents	No distinction made between maternal and paternal smoking; independent of race and parental employment status
O'Connor et al. (1987)	292 subjects aged 6 to 21 yr. in Boston, Massachusetts	Parental questionnaire	Bronchial response to cold air	Significantly increased response in asthmatics whose mothers smoked	No increase in non-asthmatics whose mothers smoked
Murray and Morrison (1989)	415 children aged 1 to 17 yr. with asthma in Vancouver, Canada	Parental questionnaire	Asthma symptom score for severity of asthma	Higher scores ($p < .01$) in children of smoking mothers	Stronger effect in boys and older children
Krzyzanowski et al. (1990)	298 children aged 5 to 15 yr. in Tucson, Arizona	Parental questionnaire	Parental reports of asthma in their children	OR = 9.0 (2.4, 34.0) for children exposed to ETS and formaldehyde vs. nonexposed	Small sample
Sherman et al. (1990)	770 children aged 5 to 9 yr. followed for 11 yr. in Boston, Massachusetts	Parental and subject questionnaire	Physician diagnosis of asthma	No effect of parental smoking on prevalence or incidence of asthma	No effort to assess effect of heavy smoking by parents; no control for socioeconomic status
Weitzman et al. (1990)	4331 children aged 0 to 5 yr. (U.S. National Health Interview Survey)	Maternal questionnaire	Asthma for at least 3 mo. at time of questionnaire	OR = 2.1 (1.3, 3.3) for children whose mothers smoked ≥ 10 cig./day	Independent of race, sex, family size, presence of both parents, and number of rooms

Study	Population	Exposure measure	Outcome	Result	Comments
Oldigs et al. (1991)	11 asthmatic children	Direct exposure to ETS for 1 hour	Changes in lung function	No effect	No assessment of effect of chronic exposure
Martinez et al. (1992)	774 children aged 0 to 5 yr. followed for several years in Tucson, Arizona	Parental questionnaire	Physician diagnosis of asthma	OR = 2.5 (1.4, 4.6) for children of low maternal education whose mothers smoked $\geq$ 10 cig./day	No effect among children of better educated mothers
Ehrlich et al. (1992)	228 children; 72 with acute asthma; 35 with nonacute asthma and controls	Cotinine levels in urine of children; smoking by maternal caregiver	Emergency room and asthma clinic visits	Higher levels of cotinine in asthmatics OR = 1.9 (1.0, 3.4)	Similar cotinine levels in acute and nonacute asthmatics
Chilmonczyk et al. (1993)	199 children aged 8 mo. to 13 yr. and with asthma in Portland, Maine	Cotinine levels in urine of children	Number of acute exacerbations of asthma in the previous year	RR = 1.7 (1.4, 2.1)	Similar results using parental reports of smoking
Holberg et al. (1993)	809 infants in a large health maintenance organization followed for first 3 yr. of life	Questionnaires	Rate of wheezing lower respiratory tract illness	OR = 3.57 (1.21, 10.54) in third year of life for smoking caregiver in day-care center	Controlling for maternal smoking, number of unrelated children present. No effect in 1st or 2nd years of life.
Rylander et al. (1995)	199 children < 4 yr./old admitted to hospital in Stockholm with wheezing, 351 controls	Parental questionnaire and cotinine levels in urine	Hospitalization for wheezing	OR = 1.8 (1.3, 2.6) if both parents smoked; OR = 2.1 (1.1, 4.6) for infants $\leq$ 18 mo. with cotinine $\geq$ 5 µg/L	No effect of cotinine levels seen with children > 18 mo.

[a] Adapted from: U.S. Environmental Protection Agency, 1992

[b] 95% confidence intervals in parentheses.

Table 9-4. Epidemiologic studies of effects of smoking on incidence of sudden infant syndrome (SIDS) [a]

Authors	Population Studied	ETS Exposure Assessment	Results[b]	Observations
Steele and Langworth (1966)	80 infants who died of SIDS; 157 matched controls in Ontario, Canada	Maternal report from hospital record at birth	OR = 2.1 (1.1, 3.8) when mother smoked 1 to 19 cig./day; OR = 3.6 (1.7, 7.9) when mother smoked ≥ 20 cig./day	No control for socioeconomic status or maternal age
Naeye et al. (1976)	59,379 infants born in several U. S. cities	Maternal report from hospital record at birth	OR = 1.6 (1.0, 2.4) for any maternal smoking; OR = 2.6 (1.7, 4.0) for mothers smoking ≥ 6 cig./day	Controlling for place of birth, date of delivery, gestational age, sex, race, and socioeconomic status
Bergman and Wiesner (1976)	100 cases of SIDS; 100 matched controls in King County, Washington	Maternal questionnaire answered after death (or at equivalent age for controls)	OR = 2.4 (1.2, 4.8); effect only significant for mothers ≤ 25 yr. (OR = 4.4 [1.7, 11.2])	Independent of maternal education, race, sex, and birth date
Lewak et al. (1979)	44 cases of SIDS	Maternal questionnaire	OR = 4.4 (2.1, 9.2)	No control for possible confounding factors
Malloy et al. (1988)	305,000 births in Missouri	Maternal reports on birth certificate	OR = 1.8 (1.4, 2.2)	Controlling for marital status, maternal age, education, parity, and birthweight
Hoffman et al. (1988)	800 SIDS cases; 1600 controls (NICHD cooperative study)	Maternal questionnaire	OR = 3.4 (p < .005)	Controlling for age, birthweight, and race
Haglund and Cnattingius (1990)	279,000 births in Sweden	Maternal questionnaire	OR = 1.8 (1.2, 2.6). Heavy-smoking mother: OR = 2.7 (1.9, 3.9)	Independent of birthweight, maternal age, social status, parity, sex, and type of birth

Study	Description	Method	OR[b]	Comments
Mitchell et al. (1991)	162 SIDS cases; 3 to 4 times as many controls	Parental questionnaire	Cig./day OR 1 to 9 1.9 (1.0, 3.5) 10 to 19 2.6 (1.5, 4.7) ≥20 5.1 (2.9, 9.0)	Independent of prenatal care, maternal age, education, marital status, sex, neonatal problems, parity, birthweight, race, season of death, and breastfeeding
Malloy et al. (1992)	636 SIDS cases in Missouri, 757 SIDS cases in NICHD Epidem. Study and 1541 controls	Maternal questionnaire	OR = 2.86 (2.32, 3.50) for ≥ 1 pack/day in Missouri; OR = 2.60 (1.93, 3.52) for ≥ 20 cigs/day in NICHD	Adjusted for maternal age, race, parity, education, marital status, and sex of infant
Schoendorf and Kiely (1992)	435 cases of SIDS infants weighing ≥ 2500 g at birth, 6098 controls	Maternal questionnaire	OR = 2.4 (1.49, 3.83) among black infants. OR = 2.2 (1.29, 3.78) among white infants for passive exposure	Controlling for maternal age, education level and marital status
Mitchell et al. (1993)	485 SIDS cases; 1800 controls	Parental interview	OR = 4.09 (3.28, 5.11) for maternal smoking during pregnancy	Controlling for socioeconomic status and birthweight. Father's smoking increases risk when mother smokes, but not if she does not.
Taylor and Sanderson (1995)	649 SIDS cases in NMIHS[c]	Maternal questionnaire	OR 2.03 (1.64, 2.52) for maternal smoking during pregnancy	Population-attributable risk percentage for maternal smoking as a risk factor for SIDS was 30%

[a] Adapted from: U.S. Environmental Protection Agency, 1992

[b] 95% confidence intervals in parentheses.

[c] NMIHS is the National Maternal and Infant Health Survey.

those persons who have smoked within the past 8 hours, and false-positive results will be obtained if persons have been exposed to wood stoves. In addition, a breath sample cannot be easily obtained from young children.

Thiocyanate

Thiocyanate has been frequently used as a biochemical marker of chronic tobacco smoke exposure because of its long half life (about 2 weeks). It is produced by the detoxification of hydrogen cyanide gas in cigarette smoke and can be measured in urine and saliva, thus having the additional advantage of being noninvasive. However, false-positive results may be obtained if the study participant has eaten certain foods (cabbage, turnips, garlic, mustard, horseradish, and almonds). Industrial exposure to cyanides will also result in positive thiocanate determinations (Bliss et al, 1984).

Nicotine

Only nicotine and cotinine have adequate sensitivity and specificity for the low-level determinations needed to study passive exposure to tobacco smoke. However, nicotine's short half life (about 30 to 110 minutes) makes it useful only for detection of very recent tobacco smoke exposure. Also, the amount of nicotine excreted in the urine is dependent on urinary pH (more nicotine being excreted at acidic pH's, when nicotine is almost entirely ionized and cannot be reabsorbed through the kidney tubules). Also, nicotine excretion is dependent on urinary volume.

Cotinine

Measurement of cotinine, a major metabolite of nicotine, has several advantages over the other biochemical methods. Cotinine is specific for tobacco exposure, is produced only in vivo, has a long circulating half-life (averaging 19 to 40 hours in adults, compared to nicotine's half-life of 30 to 110 minutes in adults), and can be measured at very low concentrations (Pirkle et al., 1996).

Cotinine is formed from the nicotine that passive smokers breathe in from the indoor environment. Hinds and First (1975) reported levels of nicotine ranging from 1 $\mu g/m^3$ to 10.3 $\mu g/m^3$ in indoor public places. Muramatsu et al. (1984) found the nicotine concentration in three houses to be between 7.61 and 14.60 $\mu g/m^3$ and in four cars to be between 7.73

and 83.13 $\mu g/m^3$. Hammond (1995) found a median nicotine concentration of 8.6 $\mu g/m^3$ in open offices at worksites that allowed smoking.

Cotinine can be measured by radioimmunoassay (Langone et al., 1973), gas-liquid chromatography (Benowitz et al., 1983), or liquid chromatography (Machacek et al., 1986) in many different body constituents, including blood (Langone et al., 1975; Pattishall et al., 1985; Williams et al., 1979), urine (Greenberg et al., 1984; Matsukura et al., 1984; Wald et al., 1984; Forastiere et al., 1993), saliva (Abrams et al., 1987; Brunnemann et al., 1987; Coultas et al., 1987; Greenberg et al., 1984; Haley et al., 1983, Hatsukami et al., 1987; Hoffmann et al., 1984; Jarvis et al., 1983, 1984, 1985, 1987a,b), amniotic fluid (Luck et al., 1985; Van Vunakis et al., 1974), cervical mucus (Sasson et al., 1985), and hair (Haley and Hoffmann 1985; Nafstad et al., 1995). The choice depends on availability and acceptability to the study participants. In general, blood cotinine measurements have been chosen only when venipuncture will be performed for another purpose. Urine collection is easier, so urine cotinine is often measured, except in worksites where there may be heightened concern about urine testing to detect illicit drug use. In such settings, saliva cotinine measurements may be preferable.

For researchers using cotinine as a biochemical marker of tobacco smoke exposure, interpreting the results of the cotinine determination can be difficult. Because few exposure chamber studies have been performed to determine the dose-response relationship (Goldstein et al., 1987), it may be difficult to determine what cotinine concentrations represent meaningful exposures to tobacco smoke. However, distinguishing between active and passive smoking on the basis of a cotinine measurement may be difficult. Several investigators attempted to define the optimal cutoff for saliva cotinine in discriminating smokers from nonsmokers. Jarvis et al. (1987b) suggested a cutoff of 14.2 ng/mL. With this cutoff, (using self-reported smoking as the gold standard) they determined saliva cotinine had a sensitivity of 96% and a specificity of 99%. Abrams et al. (1987), using a cutoff of 10 ng/mL, determined that saliva cotinine had a sensitivity of 95% and a specificity of 91%. Pierce et al. (1987) carried out a validation study on self-reported smoking for 1172 people (36% of whom were smokers) in Australia in 1983. Using 44 ng/mL as the cutoff for classifying a person as a smoker, they determined that the sensitivity of cotinine was 88.1% and the specificity was 96%.

Ideally, a receiver operating characteristic (ROC) curve, a simple empirical description of the decision threshold effect (Metz, 1978) would be used to determine the optimal cutoff. A ROC curve is a graph of sensitivity, or the true-positive fraction, against the complement of specificity, the false-positive fraction, for all possible cutoffs. A low cutoff would probably be chosen to maximize sensitivity in a study of smoking behavior. Further studies are needed to determine what levels of cotinine are associated with various adverse health outcomes.

Cotinine Concentrations in Nonsmokers

Table 9-5 summarizes the results of 13 studies of saliva cotinine concentrations in nonsmokers. Ten investigators collected data from child, adolescent, or adult nonsmokers in natural environments; these studies report mean (or median) cotinine concentrations below 10 ng/mL in nonsmokers. Three studies were performed under more controlled conditions. Jarvis et al. (1983) studied seven nonsmoking office workers at 11:30 AM on a normal working day and again at 7:45 PM after 2 hours' exposure to tobacco smoke in a pub. Tobacco smoke exposure during working hours was not controlled, whereas exposure in the pub was provided by several smoking colleagues of the subjects who were recruited to socialize with them. Hoffmann et al. (1984) exposed 10 nonsmoking adults to sidestream smoke from two concurrently smoked cigarettes in a 16-m^2 chamber. Johnson et al. (1985) exposed 10 adult nonsmokers who did not have a smoker in their households to a single, 3-hour exposure to sidestream smoke from 24 packs of cigarettes. Because of the extremely high exposure, the cotinine concentrations reported in this study are much higher than under natural conditions.

The available data suggest a separation of saliva cotinine concentrations into four categories as shown in Table 9-6. Passive smokers usually have cotinine concentrations in saliva and blood below 5 ng/mL, but heavy passive exposure can result in levels of 10 ng/mL or more. Levels between 10 ng/mL and 100 ng/mL may result from infrequent active smoking or regular active smoking with low nicotine intake. Levels above 100 ng/mL are probably the result of regular active smoking.

The literature to date does not support the use of cotinine concentration as a continuous exposure variable in epidemiologic analyses; rather, broad categorizations of cotinine concentrations are more appropriate in view of the large intra-individual differences in cotinine concentrations seen with reportedly similar exposures to tobacco smoke.

Despite the fact that biochemical markers such as cotinine measurements have been used in studies of passive smoking for the past decade, they have not yet been shown to be better than questionnaires in classifying exposure. One reason is that cotinine measurements vary depending on the child's exposure in the past week. Thus, if the sample is collected

Table 9-5. Saliva cotinine concentrations (ng/mL) in nonsmokers

First Author	Year	N	Age, y	Exposure	Mean (SD)	Range	Method
Abrams	1987	30	Adult	?	0.3 (1.6)	0–9	RIA
Coultas	1987	181	18–29	0	1.6 (2.8)		RIA
				1 cig/day	2.9 (4.2)		RIA
				>1 cig/day	3.0 (5.7)		RIA
		398	30–64	0	1.7 (3.1)		RIA
				1 cig/day	3.4 (4.7)		RIA
				>1cig/day	6.0 (5.7)		RIA
Greenberg	1984	13	Infant	None	median 0	0–3	RIA
		27	Infant	Some	median 9	0–25	RIA
Haley	1983	18	Adult	None	nondetectable		RIA
Hoffmann	1988	10	Adult	2 cigs in chamber	Peak 5 2 hr p exp.		RIA
Jarvis	1987a	330	11–16	No	1.97		GLC
			11–16	Yes	4.88		GLC
Jarvis	1983	7	Adult	None	1.50		GLC
		7	Adult	Some	8.04		GLC
Jarvis	1985	269	11–16	None	0.44 (0.68)		GLC
		96	11–16	Father	1.31 (1.21)		GLC
		76	11–16	Mother	1.95 (1.71)		GLC
		128	11–16	Both	3.38 (2.45)		GLC
Jarvis	1984	46	Adult	None	0.73		GLC
		27	Adult	Little	2.20		GLC
		20	Adult	Some	2.80		GLC
		7	Adult	a lot	2.63		GLC
Jarvis	1987b	100	Adult	?	1.7 (2.3)		GLC
Johnson	1985	10	Adult	24 pks/3 hr in chamber	Maximum 19.7 (4.58)	14–29	RIA
Langone	1988	36	4–5	None	0.81 (3.3)	0–19	RIA
		30	4–5	Parent(s)	4.67 (6.0) 0	0–30	RIA
Lee	1983	340	Adult	?	1.64 (males)		GLC
		448	Adult	?	1.16 (females)		GLC

RIA=Radiommuniossay

GLC=Gas-liquid chromatography

when the child has recently been in a smoke-filled environment (such as a waiting room or restaurant) it may be higher than if it is collected after the child has been in a smoke-free setting. The investigator needs to determine if the child's activities for the week before the sample collection are typical or atypical.

The normal variation in people's activities leads to variation in cotinine levels, which may be higher at certain times of day than others. Children of different ages may metabolize cotinine at different rates. And there is evidence that black children have higher cotinine concentrations than

Table 9-6. Categorizations of saliva cotinine concentration

Category	Cotinine (ng/mL)	Probable Nicotine Use	Probable Passive Exposure
A	N.D.[a]	None	None
B	<10	None	Yes
C	10–100	Infrequent[b]	Yes[c]
D	>100	Regular	Yes[c]

[a] Non-detectable.

[b] Or regular use with low nicotine intake.

[c] Active smokers are exposed to the sidestream smoke from their own cigarettes.

white children (Pattishall et al., 1985). Drugs are another source of variation; it is important to get a good history of the medications being used, because these may influence the metabolism and excretion of cotinine. Diet has been suggested as another source of variation; however, it is unlikely that diet is an important influence on cotinine concentrations in children (Pirkle et al., 1996).

Some investigators have reported that questionnaire ascertainment of environmental tobacco smoke exposure is more reliable than using cotinine measurements (Emerson et al., 1995). This may be, in part, due to the multiple sources of variability mentioned above.

Measurement of cotinine also reflects exposure to nicotine through routes other than inhalation (such as chewing nicotine gum or using smokeless tobacco). Snuff dipping may result in saliva cotinine concentrations of 0.54 ng/mL to 3.94 ng/mL (Brunnemann et al., 1987), comparable to levels found in passive smokers, and chewing tobacco may elevate saliva cotinine concentrations to levels comparable to those of active smokers (Hatsukami et al., 1987, Palladino et al., 1986).

Additional studies are required to determine the validity of any cotinine categorizations. We must critically evaluate whether by using saliva cotinine as a marker of tobacco smoke exposure we are able to reduce misclassification bias in epidemiologic studies.

Summary

This chapter has reviewed the health effects of environmental tobacco smoke on children. There is strong evidence that passive smoking is associated with higher rates of lower respiratory tract illness in the first year of life, middle ear disease during childhood, and more severe asthma attacks among asthmatic children. This evidence is based on studies that have incorporated multiple measures of exposure, including parental questionnaires and cotinine measurements.

These associations are likely to be casual associations, based on the fulfillment of a number of Hill's criteria for causation (Hill, 1965). The conclusions have been reached by both case-control and cohort studies, conducted by different scientists in different countries at different times. Many, but not all, investigators have demonstrated a dose-response effect. The relationship is biologically plausible based on tobacco smoke's ability to impair the function of cilia and to alter the phagocytic antibacterial defenses of the respiratory tract.

Hill's criterion for experiment ("does an experiment to reduce the exposure result in a reduction of the disease?") is often difficult to fulfill in environmental epidemiology. However, this criterion may be easier to fulfill with exposures and diseases that occur during childhood than with diseases that occur during the adult years. Randomized controlled trials are needed to determine whether interventions to reduce children's exposure to environmental tobacco smoke result in decreased rates of lower respiratory tract illness, middle ear disease, and asthma among children.

Although there is a growing body of evidence linking exposure to environmental tobacco smoke to sudden infant death syndrome, the evidence for causality is somewhat less compelling. Arguments in favor include the fact that the studies have been conducted by many different scientists in different countries at different times. Some investigators have found a dose-response effect. An argument against a casual interpretation is that the relationship between exposure to ETS and SIDS has not yet been shown to be biologically plausible. Future studies will require better assessment of exposure to ETS; investigators should incorporate additional measures of ETS exposure such as personal air monitors and urine cotinine measurements from parents and infants.

Improved methods are needed to strengthen the assessment of environmental tobacco smoke exposure in studies of children's health. This is especially important as rates of smoking decline and children are exposed to lower levels of environmental tobacco smoke. It is important that more sensitive methods of exposure measurement be utilized in order to reduce misclassification in epidemiologic studies, which tends to bias these studies toward finding no effect. Currently, the most sensitive assay method for cotinine is high-performance liquid-chromatography atmospheric pressure chemical ionization in tandem with mass spectrometry. The detection limit for this method is 0.05 ng/mL. Improving the sensitivity of personal monitoring for air nicotine can be accomplished by increasing the period of time over which the air is monitored. These modified methods should be used in future studies of children's exposure to environmental tobacco smoke to strengthen the evidence linking passive smoking to adverse health outcomes in children.

References

Abrams DB, Follick MJ, Biener L, Carey KB, Hitti J. 1987. Saliva cotinine as a measure of smoking status in field settings. Am J Public Health 77: 846–848.

American Academy of Pediatrics. 1986. Involuntary smoking—a hazard to children. Pediatrics 77:755–757.

Anderson LJ, Parker RA, Strikas RA, et al. 1988. Day-care center attendance and hospitalization for lower respiratory tract illness. Pediatrics 82:300–308.

Benowitz NL, Kuyt F, Jacob P, III, Jones RT, Osman AL. 1983. Cotinine disposition and effects. Clin Pharmacol Ther 34: 604–611.

Berg AT, Shapiro ED, Capobianco LA. 1991. Group day care and the risk of serious infectious illnesses. Am J Epidemiol 133:154–163.

Bergman AB, Wiesner BA. 1976. Relationship of passive cigarette smoking to sudden infant death syndrome. Pediatrics 58:665–668.

Black N. 1985. The aetiology of glue ear—a case-control study. Int J Pediatr Otorhinolaryngol 9:121–133.

Bliss RE, O'Connell KA. 1984. Problems with thiocyanate as an index of smoking status: a critical review with suggestions for improving the usefulness of biochemical measures in smoking cessation research. Health Psychol 3:563–581.

Burchfiel CM, Higgins MW, Keller JB, et al. 1986. Passive smoking in childhood: respiratory conditions and pulmonary function in Tecumseh, Michigan. Am Rev Respir Dis 133:966–973.

Breese-Hall C, Hall JH, Gala CL, et al. 1984. Long-term prospective study in children after respiratory syncytial virus infection. J Pediatr 105:358–364.

Brunnemann, KD, Hornby, AP, Stich, HF. 1987. Tobacco-specific nitrosamines in the saliva of Inuit snuff dippers in the Northwest Territories of Canada. Cancer Lett 37: 7–16.

Cameron P. 1967. The presence of pets and smoking as correlates of perceived disease. J Allergy 40:12.

Centers for Disease Control and Prevention. 1994. Cigarette smoking among adults—United States, 1992, and changes in the definition of current cigarette smoking. MMWR 43:342–346.

Chen Y, Li W, Yu S. 1986. Influence of passive smoking on admissions for respiratory illness in early childhood. BMJ 293:303–306.

Chen Y, Li W, Yu S, Qian W. 1988. Chang-Ning epidemiological study of children's health: I. Passive smoking and children's respiratory diseases. Int J Epidemiol 17:348–355.

Chen Y. 1989. Synergistic effect of passive smoking and artificial feeding on hospitalization for respiratory illness in early childhood. Chest 95:1004–1007.

Chilmonczyk BA, Salmun LM, Megathlin KN, et al. 1993. Association between exposure to environmental tobacco smoke and exacerbations of asthma in children. N Engl J Med 328:1665–1669.

Colley JRT, Holland WW, Corkhill RT. 1974. Influence of passive smoking and parental phlegm on pneumonia and bronchitis in early childhood. Lancet 2:1031–1034.

Corbo GM, Fuciarelli F, Foresi A, De Benedetto F. 1989. Snoring in children: association with respiratory symptoms and passive smoking. BMJ 299:1491–1494.

Coultas DB, Howard CA, Peake GT, Skipper BJ, et al. 1987. Salivary cotinine levels and involuntary tobacco smoke exposure in children and adults in New Mexico. Am Rev Respir Dis 136: 305–309.

Coultas DB, Howard CA, Peake, GT, Skipper BJ, et al. 1988. Discrepancies between self-reported and validated cigarette smoking in a community survey of New Mexico Hispanics. Am Rev Respir Dis 137: 810–814.

Dockery DW, Spengler JD. 1981. Indoor-outdoor relationship of respirable sulfates and particles. Atmos Environ 15: 335–343.

Ehrlich R, Kattan M, Godbold J, et al. 1992. Childhood asthma and passive smoking. Urinary cotinine as a biomarker of exposure. Am Rev Respir Dis 145: 594–599.

Emerson JA, Hovell MF, Meltzer SB, et al. 1995. The accuracy of environmental tobacco smoke exposure measures among asthmatic children. J Clin Epidemiol 48:1251–1259.

Etzel RA, Pattishall EN, Haley NJ, et al. 1992. Passive smoking and middle ear effusion among children in day care. Pediatrics 90:228–232.

Evans D, Levison J, Feldman CH, et al. 1987. The impact of passive smoking on emergency room visits of urban children with asthma. Am Rev Respir Dis 135:567–572.

Ey JL, Holberg CJ, Aldous MB et al. 1995. Passive smoke exposure and otitis media in the first year of life. Pediatrics 95:670–677.

Feldman J, Shenker IR, Etzel RA, et al. 1991. Passive smoking alters lipid profiles in adolescents. Pediatrics 88:259–264.

Fergusson DM, Horwood LI, Shannon FT. 1980. Parental smoking and respiratory illness in infancy. Arch Dis Child 55:358–361.

Fleming DW, Cochi SL, Hightower AW, Broome CV. 1987. Childhood upper respiratory tract infection: to what degree is incidence affected by day-care attendance? Pediatrics 79:55–60.

Forastiere F, Agabiti N, Dell'Orco V et al. 1993. Questionnaire data as predictors of urinary cotinine levels among nonsmoking adolescents. Arch Environ Health 48:230–234.

Goldstein GM, Collier A, Etzel R, Lewtas J, Haley N. 1987. Elimination of urinary cotinine in children exposed to known levels of side-stream cigarette smoke. Proceedings of the 4th International Conference on Indoor Air Quality and Climate, Berlin; 61–67.

Greenberg RA, Haley NJ, Etzel RA, Loda FA. 1984. Measuring the exposure of infants to tobacco smoke. N Engl J Med 310: 1075–1078.

Haglund B, Cnattingius S. 1990. Cigarette smoking as a risk factor for sudden infant death syndrome: a population-based study. Am J Public Health 80: 29–32.

Haley NJ, Axelrad CM, Tilton KA. 1983. Validation of self-reported smoking behavior: biochemical analyses of cotinine and thiocyanate. Am J Public Health 73:1204–1207.

Haley NJ, Hoffmann D. 1985. Analysis for nicotine and cotinine in hair to determine cigarette smoker status. Clin Chem 31:1598–1600.

Hammond SK, Sorenson G, Youngstrom R, Ockene JK. 1995. Occupational exposure to environmental tobacco smoke. JAMA 274:956–960.

Harlap S, Davies AM. 1974. Infant admissions to the hospital and maternal smoking. Lancet 1:529–532.

Hatsukami DK, Gust SW, Keenan RM. 1987. Physiologic and subjective changes from smokeless tobacco withdrawl. Clin Pharmacol Ther 41: 103–107.

Hill AB. 1965. The environment and disease: association or causation. Proc R Soc Med 58:295–300.

Hinds WC, First MW. 1975. Concentrations of nicotine and tobacco smoke in public places. N Engl J Med 292: 844–845.

Hinton AE. 1989. Surgery for otitis media with effusion in children and its relationship to parental smoking. J Laryngol Otol 103:559–561.

Hoffman HJ, Damus K, Hillman L, Krongrad E. 1988. Risk factors for SIDS. Results of the National Institute of Child Health and Human Development SIDS Cooperative Epidemiological Study. Ann NY Acad Sci 533:13–30.

Hoffmann D, Haley NJ, Adams JD, Brunnemann KD. 1984. Tobacco sidestream smoke: uptake by nonsmokers. Prev Med 13: 608–617.

Holberg CJ, Wright AL, Martinez FD et al. 1993. Child day care, smoking by caregivers, and lower respiratory tract illness in the first 3 years of life. Pediatrics 91:885–892.

Iversen M, Birch L, Lundqvist GR, et al. 1985. Middle ear effusion in children and the indoor environment: an epidemiological study. Arch Environ Health 40:74–79.

Jarvis MJ, McNeill AD, Russell MAH, West RJ, Bryant A, Feyerabend C. 1987a. Passive smoking in adolescents: one-year stability of exposure in the home. Lancet 1: 1324–1325.

Jarvis MJ, Russell MAH, Feyerabend C. 1983. Absorption of nicotine and carbon monoxide from passive smoking under natural conditions of exposure. Thorax 38: 829–833.

Jarvis MJ, Russell MAH, Feyerabend C, Eiser JR, Morgan M, Gammage P, Gray EM. 1985. Passive exposure to tobacco smoke: saliva cotinine concentrations in a representative population sample of non-smoking schoolchildren. BMJ 291: 927–929.

Jarvis M, Tunstall-Pedoe H, Feyerabend C, Vesey C, Saloojee Y. 1984. Biochemical markers of smoke absorption and self-reported exposure to passive smoking. J Epidemiol Community Health 38:335–339.

Jarvis MJ, Tunstall-Pedoe H, Feyerabend C, Vesey C, Saloojee, Y. 1987b. Comparison of tests used to distinguish smokers from nonsmokers. Am J Public Health 77: 1435–1438.

Johnson LC, Letzel H, Kleinschmidt J. 1985. Passive smoking under controlled conditions. Int Arch Occup Environ Health 56: 99–110.

Kraemer MJ, Richardson MA, Weiss NS, et al. 1983. Risk factors for persistent middle-ear effusions. JAMA 249:1022–1025.

Krzyzanowski M, Quackenboss JJ, Lebowitz MD. 1990. Chronic respiratory effects of indoor formaldehyde exposure. Environ Res 52:117–125.

Langone JJ, Cook G, Bjercke RJ, Lifschitz MH. 1988. Monoclonal antibody ELISA for cotinine in saliva and urine of active and passive smokers. J Immunol Methods 114: 73–78.

Langone JJ, Gijika HB, Van Vunakis H. 1973. Nicotine and its metabolites: radioimmunoassays for nicotine and cotinine. Biochemistry 12: 5025–5030.

Langone JJ, Van Vunakis H, Hill P. 1975. Quantitation of cotinine in sera of smokers. Res Commun Mol Pathol Pharmacol 10:21–28.

Lashner BA, Shaheen NJ, Hanauer SB, et al. 1993. Passive smoking is associated with an increased risk of developing inflammatory bowel disease in children. Am J Gastroenterol 88:356–359.

Lee PN. 1983. Does breathing other people's tobacco smoke cause lung cancer? BMJ 293: 1503–1504.

Lefcoe NM, Inculet II. 1971. Particulates in domestic premises. Arch Environ Health 22:230–238.

Lewak N, van den Berg BJ, Beckwith JB. 1979. Sudden infant death syndrome risk factors. Clin Pediatr (Phila) 18:404–411.

Luck W, Nau H, Hansen R, Steldinger R. 1985. Extent of nicotine and cotinine transfer to the human fetus, placenta and amniotic fluid of smoking mothers. Dev Pharmacol Ther 8:384–395.

Machacek DA, Jiang N-S. 1986. Quantification of cotinine in plasma and saliva by liquid chromatography. Clin Chem 32: 979–982.

Malloy MH, Hoffman HJ, Peterson DR. 1992. Sudden infant death syndrome and maternal smoking. Am J Public Health 82:1380–1382.

Malloy MH, Kleinman JC, Land GH, Schramm WF. 1988. The association of maternal smoking with age and cause of infant death. Am J Epidemiol 128: 46–55.

Marbury MC, Hammond SK, Haley NJ. 1993. Measuring exposure to environmental tobacco smoke in studies of acute health effects. Am J Epidemiol 137: 1089–1097.

Margolis PA, Greenberg RA, Keyes LL, et al. 1992. Lower respiratory illness in infants and low socioeconomic status. Am J Public Health 82:1119–1126.

Martinez FD, Cline M, Burrows B. 1992. Increased incidence of asthma in children of smoking mothers. Pediatrics 89:21–26.

Matsukura S, Taminato T, Kitano N, et al. 1984. Effects of environmental tobacco smoke on urinary cotinine excretion in nonsmokers. N Engl J Med 311: 828–832.

McConnochie KM, Roghmann KJ. 1986. Parental smoking, presence of older siblings, and family history of asthma increase risk of bronchiolitis. Am J Dis Child 140:806–812.

Metz, CE. 1978. Basic principles of ROC analysis. Semin Nucl Med 8:283–298.

Mitchell EA, Scragg R, Stewart AW, et al. 1991. Results from the first year of the New Zealand cot death study. N Z Med J 104:71–76.

Mitchell EA, Ford RPK, Stewart AW, et al. 1993. Smoking and the sudden infant death syndrome. Pediatrics 91:893–896.

Muramatsu M, Umemura S, Okada T, Tomita H. 1984. Estimation of personal exposure to tobacco smoke with a newly developed nicotine personal monitor. Environ Res 35:218–227.

Murray AB, Morrison BJ. 1989. Passive smoking by asthmatics: its greater effect on boys than on girls and on older than on younger children. Pediatrics 84: 451–459.

Murray AB, Morrison BJ. 1993. The decrease in severity of asthma in children of parents who smoke since the parents have been exposing them to less cigarette smoke. J Allergy Clin Immunol 91:102–110.

Naeye RL, Ladis B, Drage JS. 1976. Sudden infant death syndrome: a prospective study. Am J Dis Child 130:1207–1210.

Nafstad P, Botten G, Hagen JA et al. 1995. Comparison of three methods for estimating environmental tobacco smoke exposure among children aged between 12 and 36 months. Int J Epidemiol 24:88–94.

National Research Council. 1986. Environmental Tobacco Smoke: Measuring Exposures and Assessing Health Effects. National Academy Press, Washington, D.C.: p. 2.

O'Connor GT, Weiss ST, Tager IB, Speizer FE. 1987. The effect of passive smoking on pulmonary function and non-specific bronchial responsiveness in a population based sample of children and young adults. Am Rev Respir Dis 135: 800–804.

Ogston SA, Florey C du V, Walker CM. 1987. Association of infant alimentary and respiratory illness with parental smoking and other environmental factors. J Epidemiol Community Health 41:21–25.

Oldigs M, Jorres R, Magnussen H. 1991. Acute effects of passive smoking on lung function and airway responsiveness in asthmatic children. Pediatr Pulmonol 10:123–131.

Owen MJ, Baldwin CD, Swank PR, et al. 1993. Relation of infant feeding practices, cigarette smoke exposure, and group child care to the onset and duration of otitis media with effusion in the first two years of life. J Pediatr 123:702–711.

Palladino G, Brunnemann KD, Adams JD, Haley NJ, Hoffmann D. 1986. Snuff-dipping in college students: a clinical profile. Mil Med 151: 342–346.

Pattishall EN, Strope GL, Etzel RA, et al. 1985. Serum cotinine as a measure of tobacco smoke exposure in children. Am J Dis Child 139:1101–1104.

Pierce JP, Dwyer T, DiGiusto E, Carpenter T, et al. 1987. Cotinine validation of self-reported smoking in commercially run community surveys. J Chron Dis 40:689–696.

Pirkle JL, Flegal KM, Bernert JT, et al. 1996. Exposure of the U.S. population to environmental tobacco smoke: the Third National Health and Nutrition Examination Survey, 1988–1991. JAMA 275:1233–1240.

Rantakallio P. 1978. Relationship of maternal smoking to morbidity and mortality of the child up to the age of five. Acta Paediatr Scand 67:621–631.

Reed BD, Lutz LJ. 1988. Household smoking exposure—association with middle ear effusions. Fam Med 20:426–430.

Reese AC, James IR, Landau LI, LeSouef PN. 1992. Relationship between urinary cotinine levels and diagnosis in children admitted to hospital. Am Rev Respir Dis 146:66–70.

Rylander E, Pershagen G, Eriksson M, Bermann G. 1995. Parental smoking, urinary cotinine, and wheezing bronchitis in children. Epidemiology 6:289–293.

Sandler RS, Sandler DP, McDonnell CW, et al. 1992. Childhood exposure to environmental tobacco smoke and the risk of ulcerative colitis. Am J Epidemiol 135:603–608.

Sasson IM, Haley NJ, Hoffmann D, Wynder EL, Hellberg D, Nilson S. 1985. Cigarette smoking and neoplasia of the uterine cervix: smoke constituents in cervical mucus. N Engl J Med 312: 315–316.

Schoendorf KC, Kiely JL. 1992. Relationship of sudden infant death syndrome to maternal smoking during and after pregnancy. Pediatrics 90:905–908.

Sepkovic DW, Haley NJ. 1985. Biomedical applications of cotinine quantitation in smoking related research. Am J Public Health 75: 663–665.

Sherman CB, Tosteson TD, Tager IB, et al. 1990. Early childhood predictors of asthma. Am J Epidemiol 132:83–95.

Spengler JD, Dockery DW, Turner WA, et al. 1981. Long-term measurements of respirable sulfates and particles inside and outside homes. Atmospheric Environment 15:23–30.

Steele R, Langworth JT. 1966. The relationship of antenatal and postnatal factors to sudden unexpected death in infancy. Can Med Assoc J 94:1165–1171.

Strachan DP, Jarvis MJ, Feyerabend C. 1989. Passive smoking, salivary cotinine concentrations, and middle ear effusion in 7 year old children. BMJ 298: 1549–1552.

Tager IB, Weiss ST, Munoz A, et al. 1983. Longitudinal study of the effects of maternal smoking on pulmonary function in children. N Engl J Med 309: 699–703.

Tainio VM, Savilahti E, Salmenpera L, et al. 1988. Risk factors for infantile recurrent otitis media: atopy but not type of feeding. Pediatr Res 23:509–512.

Takasaka T. 1990. Incidence, prevalence, and natural history of otitis media in different geographic areas and populations. Ann Otol Rhinol Laryngol 99: 13–14.

Taylor JA, Sanderson M. 1995. A reexamination of the risk factors for the sudden infant death syndrome. J Pediatr 126:887–891.

Teele DW, Klein JO, Rosner B. 1989. Epidemiology of otitis media during the first seven years of life in children in greater Boston: a prospective, cohort study. J Infect Dis 160:83–94.

U.S. Department of Health and Human Services. 1989. Reducing the health consequences of smoking: 25 years of progress. A report of the Surgeon General. U.S. Department of Health and Human Services, Public Health Service, Centers for Disease Control, Center for Chronic Disease Prevention and Health Promotion, Office on Smoking and Health, Rockville, Maryland. DHHS Publication No. (CDC) 89-8411.

U.S. Department of Health and Human Services. 1987. The health consequences of involuntary smoking. A report of the Surgeon General. U.S. Department of Health and Human Services, Public Health Service, Centers for Disease Control, Center for Health Promotion and Education, Office on Smoking and Health, Rockville, Maryland. DHHS Publication No. (CDC) 87-8398.

U.S. Environmental Protection Agency. 1992. Respiratory health effects of passive smoking: lung cancer and other disorders. Office of Research and Development, Office of Air and Radiation, Washington, D.C.: EPA/600/6-90/006F.

Van Vunakis H, Langone JJ, Milunsky A. 1974. Nicotine and cotinine in the amniotic fluid of smokers in the second trimester of pregnancy. Am J Obstet Gynecol 120:64–66.

Wald NJ, Boreham J, Bailey A, Ritchie C, Haddow JE, Knight G. 1984. Urinary cotinine as marker of breathing other people's tobacco smoke. Lancet 1: 230–231.

Wall MA, Johnson J, Jacob P, Benowitz NL. 1988. Cotinine in the serum, saliva, and urine of nonsmokers, passive smokers, and active smokers. Am J Public Health 78: 699–701.

Ware JH, Dockery DW, Spiro A, et al. 1984. Passive smoking, gas cooking, and respiratory health of children living in six cities. Am Rev Respir Dis 129: 366–374.

Weitzman M, Gortmaker S, Klein Walker D, Sobol A. 1990. Maternal smoking and childhood asthma. Pediatrics 85:505–511.

Willatt DJ. 1986. Children's sore throats related to parental smoking. Clin Otolaryngol 11:317–321.

Williams CL, Eng A, Botvin GJ, Hill P, Wynder EL. 1979. Validation of students' self-reported cigarette smoking status with plasma cotinine levels. Am J Public Health 69: 1272–1274.

Woodward A, Douglas RM, Graham NMH, Miles H. 1990. Acute respiratory illness in Adelaide children: breast feeding modifies the effect of passive smoking. J Epidemiol Community Health 44:224–230.

Wright AL, Holberg C, Martinez FD, Taussig LM. 1991. Relationship of parental smoking to wheezing and nonwheezing lower respiratory tract illnesses in infancy. J Pediatr 118: 207–214.

Environmental Tobacco Smoke II: Lung Cancer

10

ANNA H. WU

WORLDWIDE, environmental tobacco smoke (ETS) exposure is among the leading environmental health concerns, based on the high prevalence of exposure and on the severity of the diseases with which it has been associated. Lung cancer is the outcome that the general public most strongly associates with ETS.

Exposures to tobacco smoke for nonsmokers are very low compared to those of active smokers. The median levels of serum cotinine for ETS-exposed nonsmokers in the Third National Health and Nutrition Examination Survey (NHANESIII) was approximately 0.5 ng/ml, with an upper limit of about 10 to 15 ng/mL. Active smokers had a median serum cotinine level of approximately 180 ng/mL. This large discrepancy between cotinine levels for nonsmokers and smokers has led some to believe that ETS could have little if any health effect. If ETS is measured in "active smoking equivalents" based on cotinine, then most ETS exposures are equivalent to less than a single cigarette per day. Yet there is a strong body of evidence linking ETS with lung cancer.

As this chapter points out, cotinine is probably not a good marker of the relevant exposure. There are a number of carcinogenic biomarkers with higher relative levels in ETS-exposed nonsmokers compared with active smokers than cotinine, which is not itself carcinogenic.

This chapter reviews the evidence from a very large number of epidemiologic studies linking ETS to lung cancer. These studies are mostly case-control studies of never-smoking women, in which exposure is usually defined as being married to a smoker. The case-control design has been motivated by the fact that lung cancer is a rare disease among never-smokers. Women have been studied predominantly because a much higher percentage of women than men have never smoked. Exposure defined by marriage to a smoker has been used because it is relatively easily and accurately ascertained via questionnaires. Furthermore, numerous exposure assessments have indicated that spousal smoking is a good marker of overall ETS exposure, although significant exposure takes place at work and in social settings. The weight of the evidence from lung cancer studies is that there is a small but consistent excess of lung cancer, on the order of 20% to 30%, among never-smoking women married to smokers versus never-smoking women married to nonsmokers.

This chapter covers the questions that have been raised as to whether this overall finding represents a causal relation. Relatively few potential confounding variables could explain these findings. Biases arising from selective recall or misclassification of never-smoking status also seem unlikely to explain the findings. While the overall increase is relatively well established, controversy continues to surround other issues, such as whether workplace exposure contributes substantially to lung cancer, or which biomarkers are useful for exposure assessment.

The first epidemiologic studies of ETS and lung cancer (Hirayama, 1981; Trichopoulos et al., 1981) showed that nonsmokers married to smokers had a significantly higher risk of lung cancer than nonsmokers married to nonsmokers. Some 30 epidemiologic studies have since been published. Although most of the individual studies demonstrated a small increased risk, few of the studies had statistically significant results, in part because all the studies published in the 1980s had small sample sizes that lacked sufficient statistical power to detect a significant association. As a result, meta-analysis was used to pool results of comparable studies in order to gain a more accurate estimate of the association between ETS and lung cancer. The individual studies have been reviewed extensively and numerous meta-analyses have been published (U.S. Surgeon General, 1986; National Research Council [NRC], 1986; Arundel et al., 1987; Letzel et al., 1988; Vainio and Partensen, 1989; Wu-Williams and Samet, 1989; Repace and Lowry 1990; Spizer et al., 1990; Fleiss and Gross, 1991; EPA, 1992; Kilpatrick, 1992; Katzenstein, 1992; Pershagen, 1992; Wells, 1991a,b, 1993).

The most recently published meta-analysis on lung cancer and ETS was conducted by the U.S. Environmental Protection Agency (EPA, 1992). The EPA report covered a total of 30 epidemiologic studies (four prospective follow-up and 26 case-control studies) from eight countries. Most studies of lung cancer and ETS exposure among never-smokers have been case-control studies because lung cancer is very rare among never-smokers. A cohort study would require large sample sizes and relatively long follow-up to have much statistical power, but such studies have the advantage of ascertaining exposure to ETS prospectively.

All the studies reviewed in the EPA report examined risk of lung cancer in nonsmokers in relation to spouses' smoking habits. Each study was examined in detail and then all were analyzed collectively. Because no studies were exactly alike and the individual studies varied in sample size and had different methodologic strengths and weaknesses, the EPA ranked studies in four tiers of quality and gave special weight to the 15 studies in the two highest tiers. There is, however, no consensus regarding the use of quality scores to weigh the studies included in a meta-analysis (Greenland, 1994a,b; Olkin, 1994). The EPA authors also calculated pooled risk estimates for ETS by country because ETS exposure is likely to be variable across countries due not only to different chemical composition of tobacco smoke but also to widely differing social customs and corresponding levels of exposure.

Combined results by country showed statistically significant associations for Greece (two studies; OR=2.01, 90% CI=1.42, 2.84), Hong Kong (four studies; OR=1.48, 90% CI=1.21, 1.81), Japan (five studies, OR=1.41, 90% CI=1.18, 1.69), and the United States (11 studies, OR=1.19, 90% CI=1.04, 1.35). The pooled result of the four western European studies was also elevated although the result did not reach statistical significance (three countries; OR=1.17, 90% CI=0.84, 1.62). The combined results of the Chinese studies did not show an association between ETS and lung cancer (OR=0.95, 90% CI=0.81, 1.12) (Table 5-9, EPA report); however, two of the four Chinese studies were designed mainly to determine the lung cancer effects of high levels of other indoor air pollutants indigenous to those areas, which would obscure a smaller ETS effect. The EPA report concluded that ETS is a human lung carcinogen, responsible for approximately 3000 lung cancer deaths per year in U.S. nonsmokers.

Despite careful considerations of many methodologic issues of concern in the meta-analysis on ETS and lung cancer (e.g., measurement of ETS exposure, misclassification bias of nonsmoker status and disease status, adjustment for potential confounders), the EPA report drew criticisms. Some of the debate centered around issues that were specific to the study of ETS and lung cancer, including misclassification bias of smokers as nonsmokers and the extent of such misclassification (Gori 1993, 1994a,b). On the other hand, other issues were generic to meta-analysis techniques and they include possible publication bias of positive studies and difficulty in obtaining adjusted risk estimates (Gori 1993, 1994a,b) for meta-analysis.

The EPA scientists responded to these criticisms (Farland et al., 1994; Jinot and Bayard, 1994). In addition, Bero et al. (1994) reviewed in detail the issue of publication bias and concluded that there is no publication bias against studies showing no association with ETS in the peer-reviewed literature.

Since the publication of the EPA report, results are available from three large population-based case-control studies, one hospital-based case-control study, and one cohort study conducted in the United States. Florida (Stockwell et al., 1992), Missouri (Brownson et al., 1992), and five geographic areas in the United States—New Orleans, Louisiana; Atlanta, Georgia; Houston, Texas; Los Angeles County, and San Francisco Bay Area (referred to as the U.S. multicenter study) (Fontham et al., 1991, 1994)—were the study areas of the population-based case-control studies; six hospitals located in four U.S. cities (New York City, Chicago, Detroit, and Philadelphia were included in the hospital-based case-control study (Kabat et al., 1995). The cohort study, referred to as the Cancer Prevention Study (CPS)-II, was conducted by the American Cancer Society involving participants in all 50 states (Cardenas et al., in press). This chapter will review these five new U.S. studies, comparing similarities and differences in their results and study methods, and summarize their results. Next, we will examine some of the major issues in studies of ETS and lung cancer. Finally, we will describe the accumulating information on internal doses of ETS exposure based on various markers of exposure (cotinine, aminobiphenyl [ABP]-adducts, polycyclic aromatic hydrocarbon [PAH]-adducts). This information reinforces the difficulties in using biomarkers to estimate past ETS exposure and to determine the lung cancer risk for never-smokers exposed to ETS via the use of "cigarette equivalent" doses, based on comparing the biomarkers levels between ETS-exposed never-smokers and active smokers.

U.S. Studies Available Since 1991—Four Case-Control Studies and one Cohort Study

Sample size

Table 10-1 summarizes the study methods of the case-control and cohort studies conducted in the United States and published since 1991. One important advantage of the three population-based case-control studies is that the sample sizes were substantially larger than previously published case-control studies in the United States (Correa et al., 1983; Buffler et al., 1984; Kabat and Wynder, 1984; Dalager et al., 1986; Wu et al., 1985; Garfinkel et al.; 1985; Humble et al., 1987; Brownson et al., 1987; Janerich et al., 1990). The largest was the U.S. multicenter study, with about 3 to 4 times as many lung cancer cases and controls as the Florida study and about 30% more cases and 10% more controls than the Missouri study. The sample size of 653 cases and 1253 controls in the U.S. multicenter study can be compared to a total of 470 cases and 1218 controls accumulated in all the other nine U.S. case-control studies combined (excluding the first 3 years of the U.S. Multicenter study (Fontham et al., 1991) that were included in the EPA report. The large sample sizes of the three population-based case-control studies provided sufficient statistical power to examine a relatively weak ETS association, and also permitted adjustment for potential confounders (e.g., dietary habits, occupation, family and personal histories) that were seldom considered in previous studies. The hospital-based case-control study conducted by Kabat et al. (1995) included 110 never-smoking lung cancer patients and 304 never-smoking hospital patient controls. This study had an approximately 30% power to detect a significant association if the OR for lung cancer is 1.5 in relation to spousal smoking (assuming a prevalence of 60% of control husbands who smoked and 30% of control wives who smoked, an alpha of 0.05, and a 2-sided test). The OR for lung cancer in relation to spousal smoking is about 1.20 according to the EPA report.

The CPS-II cohort study included a considerably larger number of lung cancer deaths among nonsmoking subjects compared to published prospective studies of lung cancer and ETS in the United States three cases in one study (Butler, 1990) and 153 cases in a second study (Garfinkel, 1985). However, even in this large cohort study, there were only 255 lung cancer deaths available for analysis; approximately 1000 expected cases are needed to achieve 80% statistical power (assuming an RR of 1.2, alpha of 0.05, 2-sided testing, and 60% of nonsmoking women who were exposed).

Sources of lung cancer patients and controls

Three of the four case-control studies were population-based studies in which lung cancer patients were identified from the cancer registries and hospitals covering a specific study area. The use of population-based cases avoids the possibility of selection bias associated with cases from selected hospitals. The use of population-based controls instead of other patients as controls is also important because ETS exposure of patients with certain diagnoses may be higher and not representative of the exposure distribution of the source population from which cases were drawn. In the hospital-based case-control study, approximately 30%

Table 10-1. Study characteristics of the U.S. case-control and cohort studies published since 1991

	Case-Control Studies				Cohort Study, Cardenas et al. in press
	Stockwell et al. 1992	Brownson et al. 1992	Fontham et al. 1994	Kabat et al. 1995	
Area	Central Florida	Missouri	5 US metropolitan areas	4 US cities	50 U.S. states
Accrual Period	1987–91	1986–91	1985–91	1983–90	1982–89
Sample size (lifetime nonsmokers)					
cases	210 (F)	430 (F)	653 (F)	69 (F), 41 (M)	150(F), 97 (M)
controls	301 (F)	1166 (F)	1253 (F)	187 (F), 117 (M)	192,234 (F) 281,536 (M) [a]
Source of cases	Florida Cancer Registry	Missouri Cancer Registry	All hospital/registries in specific geographic areas	6 hospitals in the 4 cities	Identified by 3 direct mailed inquiries & linkage with NDI
Source of controls	RDD	DMV, HCFA	RDD, HCFA	Other hospital patients	NA
Percent of self-respondent					
cases	33	34 [b]	63	100	100
controls	100	100	100	100	100

Data collection	In-person, telephone, mailed questionnaires	Telephone	In-person	In-person	Mailed questionnaire
Histologic confirmation	100%	76%[c]	100%[c]	100%	47%
Percent of adenocarcinoma	61%	66%	76%	NA	70%
Definition of lifetime nonsmoker	Smoked total <6mo. or <100 cigarettes in lifetime	Not described	<100 cigarettes, no use of other tobacco for >6 mo.	<365 cigarettes over lifetime	Not described
Verification of nonsmoking status	Multistep—medical record, physician, at initial contact & interview	At interview	Multistep—medical record, physician, at initial contact & interview	At interview	Spouses' own report of tobacco use
Biological markers	None	None	Urinary cotinine	None	None

[a] In the Cardenas et al. (in press) study, number of lung cancer death in never-smokers is shown under cases and persons never smoked enrolled in the cohort is shown under controls.

[b] Presented for nonsmokers and ex-smokers combined.

[c] Confirmed by independent histologic review.

Abbreviations: F—females, M—males, NA—not available, NDI—National Death Index, RDD—random digit dialing, DMV—Department of Motor Vehicles, HCFA—Health Care Financing Administration.

of the control patients were diagnosed with cancers (stomach/intestine, genitourinary tract, or lymphatic and hematopoietic system) that may be positively associated with tobacco use (Austin and Cole 1986; Brownson et al., 1993; Forman, 1991; Wu-Williams et al., 1990; Yu et al., 1986). Thus, the prevalence of ETS exposure among some controls in this study may be higher than the general population, leading to a bias toward the null.

Lung cancer deaths in the CPS-II study was determined by active inquiries of the vital status of study subjects in 1984, 1986, and 1988 and by automated linkage using the National Death Index through December 31, 1989 (Cardenas et al., in press). Because the follow-up of the cohort was uniform irrespective of the ETS exposure status, problems of selection bias (a concern of case-control studies) is not applicable in this cohort study design. In addition, for the subset of subjects who resided in areas with an existing SEER (Surveillance, Epidemiology, and End Results) tumor registry, the diagnosis of lung cancer was verified over 90% of the time. The percentage of adenocarcinoma of the lung in this study (70%) is also compatible with the proportion of this cell type reported in other studies of lung cancer in nonsmokers (Table 10-1).

Recall bias

It is important to minimize differential recall between lung cancer cases and controls. This issue was addressed in the U.S. multicenter study (Fontham et al., 1991) and the study by Kabat et al. (1995). In the first 3 years of the U.S. multicenter study (Fontham et al., 1991), a colon cancer control group was interviewed as a second control group because there is no known association between active or passive smoking and risk of colon cancer, and it provided an opportunity to examine the issue of recall bias associated with a recent diagnosis of cancer. The findings on ETS were comparable when lung cancer patients were compared to population controls and to colon cancer controls, suggesting that recall bias resulting from having a diagnosis of cancer was not a likely explanation of the observed association. In the study by Kabat et al. (1995), cases and controls were interviewed while they were hospitalized. Because control patients had diagnoses of various cancer and noncancer outcomes, the concern of selective recall bias associated with being ill or hospitalized is minimized in this study. In the CPS-II cohort study, ETS exposure status (i.e., spousal smoking) was determined for all subjects at the time of enrollment, eliminating any possibility of selective recall bias.

Misclassification of smokers as nonsmokers

In the 1986 National Research Council report and a subsequent paper, Wald et al. (1986) pointed out that because smokers tend to marry smokers, if a study contains subjects who are classified as nonsmokers when they are not, they are more likely to be classified as exposed to ETS and thus the estimate of relative risk of exposure to ETS will be exaggerated due to the association of lung cancer with active smoking for this group of deceivers. Wald et al. (1986) estimated the proportion of ever-smokers who are misclassified as lifelong nonsmokers to be about 7%. This estimate was based on the percent of self-reported nonsmokers (2.1%) who have levels of nicotine and cotinine in the range of those of smokers and the percent of smokers who on subsequent re-interview claimed to have never smoked (4.9%). Lee (1986, 1989, 1991a–c) has argued that the true extent of this misclassification bias is higher, about 12%. The actual level of misclassification in any individual study is likely to vary and may be dependent on the methods that are used to enroll lifetime nonsmokers and the definition of a lifetime nonsmoker. Definitions of nonsmokers and verification of nonsmoking status for the four case-control studies are shown in Table 10-1. Verification by multiple sources, as was done in two of the four studies, will tend to decrease misclassification.

Biomarker confirmation of current nonsmoking status

The U.S. multicenter study was the only case-control study in which subjects' current nonsmoking status was corroborated by measurement of urinary cotinine levels. Cotinine, a sensitive and specific biologic marker of tobacco exposure in the previous 72 hours (Haley et al., 1983) was measured on 81% of self-respondent cases and 83% of controls. Levels of urinary cotinine exceeding 100 ng/mg or higher were found in 0.6% of cases and 2.3% of controls, indicating a very low percentage of misclassification of smokers as nonsmokers (Fontham et al., 1994) and compatible with the estimate used by Wald et al. (1986). The low level of misclassification of smokers as nonsmokers in the U.S. multicenter study may be attributed to the strict definition of nonsmokers used in the study as well as the multistep procedure used to identify lifetime nonsmokers. This cotinine test is particularly useful for control subjects; case subjects who were former smokers are likely not to have been currently smoking because of their disease. Although the urinary cotinine/creatinine concentration only assesses current smoking (there are currently no biomarkers that allow assessment of past tobacco exposure), this provided an additional verification of the current nonsmoking status.

Summary of results from the four case-control and one cohort studies

Table 10-2 summarizes the findings from these studies on the association between ETS exposure from spouses and risk of lung cancer. In all five studies, the risk of lung cancer in nonsmokers was increased in relation to spousal smoking; the results were statistically significant in two studies. In the Missouri study, although there was no increased risk of lung cancer in the ever-exposed category for spousal ETS (adjusted OR = 1.0; 95% CI = 0.8, 1.2), an OR of 1.3 (95% CI = 1.0, 1.7) was obtained for the highest exposure category to spouses' smoking (greater than 40 pack-years). In the hospital-based study (Kabat et al., 1995), the OR for lung cancer in men was 1.60 (95% CI = 0.67, 3.82) in relation to wives' smoking; the OR for lung cancer in women was 1.08 (95% CI = 0.60, 1.94) in relation to husbands' smoking. We calculate that the OR for lung cancer is 1.19 (95% CI = 0.76, 1.87) in association with spousal smoking for men and women combined. In the CPS II study, the risk of lung cancer was 1.17 (95% CI = 0.84, 1.64) for nonsmoking men whose wives smoked and 1.05 (95% CI = 0.62, 1.75) for nonsmoking women whose husbands smoked. The risk of lung cancer among nonsmoking women was higher when their husbands continued to smoke (RR = 1.27, 95% CI = 0.85, 1.89) or smoked more than 35 pack-years of cigarettes during the marriage (RR = 1.53, 95% CI = 0.85, 2.77). In the Florida and the U.S. multicenter studies, ever-exposure to ETS from spouses and increasing levels of ETS exposure from spouses were associated with significant increased risks of lung cancer. The finding from the U.S. multicenter study was closest to the pooled estimate from the EPA report; ORs of 1.3 (95% CI = 1.0 to 1.6) for ever-exposed to smoking spouses and 1.8 (95% CI = 1.0, 3.3) for 80 or more pack-years exposure to spouses' smoking. The finding from the Florida study was among the strongest reported for the U.S. studies: ORs of 1.6 (95% CI = 0.8 to 3.0) for ever-exposed to smoking spouses and 2.4 (95% CI = 1.1, 5.3) for 40 or more smoke-years in adulthood. Overall, the results from these five new U.S. studies published since 1991 are certainly compatible with the pooled estimate of the EPA report.

Issues in Studies of ETS and Lung Cancer

Self-respondent versus surrogate respondents

Lee (1993) suggested that the use of only self-respondent control subjects, in studies where cases often have died and interviews are done with next-of-kin, may introduce a type of information bias. However, there is evi-

Table 10-2. Association between risk[a] of lung cancer in lifetime nonsmokers and exposure to spouses' smoking

Stockwell et al., 1992	
Spouse smoked	Adjusted OR[b]
yes	1.6 (0.8–3.0)
Smoking in adult household (spouse and others)	
<22	1.6 (0.8–3.2)
23–39	1.4 (0.7–2.9)
40+	2.4 (1.1–5.3)

Brownson et al., 1992	
Spouse smoked	Adjusted OR[c]
ever	1.0 (0.8–1.2)
Cigarette pack-years	
0–15	0.7 (0.5–1.1)
15–40	0.7 (0.5–1.0)
40+	1.3 (1.0–1.7)

Fontham et al., 1994	
Spouse smoked	Adjusted OR[d]
any type of tobacco	1.29 (1.04–1.60
cigarettes	1.18 (0.96–1.46)
cigars	1.25 (0.92–1.71)
pipes	1.19 (0.88–1.60)
Pack-years of spouses's smoking	Adjusted OR[d]
<15.0	1.08 (0.86–1.39)
15.1–39.9	1.04 (0.76–1.42)
40.0–79.9	1.36 (0.97–1.91)
80.0+	1.79 (0.99–3.25)

dence that dead controls would be unrepresentative of the general population because exposures associated with premature death (i.e. tobacco, alcohol, use of other drugs, diagnoses of certain medical conditions) are over-represented in dead controls compared with living controls (Rogot and Reid, 1975; Gordis, 1982; Mclaughlin et al., 1985). On this basis, it is reasonable to assume that exposure to ETS may be over-represented if dead controls were used. In some studies in which most cases are decedents, proxy interviews for live controls may be desirable, particularly in situations when the information about the exposure of interest is obtained by interview and there is evidence that a proxy report for the case is considerably less accurate than the control's self-report of the same exposure variables (Wacholder et al., 1992). However, it is un-

Table 10-2. (*continued*)

Kabat et al., 1995

	Males Adjusted OR[e]	Females Adjusted OR[e]
Spouse smoked		
yes	1.60 (0.67–3.82)	1.08 (0.60–1.94)
Amount smoked by spouse		
1–10 cigarettes/day	0.74 (0.24–2.23)	0.82 (0.42–1.61)
11 + cigarettes/day	7.48 (1.35–41.36)	1.06 (0.49–2.30)

Cardenas et al., in press

	Males Adjusted OR[f]	Females Adjusted OR[f]
Spouse smoked		
yes	1.05 (0.62–1.75)	1.17 (0.84–1.64)
Pack-years of exposure		
1–16	not available	1.06 (0.51–2.14)
17–35		1.34 (0.70–2.53)
36+		1.53 (0.85–2.77)

[a] All risk estimates were calculated using subjects married to never-smoking spouses as the reference group. The exception is the study by Stockwell et al. (1992) in which the baseline group was women who had no household ETS exposure; 95% CI are in parentheses.

[b] Adjusted for age, race, and education.

[c] Adjusted for age, and previous lung disease.

[d] Adjusted for age, race, study area, education, fruits, vegetables, and supplemental vitamin index, dietary cholesterol, family history of lung cancer, and employment in high-risk occupations.

[e] Adjusted for age, years of education and type of hospital.

[f] Adjusted for age, gender, education, dietary factors, and previous lung disease.

clear whether this type of control is suitable for studies on ETS. In studies of ETS, the surrogate respondent may be a spouse or other family members (Table 10-3), and the surrogate's reporting of ETS may be more accurate than the self-respondent's assessment of the spouses' smoking (i.e., if the respondent is the spouse and assuming there is no under-or over-reporting by the spouse).

Most of the case-control studies on ETS and lung cancer have included some percentage of case patients for whom information was obtained from a surrogate respondent. In the U.S. multicenter study, the odds ratios associated with ETS exposure during adult life were similar for self- and surrogate respondents (Fontham et al., 1991, 1994) but there were appreciable differences for ETS exposure during childhood (Fontham et al., 1994). However, in the Florida study (Stockwell et al., 1992) as well as two other U.S. studies (Garfinkel et al., 1985; Janerich et al., 1990), odds ratios obtained from surrogates differed from those of self-respondents even for adult ETS exposure; the ORs also differed depending on the

Table 10-3. Odds ratios for lung cancer in nonsmokers in relation to exposure to ETS by respondent type

Garfinkel et al., 1985

Respondent type	Smoke Exposure		Husband's Smoking Habits	
	Last 5 yr	Last 25 yr	Total	At home
Self (n=16)	1.96	0.91	0.83	1.00
Husband (n=34)	1.00	0.46	0.77	0.92
Children (n=48)	0.92	1.41	3.57	3.19
Other (n=36)	2.23	2.23	1.58	0.77

Janerich et al., 1990

Respondent type		Spouse Smoked				
	No/yes	Smoke-yr		Pack-yr		
		1–24	25+	1–24	25–49	50+
Self (n=129)	0.93	0.78	1.07	0.71	0.98	1.10
Surrogate (n=59)	0.44	0.33	0.33	0.16	0.68	0.20

Stockwell et al., 1992

Respondent type	Adulthood (husband and others)			All lifetime household exposure		
	<22	22–39	40+ (yr)	<22	22–39	40+ (yr)
Self (n=70)	3.4	3.6+	4.7+	2.0	4.4[a]	4.1[a]
Husband (n=48)	3.1	1.8	4.2	3.2	1.0	3.5
Other surrogate (n=92)	0.8	0.8	1.5	0.6	0.6	1.5

[a]95% confidence intervals exclude 1.0.

relationship of the surrogate respondent to the self-respondent (Stockwell et al., 1992, Garfinkel et al., 1985) (Table 10-3). These results suggest some heterogeneity in risk estimates by respondent types although there is no consistent pattern. The error introduced by surrogate respondents may be random, biasing the results toward the null.

This variability in a surrogate's knowledge regarding ETS exposure of an index subject is also evident in a cross-sectional study (Cummings et al., 1989). In this study, healthy nonsmoker subjects who attended a free cancer checkup clinic and suitable surrogates selected for each subject were asked about the subject's exposure to ETS during childhood and adult life, including exposures at home and at work. There was generally good agreement (kappa of about 0.7) between subjects and their siblings regarding subjects' exposure to ETS at home during childhood, and about their parents' smoking habits. The level of agreement between subjects and their spouses regarding subjects' exposure to smoke at home during adult life was modest (kappa = 0.54) but the agreement was considerably higher regarding spouses' smoking habits (kappa = 0.79). The level of agreement was generally lower when children and other relatives of subjects (kappa of about 0.2 to 0.4) were asked the same questions regarding subjects' exposures at home during adult life. These results show that a surrogate's knowledge of the ETS exposure of an index subject is variable, dependent on their relationship and the period of exposure of interest. It is likely that the quality of information on ETS exposure and other risk factors is higher in studies in which a high percentage of interviews is conducted with self-respondents.

Adjustment for potential confounders

Another criticism of the lung cancer studies showing a small increased risk associated with ETS is that confounding factors may have influenced the observed associations (Mantel, 1983; Katzenstein, 1992; Layard, 1993). In particular, it is been suggested that nonsmokers living with smokers have lower dietary intakes of specific micronutrients (Koo et al., 1988; Sidney et al., 1989; Le Marchand et al., 1991; Matanoski et al., 1995), including beta-carotene, which may be protective for lung cancer. However, there is little evidence of confounding by dietary factors in case-control (Fontham et al., 1994; Kalandidi et al., 1990) or cohort studies of ETS and lung cancer (Cardenas et al., in press). Fontham et al. (1994) reported similar trends of increased risk of lung cancer associated with increasing smoke-years of exposure at all levels of dietary factors (including index of fruits, vegetables and supplemental vitamin use and dietary cholesterol). Furthermore, report from the first randomized trial of supplementation with antioxidant vitamins indicated no protection against lung cancer (Alpha-Tocopherol, Beta-Carotene Cancer Prevention Study Group, 1994). Other factors including employment in high-risk occupations (Fontham et al., 1994; Cardenas et al., in press) and previous lung diseases (Brownson et al., 1992; Wu et al, 1995; Cardenas et al., in press) were examined in case-control and cohort studies, and they did not confound the ETS and lung cancer association.

Measurement of ETS exposure

Because of the importance of obtaining a comprehensive measure of lifetime ETS exposure (Cummings et al., 1989), all four case-controls studies (Brownson et al., 1992; Stockwell et al., 1992; Fontham et al., 1994; Kabat et al., 1995) included questions to assess ETS exposure from spouses and other household members (childhood and adulthood), at the workplace and at other social settings. In addition to including questions covering all sources of exposure, it is equally important to develop study instruments that are valid and reliable. Validated questionnaires have been developed to measure ETS exposure—in particular, to assess current exposure to ETS (Coghlin et al., 1989). Coghlin et al. (1989) found a very high correlation (over 0.90) between ETS exposure measured by passive monitors of nicotine and a questionnaire-derived ETS exposure index that included responses regarding the number of smokers, number of hours of exposure, and proximity to exposure in a recent week.

There is also generally good agreement in the responses on ETS exposure when subjects themselves were asked on two different occasions whether specific household members smoked although the level of agreement diminished on quantitative aspects of smoking by household members (Pron et al., 1986; Coultas et al., 1989; Brownson et al., 1993a). Pron et al. (1986) also reported higher concordance level in subjects' report of residential than workplace ETS exposure. Although there was generally high concordance on exposure to ETS during childhood and parents' smoking habits (Coultas et al., 1989; Brownson et al., 1993a), this high level of agreement was based on responses reported by the subjects themselves. Thus the failure in most studies in obtaining clearer associations between the risk of lung cancer and ETS exposure form sources other than spouses may be partly explained by the fact that such exposures are reported less reliably.

Workplace ETS exposure

In addition to ETS exposure inside the home, ETS exposure outside the home may be equally important. ETS exposure at the workplace represents one important source of ETS exposure outside the home (Biggerstaff et al., 1994; LeVois and Layard, 1994; Repace and Lowrey, 1993).

Table 10-4 summarizes case-control studies that included questions on ETS exposure at the workplace. Indicators of workplace ETS exposure were varied (the actual questions asked were not provided and we deduced what was asked based on the variables presented in the results section). In some studies, the indicators of workplace ETS exposure were limited to the most recent job or the last job, at other specific times or the timing of the question was not specified. In one study, number of smokers at work (lifetime) and amount of time working with smokers was assessed. In another study, ETS exposure at each workplace of at least 3 months was asked. In three other studies, lifetime occupational history was asked and exposure to ETS was assessed for each job. Janerich et al. (1990) did not find any association between exposure to tobacco smoke in the workplace and risk but they acknowledged they did not have enough information about the level of exposure in the workplace to assess

Table 104. Studies on ETS exposure at the workplace among lifetime nonsmoking subjects

Study	Years of Study	Cases/Controls	Questions on ETS at Work	ETS Exposure (%) in Controls (ever-exposed)	Odds Ratio (ever-exposed)
Studies in United States					
Kabat (1984)	1961–80	25/25 (M) 54/53 (F)	Current or last job	44% 58%	0.98 (0.8, 1.0) 1.00 (0.5, 2.1)
Garfinkel (1985)	1971–81	134/402	Number hr/day exposed to smoke at work, past 5 & 25 yr	Past 5 yr: 17% Past 25 yr: 47%	0.88 (0.7, 1.2) 0.93 (0.7, 1.2)
Wu (1985)	1981–82	29/62	Number yr exposed at each job	52%	1.3 (0.5, 3.3)
Janerich (1990)	1982–84	191/191	Number smokers at work (lifetime), amount of time working with smokers	NA	NA
Brownson (1992)	1986–91	430/1166	Current/most recent job, exposed to others' smoke	NA	NA

Study	Years	Cases/Controls	Exposure	%	RR (CI)
Stockwell (1992)	1987–91	210/301	Not described	NA	NA
Fontham (1994)	1985–91	653/1253	Number yr exposed at each job (lifetime yr of exposure at work)	61%	1.39 (1.1, 1.7)
Kabat (1995)	1983–90	41/117 (M) 58/149 (F)	For 4 jobs that lasted 1 year or more	56% (M) 57% (F)	1.02 (0.50–2.09) 1.15 (0.62–2.13)
Studies in United Kingdom and Greece					
Lee (1986)	1977–82	10/98 (M) 15/158 (F)	Timing not specified; rated exposure as no, little, a lot	59% 28%	1.61 (0.4, 6.6) 0.63 (0.2, 2.3)
Kalandidi (1990)	1987–89	91/120	Current/last job number smokers at work	9%	1.39 (0.8, 2.5)
Studies in Asia					
Koo (1987)	1981–83	80/136	Any ETS exposure at work (all jobs)	9%	0.91
Shimizu (1988)	1982–85	90/163	Most recent/ current job, any smokers at work	35%	1.2
Wu-Williams (1990)	1985–87	417/602	Exposure at each job (lifetime)	50%	1.1 (0.9, 1.6)

the precision of their measurements (actual results were not presented). In the study by Koo et al. (1987) in Hong Kong, there was also no association with ETS exposure at the workplace but less than 10% of nonsmoking women in this study reported they were exposed at work. In three other studies in which assessment of workplace exposure to ETS was complete, covering all jobs, and there was considerable exposure among women in the studies, the findings are generally supportive of an association between workplace ETS exposure and risk of lung cancer (Wu et al., 1985; Wu-Williams et al., 1990; Fontham et al., 1994). In particular, results from the U.S. multicenter study (Fontham et al., 1994) suggested a trend of increasing risks with increasing duration of exposure to ETS at the workplace. Compared to women who had no ETS exposure at the workplace, women who reported exposure 1–15, 16–30, and 30 or more years showed adjusted odds ratios of 1.30, 1.40, and 1.86, respectively (p for trend=.001).

In addition to the incomplete assessment of ETS workplace exposure in some studies, it is likely that surrogate respondents may be less able to provide information on the subjects' exposure to ETS at the workplace. This may be a particularly important problem in studies in which the proportion of surrogate respondents was high (Brownson et al., 1992; Stockwell et al., 1992).

Despite some of the above-mentioned difficulties in obtaining histories of lifetime ETS exposure at the workplace, this source of ETS exposure is as likely to increase the risk of lung cancer as ETS exposure from spouses. The workplace has been a major source of exposure to ETS outside the home (Cummings et al., 1990; Emmons et al., 1992; Siegel, 1993) although increasingly companies are restricting smoking in the workplace. In the IARC 10-country collaborative study that correlated urinary cotinine levels to self-reported recent exposure to ETS from spouses, workplace, and other social settings, Riboli et al. (1990) found that exposure to ETS at the workplace was a significant predictor of cotinine levels similar to ETS exposure from spouses. In this study, self-reported exposure to ETS from the husband would predict an increase of 6.2 ng cotinine (adjusted for creatinine) above the baseline level whereas exposure to ETS at work would predict about half of the increase in cotinine levels as from husbands.

The levels of ETS exposure in the workplace are likely to vary, dependent to a large extent on whether there is any restriction of tobacco smoke and the room conditions of the workplace if tobacco smoking is allowed. According to a risk assessment of the risk of ETS exposure in the workplace conducted by Repace and Lowry (1993), they estimated that exposure to 2.3 µg/m³ nicotine for 40 years is associated with a significant increase in risk of lung cancer. This level of ETS exposure at the workplace is not uncommon, particularly in settings with no smoking restriction. For example, in a study of railroad office workers in which there is no smoking restriction, about half of the subjects who worked in the railroad offices showed exposure levels over 5 $\mu g/m^3$ nicotine (Hammond, 1995). In the Wellworks study in which distribution of ETS exposure was compared by smoking policy at the workplace, in open and closed offices in which smoking was allowed, levels of ETS exposure measured by passive samplers was over 6.8 $\mu g/m^3$ nicotine at least 50% of the time, whereas the levels of exposure were substantially less in work settings where tobacco smoke was restricted or banned (Hammond, 1995). Moreover, in another study in which levels of ETS exposure at the workplace and at homes of smokers were compared, Hammond (1995) showed that ETS exposure in workplaces that do not restrict smoking are comparable to, and often greater than, the ETS exposures of nonsmokers married to smokers.

Biomarkers of Exposure to ETS

Questionnaires have been used in epidemiologic studies to determine lifetime history of ETS exposure. However, because of well-known limitations with the questionnaire approach, there is considerable interest in identifying sensitive and specific biomarkers of exposure to ETS. To date, none of the biomarkers can measure past exposures relevant for lung cancer.

Cotinine, a major metabolite of nicotine, is currently the best marker of recent (24 to 72 hours) tobacco smoke exposure (Haley et al., 1983). Measurement of cotinine levels provides biochemical validation of reported current exposure to ETS, lending credibility to the epidemiologic findings on the association between ETS and lung cancer. In a 10-country study of nonsmokers in which self-reported exposures to ETS at home, work, and other social settings in the week preceding specimen collection were correlated with urinary cotinine levels, the correlation coefficients were 0.4 to 0.5 (Riboli et al., 1990). Correlation coefficients of about 0.3 have been reported in some studies (Cummings et al., 1990; Coultas et al., 1989). This more modest result may be due partly to the collection of information on ETS exposure only for the preceding 24 hours before specimen collection whereas exposures up to 72 hours may be relevant (Coultas et al., 1989). Cotinine levels in blood, urine, and saliva have also been measured in different population groups to determine the extent of ETS exposure among the nonsmoking population (Cummings et al., 1990; Coultas et al., 1989; Greenberg et al., 1984; Haley et al., 1989; Jarvis et al.,

1987; Matsukura et al., 1984; Perez-Stable et al., 1992; Riboli et al., 1990; Wald et al., 1990; Wagenkneckt et al., 1992).

Cotinine levels have also been used as a measure of the extent of tobacco smoke exposure in nonsmokers (i.e., in "cigarette equivalents") relative to smokers. The ratio of cotinine levels in nonsmokers exposed to ETS to the cotinine levels in smokers ranged from 0.6% to 1% in most studies (Wald and Ritchie, 1984; Jarvis et al., 1984; Darby and Pike, 1988; Wald et al., 1990; 1991; Lee 1991a; EPA, 1992). Based on the assumption that there is a direct linear relationship between the ratio of excess lung cancer risk and the cotinine ratio, excess risks of lung cancer have been estimated for nonsmokers exposed to ETS (NRC 1986; Repace and Lowry, 1990; Tweedie and Mengersen, 1992). This extrapolation approach using cotinine ratios has produced substantially lower risk estimates than epidemiologic studies (Tweedie and Mengersen, 1992) and the discrepancy between the two methods has generated considerable debate (Darby and Pike, 1988; Wald et al., 1990, 1991; Lee 1991a,b). It is not surprising that the estimation of risks using cigarette equivalents based on cotinine (or any other tobacco constituent) would yield different results given that cotinine (and nicotine) are not carcinogens and their levels in biological samples may not indicate carcinogenic uptake and metabolic activation.

Several other biomarkers of tobacco smoke exposure have been investigated in recent studies, including two classes of hemoglobin adduct and albumin adducts (Bartsch et al., 1990; Coghlin et al., 1991; Hammond et al., 1993; Crawford et al., 1994) Because the carcinogenic components of tobacco smoke may react with and covalently bind to cellular macromolecules such as hemoglobin, albumin, or DNA, the presence of carcinogen-hemoglobin (Hb) or albumin adduct in human tissues has been considered a marker for smoking-induced DNA damage. PAH-DNA adducts in lymphocytes have recently been shown to be a good predictor of lung cancer in smokers even after controlling for pack-years of tobacco use (Tang et al., 1995). However, the extent to which a specific marker will measure specific time periods of exposure will depend on the pharmacokinetics of the chemical and the persistence of the marker in the biologic sample assayed. For example, given that the erythrocyte has a 120-day lifetime and lacks a repair system, hemoglobin adduct measurements (e.g., 4-ABP hemoglobin adduct) would be a good marker of short-term exposure. On the other hand, the precise exposure period will be more difficult to determine based on adduct measurements carried out in lymphocytes (e.g., PAH-albumin adducts) because of the varying lifetimes of lymphocytes (Perera, 1991). PAH-albumin adducts are also less specific than 4-ABP adducts for ETS, as there are many sources of PAH.

Several studies of smokers and nonsmokers in which levels of 4-ABP

Table 10-5. Levels of 4-aminobiphenyl (ABP) hemoglobin (HB) adduct concentrations and PAH-albumin adduct levels in smokers and nonsmokers categorized by ETS exposure

Study	Mean Levels of Adducts	
Bartsch et al., 1990	4-ABP-Hb adducts (in pg/g Hb)	
	Slow acetylator phenotype	Fast acetylator phenotype
Black-tobacco smokers (n=16)	175.0	117.5
Nonsmokers (n=50)	31.7	19.4
Exposed to ETS[a]		
No (n=35)	30.4	12.3
Yes (n=15)	34.8	33.6
Coghlin et al., 1991; Hammond et al., 1993	4-ABP-Hb adducts (in pg/g Hb)	
Smoking pregnant women (n=15)	183	
Nonsmoking pregnant women (n=40)	22	
Exposed to ETS[b]		
No/little (n=7)	17.6	
Moderate (n=20)	20.8	
Heavy (n=9)	27.8	
Crawford et al., 1994	PAH-albumin (fmol/μg)	
Active smoking women (n=31)	0.80	
Nonsmoking women exposed to ETS[c](n=32)	0.49	
Nonsmoking women not exposed to ETS (n=24)	0.31	

[a]Exposure to ETS the day before specimen collection.

[b]Nicotine levels (μg/m^3) measured by a lightweight nicotine monitor worn by subjects during a week of the third trimester of pregnancy. Nicotine levels (μg/m^3) were <0.5, 0.5–1.9, and 2.0+ for no/little, moderate, and heavy ETS exposure, respectively.

[c]Average number of cigarettes smoked by visitors in the home.

hemoglobin adducts and PAH-albumin adducts have been measured are shown in Table 10-5. In one study (Barstch et al., 1990), 4-ABP-Hb levels as well as N-acetylation phenotype, a marker of susceptibility for bladder cancer, were both measured. Nonsmokers with self-reported exposure to ETS showed higher 4-ABP-Hb levels than nonsmokers with no reported exposure to ETS. The levels of 4-ABP-Hb among nonsmokers not exposed to ETS were 17% and 10% of those of active smokers, for slow and fast acetylators, respectively. The corresponding figures were 20% and 28% among nonsmokers with self-reported ETS exposure. In a study of pregnant women, levels of 4-ABP-Hb levels in all nonsmoking women were about 12% of those of smoking women (15% among nonsmokers with the highest ETS exposure and about 10% among nonsmokers with no or little ETS exposure) (Coghlin et al., 1991; Hammond et al., 1993). In a third study (Crawford et al., 1994), serum PAH-albumin adducts in active smoking women and nonsmoking women, categorized by any exposure to ETS, were compared. The serum PAH-albumin adduct levels in nonsmoking women exposed to ETS were 61% of those of active smokers whereas the levels in nonsmoking women not exposed to ETS were 39% of those of active smokers.

Hecht et al. (1993) also demonstrated the uptake and metabolism of the tobacco-specific lung carcinogen, NNK (4-(methylnitrosamino)-l-(3-pyridyl)-l-butanone), in a small number of nonsmokers exposed to ETS. Both NNK and its metabolite, NNAL (4-(methylnitrosamino)-l-(3-pyridyl)-l-butanol), are potent pulmonary carcinogens in rats and mice, inducing a high incidence of adenocarcinoma of the lung. In this study, levels of urinary excretion of NNAL and its glucuronide were about seven-and five-fold higher, respectively, after nonsmokers were exposed to high levels of ETS, comparable to levels occasionally encountered in a very heavily smoke-polluted bar (nicotine concentration in the exposure room of this study was up to 119 µg per cubic meter).

These results on carcinogen hemoglobin or albumin adduct levels and NNK levels only serve to illustrate the difficulty in using cigarette-equivalents based on a single tobacco constituent to estimate the risk of lung cancer in nonsmokers. Depending on the biomarker selected, widely different cigarette equivalents of tobacco smoke exposure can be obtained.

Conclusion

Since the 1981 publication of the first studies on ETS as a risk factor of lung cancer in nonsmokers, a large number of studies (more than 30) have been published, including five new U.S. studies published since 1991. The five new studies represent a concerted effort of the scientific community to conduct studies that could address previous criticisms raised regarding earlier studies of ETS and lung cancer. Despite inherent limitations of individual case-control or cohort studies and of the methods of pooled analysis such as meta-analysis, the overwhelming evidence, including results from these five individual studies suggest a small, significant increased risk of lung cancer in nonsmokers in association with spousal smoking. The data on other sources of ETS exposure (i.e., at work or social setting) are less consistent, but they also point to all sources of ETS to be deleterious to a nonsmoker's health.

It is unlikely that additional questionnaire-based case-control studies will augment considerably the already available information on ETS and lung cancer. Large cohort studies with longitudinal questionnaire assessment of ETS exposure, in conjunction with validation of ETS exposure in subsamples with nicotine monitoring would be useful; such studies would be expensive and logistically challenging to implement. As demonstrated in the CPS-II study, large sample sizes and long follow-up would be required to achieve meaningful study power because lung cancer is a rare disease among never-smokers. Identification of a biomarker of past ETS exposure could complement the information we can derive from traditional questionnaire-based case-control studies. Although at present the existence of such a biomarker seems unlikely due to the lack of persistence and specificity of such markers, recent results on the PAH-DNA adducts in lymphocytes in smokers are encouraging and suggest that continued studies to identify markers of ETS exposure are important.

References

Alpha-Tocopherol, Beta-Carotene Cancer Prevention Study Group. 1994. The effect of vitamin E and beta-carotene on the incidence of lung cancer and other cancers in male smokers. N Engl J Med 330: 1029–1035.

Arundel A, Sterling T, Weinkam J. 1987. Never smoker lung cancer risks from exposure to particulate tobacco smoke. Environ Int 13:409–426.

Austin H, Cole P. 1986. Cigarette smoking and leukemia. J Chron Dis 39:417–421.

Bartsch H, Caporaso N, Coda M, Kadlubar F, Malaveille C, Skipper P, Talaska G, Tannenbaum SR, Vineis P. 1990. Carcinogen hemoglobin adducts, urinary mutagenicity, and metabolic phenotype in active and passive cigarette smokers. J Natl Cancer Inst 82: 1826–1831.

Bero LA, Glantz SA, Rennie D. 1994. Publication bias and public health policy on environmental tobacco smoke. JAMA 272: 133–136.

Biggerstaff BJ, Tweedie RL, Mengersem KL. 1994. Passive smoking in the workplace: classical and Bayesian meta-analyses. Int Arch Occup Environ Health 66:269–277.

Brownson RC, Reif JS, Keefe TJ, Ferguson SW, Pritzl JA. 1987. Risk factors for adenocarcinoma of the lung. Am J Epidemiol 125: 25–34.

Brownson RC, Alavanja MCR, Hock ET, Loy TS. 1992. Passive smoking and lung cancer in nonsmoking women. Am J Public Health 82: 1525–1530.

Brownson RC, Alavanja MCR, Hock ET. 1993a. Reliability of passive smoke exposure histories in a case-control study of lung cancer. Int J Epidemiol 22: 804–808.

Brownson RC, Novotny TE, Perry MC. 1993b. Cigarette smoking and adult leukemia. Arch Intern Med 153: 469–473.

Buffler PA, Pickle LW, Mason TJ, Contant C. 1984. The causes of lung cancer in Texas. In: Mizell M, Correa P, eds. Lung Cancer: Causes and Prevention. Verlag Chemie International, New York: pp 83–99.

Butler WJ. 1990. Comments submitted to Environmental Protection Agency on its draft report, Health Effects of Passive Smoking: Assessment of Lung Cancer in Adults and Respiratory Disorders in Children. EPA/600/6-9-/006A.

Cardenas VM, Thun MJ, Austin H, Lally Ca, Clark SW, Greenberg RS, Heath CW Jr. Environmental tobacco smoke and lung cancer mortality in the American Cancer Society's Cancer Prevention Study II. Can Causes Control (in press).

Coghlin J, Hammond SK, Gann PH. 1989. Development of epidemiologic tools for measuring environmental tobacco smoke exposure. Am J Epidemiol 130: 696–704.

Coghlin J, Gann PH, Hammond SK, Skipper PL, Taghizadeh K, Paul M, Tannenbaum SR. 1991. 4-aminobiphenyl hemoglobin adducts in fetuses exposed to the tobacco smoke carcinogen in utero. J Natl Cancer Inst 83:274–280.

Correa P, Pickle LW, Fontham E, Lin Y, Haenszel W. 1983. Passive smoking and lung cancer. Lancet 1:595–597.

Coultas DB, Peake GT, Samet JM. 1989. Questionnaire assessment of lifetime and recent exposure to environmental tobacco smoke. Am J Epidemiol 130:338–347.

Crawford FG, Mayer J, Santella RM, Cooper TB, Ottman R, Tsai WY, Simon-Cereijido G, Wang M, Tang D, Perera FP. 1994. Biomarkers of environmental tobacco smoke in preschool children and their mothers. J Natl Cancer Inst 86:1398–1402.

Cummings KM, Markello SJ, Mahoney MC, Marshall JR. 1989. Measurement of lifetime exposure to passive smoke. Am J Epidemiol 130:122–132.

Cummings MK, Markello SJ, Mahoney M, Bhargava AK, Mcelroy PD, Marshall JR. 1990. Measurement of current exposure to environmental tobacco smoke. Arch Environ Health 45:74–79.

Darby SC, Pike MC. 1988. Lung cancer and passive smoking: predicted effects from a mathematical model for cigarette smoking and lung cancer. Br J Cancer 58:825–831.

Darby SC, Pike MC. 1990. Response to the letter from Dr. Wald. Br J Cancer 61: 337–338.

Dalager NA, Pickle LW, Mason TJ, Correa P, Fontham E, Stemhagen A, Buffler PA, Ziegler RG, Fraumeni JF, Jr. 1986. The relation of passive smoking to lung cancer. Cancer Res 46:4808–4811.

Emmons KM, Abrams DB, Marshall TJ, Etzel RA, Novotny TE, Marcus BH, Kane ME. 1992. Exposure to environmental tobacco smoke in naturalistic settings. Am J Public Health 82:24–28.

Environmental Protection Agency, Office of Health and Environmental Assessment, Office of Research and Development. 1992. Respiratory Health Effects of Passive Smoking: Lung Cancer and Other Disorders. US Environmental Protection Agancy, Washington, DC.

Farland W, Bayard S, Jinot J. 1994. Dissent (A) Environmental tobacco smoke: A public health conspiracy? A dissenting view. J Clin Epidemiol 47:335–337.

Fleiss JL, Gross AJ. 1991. Meta-analysis in epidemiology, with special reference to studies of the association between exposure to environmental tobacco smoke and lung cancer: A critique. J Clin Epidemiol 44: 127–139.

Fontham ETH, Correa P, Wu-Williams A, Reynolds P, Greenberg RS, Buffler PA,

Chen VW, Boyd P, Alterman T, Austin DF, Liff J, Greenberg SD. 1991. Lung cancer in nonsmoking women: a multicenter case-control study. Cancer Epidemiol Biomarkers Prev 1:35–43.

Fontham ETH, Correa P, Reynolds P, Wu-Williams A, Buffler PA, Greenberg RS, Chen VW, Alterman T, Boyd P, Austin DF, Liff J. 1994. Environmental tobacco smoke and lung cancer in nonsmoking women. JAMA 271:1752–1759.

Forman D. 1991. The etiology of gastric cancer. In: O'Neill IJ, Chen J, Bartsch H (eds): Relevance to Human Cancer of N-Nitroso Compounds, Tobacco Smoke and Mycotoxins. Lyon, International Agency for Research on Cancer.

Garfinkel L, Auerbach O, Joubert L. 1985. Involuntary smoking and lung cancer: a case-control study. J Natl Cancer Inst 75:463–469.

Gordis L. 1982. Should dead controls be matched to dead controls? Am J Epidemiol 115:1–5.

Gori BG. 1993. Passive smoking. Lancet 341:965.

Gori GB. 1994a. Science, policy, and ethnics: the case of environmental tobacco smoke. J Clin Epidemiol 47:325–334.

Gori GB. 1994b. Response. Reply to the preceding dissents. J Clin Epidemiol 47: 351–353.

Greenberg RA, Haley NJ, Etzel RA, Loda FA. 1984. Measuring the exposure of infants to tobacco smoke. N Engl J Med 310:1075–1078.

Greenland S. 1994a. Invited commentary: a critical look at some popular meta-analytic methods. Am J Epidemiology 140: 290–296.

Greenland S. 1994b. Quality scores are useless and potentially misleading. Reply to: "Re: A critical look at some popular analytic methods." Am J Epidemiology 140:300–301.

Haley NJ, Axelrad CM, Tilton KA. 1983. Validation of self-reported smoking behavior: biochemical analysis of cotinine and thiocyanate. Am J Public Health 73:1204–1207.

Haley JH, Colosimo SG, Axelrad CM, Harris R, Sepkovic DW. 1989. Biochemical validation of self-reported exposure to environmental tobacco smoke. Environ Res 49:127–135.

Hammond SK, Coghlin J, Gann PH, Paul M, Taghizadeh K, Skipper PL, Tannebaum SR. 1993. Relationship between environmental tobacco smoke exposure and carcinogen-hemoglobin adduct levels in nonsmokers. J Natl Cancer Inst 85:474–478.

Hammond SK. 1995. Occupational exposure to environmental tobacco smoke. OSHA Hearings on Indoor Air. Washington DC.

Hecht SS, Carmella SG, Murphy SE, Akerkar S, Brunnemann KD, Hoffman D. 1993. A tobacco-specific lung carcinogen in the urine of men exposed to cigarette smoke. N Engl J Med 329:1543–1546.

Hirayama T. 1981. Nonsmoking wives of heavy smokers have a higher risk of lung cancer: A study from Japan. BMJ 282:183–185.

Humble CG, Samet JM, Pathak DR. 1987. Marriage to a smoker and lung cancer risk. Am J Public Health 77: 598–602.

Janerich DT, Thompson WD, Varela LR, Greenwald P, Chorost S, Tucci C, Zaman M, Melamed MR, Kiely M, MnKneally MF. 1990. Lung cancer and exposure to tobacco smoke in the household. N Engl J Med 323: 632–636.

Jarvis M, Tunstall-Pedoe H, Feyerabend C, Vesey C, Kabat GC, Wynder El. 1984. Lung cancer in nonsmokers. Cancer 53: 1214–1221.

Jarvis MJ, Tunstall-Pedoe H, Feyerabend C, Vesey C, Saloojee Y. 1987. Comparison of tests used to distinguish smokers from nonsmokers. Am J Public Health 77: 1435–1438.

Jinot J, Bayard S. 1994. Dissent (B) Respiratory health effects of passive smoking: EPA's weight-of-evidence analysis. J Clin Epidemiol 47: 339–349.

Kabat GC, Wynder EL. 1984. Lung cancer in nonsmokers. Cancer 53: 1214–1221.

Kabat GC, Steelman SD, Wynder DL. 1995. Relation between exposure to environmental tobacco smoke and lung cancer in lifetime nonsmokers. Am J Epidemiol 142: 141–148.

Kalandidi A, Katsouyanni K, Voropoulou N, Bastas G, Saracci R, Trichopoulos D. 1990. Passive smoking and diet in the etiology of lung cancer among nonsmokers. Cancer Causes Control 1: 15–21.

Katzenstein AW. 1992. Environmental tobacco smoke and lung cancer risk: epidemiology in relation to confounding factors. Environ Int 18: 341–345.

Kilpatrick SJ. 1992. The epidemiology of environmental tobacco smoke (ETS) and the weight of evidence argument. Int Surg 77: 131–133.

Koo LC, Ho JHC, Saw D, Ho CY. 1987. Measurements of passive smoking and estimates of lung cancer risk among non-smoking Chinese females. Int J Cancer 39: 162–169.

Koo LC, Ho JHC, Rylander R. 1988. Life-history correlates of environmental tobacco smoke: a study on nonsmoking Hong Kong Chinese wives with smoking versus nonsmoking husbands. Soc Sci Med 26: 751–760.

Koo LC. 1989. Environmental tobacco smoke and lung cancer: is it the smoke or diet? In: Bieva CJ, Courtois M, Govaerts M, eds. Present and Future of Indoor Air Quality. Elsevier Science Publishers B.V. (Biomedical Division), Amsterdam, New York: pp 65–75.

Layard MW. 1993. Re: Environmental tobacco smoke and lung cancer risk in nonsmoking women (2nd letter). J Natl Cancer Inst 85: 748–749.

Letzel H, Blumner E, Uberla K. 1988. Meta-analyses on passive smoking and lung cancer effects of study selection and misclassification of exposure. Environ Tech Letters 9: 491–500.

Le Marchand L, Wilkens LR, Hankin JH, Haley NJ. 1991. Dietary patterns of female nonsmokers with and without exposure to environmental tobacco smoke. Cancer Causes Control 2: 11–16.

Lee PN, Chamberlain J, Alderson MR. 1986. Relationship of passive smoking to risk of lung cancer and other smoking-associated diseases. Br J Cancer 54: 97–105.

Lee PN. 1986. Misclassification as a factor in passive smoking risk. Lancet 2: 867.

Lee PN. 1989. Passive smoking and lung cancer: fact or fiction. In: Bieva CJ, Courtois M, Govaerts M, eds. Present and Future of Indoor Air Quality. Elsevier

Science Publishers B.V. (Biomedical Division), Amsterdam, New York. pp 119–128

Lee PN. 1991a. An estimate of adult mortality in the United States from passive smoking (letter). Environ Int 17: 379–381.

Lee PN. 1991b. Lung cancer and passive smoking (continued). Br J Cancer 64: 220.

Lee PN. 1991c. Lung cancer and passive smoking. Br J Cancer 63: 161–162.

Lee PN. 1993. Re: Environmental tobacco smoke and lung cancer risk in nonsmoking women. J Natl Cancer Inst 85: 748.

LeVois ME, Layard MW. 1994. Inconsistency between workplace and spousal studies of environmental tobacco smoke and lung cancer. Regul Toxicol Pharmacol 19: 309–316.

Mantel N. 1983. Epidemiologic investigations. Care in conduct, care in analysis, and care in reporting. J Cancer Res Clin Oncol 105: 113–116.

Matanoski G, Kanchanaraksa S, Lantry D, Chang Y. 1995. Characteristics of nonsmoking women in NHANES I and NHANES I epidemiologic follow-up study with exposure to spouses who smoke. Am J Epidemiol 142: 149–157.

McLaughlin JK, Blot WJ, Mehl ES, Mandel JS. 1985. Problems in the use of dead controls in case-control studies. I. General results. Am J Epidemiol 121: 131–139.

Matsukura S, Taminato T, Kitano N, Seino Y, Hamada H, Uchihashi M, Nakajima K, Hirata Y. 1984. Effect of environmental toabcco smoke on urinary cotinine excretion in nonsmokers. Evidence for passive smoking. N Engl J Med 311: 828–832.

National Research Council. 1986. Environmental tobacco smoke: measuring exposures and assessing health effects. National Academy Press, Washington, DC.

Olkin I. 1994. Invited commentary: Re: "A critical look at some popular meta-analytic methods". Am J Epidemiology 140: 297–299.

Perera FP. 1991. Validation of molecular epidemiologic methods. In: Groopman JD, Skipper PL, eds. Molecular Dosimetry and Human Cancer: Analytical, Epidemiological, and Social Considerations. CRC Press, Inc, Florida; Chap. 4.

Perez-Stable EJ, Marin G, Marin BV, Benowitz NL. 1992. Misclassification of smoking status by self-reported cigarette consumption. Am Rev Respir Dis 145: 53–57.

Pershagen G, Hrubec Z, Svensson G. 1987. Passive smoking and lung cancer in Swedish women. Am J Epidemiol 125: 17–24.

Pershagen G. 1992. Passive smoking and lung cancer. In: Samet JM, ed. Epidemiology of Lung Cancers. Marcel Dekker, Inc., New York.

Pron GE, Burch D, Howe GR, Miller AB. 1986. The reliability of passive smoking histories reported in a case-control study of lung cancer. Am J Epidemiol 127: 267–273.

Repace JL, Lowrey AH. 1990. Risk assessment methodologies for passive smoking-induced lung cancer. Risk Analysis 10: 27–37.

Repace JL, Lowrey AH. 1993. An enforceable indoor air quality standard for environmental tobacco smoke in the workplace. Risk Analysis 13: 334–355.

Riboli E, Preston-Martin S, Saracci R, Haley NJ, Trichopoulos D, Becher H, Burch D, Fontham ETH, Gao YT, Jindal SK, Koo LC, Le Marchand L, Segnan N, Shimizu H, Stanta G, Wu-Wiiliams AH, Zatonskii W. 1990. Exposure of nonsmoking women to environmental tobacco smoke: a 10-country collaborative study. Cancer Causes Control 1: 243–252.

Rogot E, Reid DD. 1975. The validity of data from next-of-kin in studies of mortality among migrants. Int J Epidemiol 4: 51–54.

Sidney S, Cann BJ, Friedman GD. 1989. Dietary intake of carotene in nonsmokers with and without passive smoking at home. Am J Epidemiol 129: 1305–1309.

Siegel M. 1993. Involuntary smoking in the restaurant workplace. A review of employee exposure and health effect. JAMA 270: 490–493.

Shimizu H, Morishita M, Mizuno K, et al. 1988. A case-control study of lung cancer in nonsmoking women. Tohoku J Exp Med 154: 389–397.

Sobue T. 1990. Association of indoor air pollution and lifestyle with lung cancer in Osaka, Japan. Int J Epidemiol 19 (suppl 1) S 62–S 66.

Spizer WO, Lawrence V, Dales R, Hill G, Archer MC, Clark P, Abenhaim L, Hardy J, Sampalis J, Pinfold SP, Morgan PP. 1990. Links between passive smoking and disease: a best-evidence synthesis. A report of the working group on passive smoking. Clin Invest Med 13: 17–42.

Stockwell HG, Goldman AL, Lyman GH, Noss CI, Armstrong AW, Pinkham PA, Candelora EC, Brusa MR. 1992. Environmental tobacco smoke and lung cancer risk in nonsmoking women. J Natl Cancer Inst 84: 1417–1422.

Trichopoulos D, Kalandid A, Spanos L. 1981. Lung cancer and passive smoking. Int J Cancer 27: 1–4.

Tang D, Santella RM, Blackwood AM, Young TL, Mayer J, Jaretzki A, Grantham S, Tsai WY, Perera FP. 1995. A molecular epidemiological case-control study of lung cancer. Cancer Epidemiol Biomarkers Prev 4: 341–346.

Tweedie RL, Mengerson KL. 1992. Lung cancer and passive smoking: reconciling the biochemical and epidemiological approaches. Br J Cancer 66: 700–705.

U.S. Surgeon General. 1986. The health consequences of involuntary smoking. United States Department of Health and Human Services, Washington, DC.

Vainio H, Partenen T. 1989. Population burden of lung cancer due to environmental tobacco smoke. Mutat Res 222: 137–140.

Wacholder S, Silverman DT, McLaughlin JK, Mandel JS. Selection of controls in case-control studies. Am J Epidemiol 135: 1029–1041.

Wagenknecht LE, Burke GL, Perkins LL, Haley NJ, Friedman GD. 1992. Misclassification of smoking status in the CARDIA Study: a comparison of self-report with serum cotinine levels. Am J Public Health 82: 33–36.

Wald N, Ritchie C. 1984. Validation of studies of lung cancer in nonsmokers married to smokers (letter). Lancet 1: 1067.

Wald NJ, Nanchahal K, Thompson SM, Cuckle HS. 1986. Does breathing other people's tobacco smoke cause lung cancer. Br Med J 293: 1217–1222.

Wald NJ, Nanchahal K, Cuckle H. 1990. Lung cancer and passive smoking. Br J Cancer 61: 337–344.

Wald NJ, Cuckle HS, Nanchahal K, Thompson SM 1991. Response to the letter from Dr. P. Lee. Br J Cancer 63: 163.

Wells N, Cuckle H, Nanchahal K, Thompson S. 1991. Response to letter from Dr Lee. Br J Cancer 64: 201.

Wells JA. 1993. An estimate of adult mortality in the United States from passive smoking: a further reply. Environ Int 19: 97–100.

Wu AH, Henderson BE, Pike MC, Yu MC. 1985. Smoking and other risk factors for lung cancer in women. J Natl Cancer Inst 74: 747–751.

Wu-Williams AH, Samet JM. 1989. Environmental tobacco smoke: exposure-response relationships in epidemiologic studies. Risk Analysis 10: 39–48.

Wu-Williams AH, Dai XD, Blot W, Xu ZY, Sun XW, Xiao HP, Stone BJ, Yu SF, Feng YP, Ershow AG, Sun J, Fraumeni JF Jr, Henderson BE. 1990. Lung cancer among women in northeast China. Br J Cancer 62: 982–987.

Wu-Williams AH, Yu MC, Mack TM. 1990. Life-style, workplace, and stomach cancer by subsite in young men of Los Angeles County. Cancer Res 50: 2569–2576.

Wu AH, Fontham ETH, Reynolds P, Greenberg RS, Buffler P, Liff J, Boyd P, Henderson BE, Correa P. 1995. Previous lung disease and risk of lung cancer among lifetime nonsmoking women in the United States. Am J Epidemiol 141: 1023–1032.

Yu MC, Mack TM, Hanisch R, Cicioni C, Henderson BE. 1986. Cigarette smoking, obesity, diuretic use, and coffee consumption as risk factors for renal cell carcinoma. J Natl Cancer Inst 77: 351–355.

Environmental Tobacco Smoke III: Heart Disease

11

KYLE STEENLAND

THIS chapter considers the evidence linking heart disease to environmental tobacco smoke (ETS). Heart disease is not so often regarded as being associated with ETS, compared with lung cancer and childhood respiratory disease. Yet there is an increasing body of epidemiologic evidence for a causal association between ETS and heart disease.

The main study design has been cohort studies of never-smokers, both men and women. This approach is feasible because heart disease is relatively common (ETS studies of lung cancer, in contrast, have largely been case-control studies of never-smokers). Exposure usually has been defined as marriage to a smoker, particularly a current smoker. The focus on exposure to a current smoker is probably appropriate as it seems likely that much of the effect of ETS on the heart is due recent exposure (in contrast to lung cancer), a temporal relation that applies to active smoking as well.

Overall, the ETS/heart disease studies are generally consistent in showing a relative risk of about 1.2 for never-smokers married to a smoker. The link between ETS and heart disease has been more controversial than the link with lung cancer because active smoking itself is much less strongly associated with heart disease than lung cancer is (relative risk of 2 versus 10 to 20). However, there is a substantial amount of evidence from experiments in both animals and humans linking ETS with measurable effects on the cardiovascular system (e.g., increased platelet aggregation, decreased oxygen supply to the heart). Some authors have also argued that the cardiovascular system either adapts to or is saturated by tobacco smoke, so that after a certain level further exposure does not appreciably increase risk.

A second issue is confounding. There are many well-established potential confounders for heart disease such as obesity, blood pressure, and cholesterol. Several studies have shown that those exposed to ETS tend to have less education and somewhat more risk factors for heart disease than those not exposed to ETS. However, a number of the epidemiologic studies have controlled for the known cardiovascular confounders.

Overall, the weight of the evidence is in favor of a causal relationship, but with a relative risk as small as 1.2, possible confounding remains an issue. This chapter argues that future advances in the epidemiology of ETS and heart disease may require a focus on intermediate end points such as carotid artery thickness, the use of prospective designs with repeated exposure assessment, and thorough evaluation of potential confounders.

The potential public health burden for an ETS–heart disease link is much higher than for the ETS–lung cancer link. Assuming causality, the estimated number of excess U.S. heart disease deaths among never-smokers attributable to exposure is on the order of 30,000 to 40,000 annually, compared with approximately 3,000 for lung cancer.

In 1992 the American Heart Association (Taylor et al., 1992) reviewed the published literature and determined that "the risk of death due to heart disease is increased by about 30% among those exposed to environmental tobacco smoke (ETS) at home and could be much higher in those exposed at the workplace, where higher levels of ETS may be present. Even though considerable uncertainty is a part of any analysis on the health effects of ETS because of the difficulty of conducting long-term studies and selecting sample populations, an estimated 35,000–40,000 cardiovascular disease–related deaths and 3,000–5,000 lung cancer deaths due to ETS exposure have been predicted to occur each year."

There have been 15 epidemiologic studies (eight cohort, seven case-control) of heart disease among never-smokers exposed to environmental tobacco smoke (ETS) (Butler, 1988; Dobson et al., 1991; Garland et al., 1985, He et al., 1989, Hirayama, 1990; Hole et al., 1989; Humble et al., 1990; Jackson et al, 1989; Lee et al., 1986, Sandler et al., 1989; Svendsen et al., 1987, He et al., 1994; LaVecchia et al., 1993; Muscat and Wynder, 1995; Steenland et al., 1996). Almost all these studies showed an increased risk of heart disease for the exposed group (usually defined as currently exposed) compared to the nonexposed group. A number of studies controlled for the main heart disease risk factors, and several showed a positive dose-response trend according to the level of presumed ETS exposure. Almost all of these studies were based on analyses of spousal smoking (i.e, never-smokers exposed to ETS from a smoking spouse compared to never-smokers not so exposed); a few also had data on ETS exposure at work. Wells (1994) reviewed 12 of these studies in 1994 and conducted a meta-analysis that showed an overall relative risk of 1.23 (1.12 to 1.35) for heart disease mortality (1.23 for women and 1.25 for men), for ETS exposure from a spouse among never-smokers. The studies published since Wells' review are consistent with this estimate.

The fact that heart disease is fairly common among never-smokers makes it amenable to study via cohort studies; most ETS studies to date have been cohort studies. This is in contrast to studies of lung cancer among never-smokers exposed to ETS, in which the great majority of studies have been case-control studies (lung cancer is very rare among never-smokers). The cohort approach has the advantage that exposure status can be defined prospectively, avoiding problems of recall bias by case subjects in case-control studies (i.e., subjects might over-report their exposure). The cohort approach has the disadvantage in that ETS exposure is typically defined at one point at time, at the beginning of follow-up, usually by self-report on a questionnaire. Those never-smokers exposed at baseline in a cohort study may subsequently become nonexposed; for example, their spouse may give up smoking. The converse is also possible, although probably less likely. If large numbers of those exposed at baseline become nonexposed during follow-up, and if exposure to ETS does in fact increase the risk of heart disease, and if such exposure acts primarily by an acute effect, then such misclassification of exposure status will bias findings toward the null. This problem could be solved, of course, by repeated longitudinal ascertainment of ETS exposure status, but such repeated ascertainment is usually prohibitively costly. If sample sizes are large enough, it is possible to assess risk ratios for exposed versus nonexposed repeatedly as follow-up time increases; decreasing rate ratios with increased follow-up time might indicate that this phenomenon is occurring.

Besides the epidemiologic evidence, various experimental and clinical studies also support an ETS–heart disease association and suggest possible mechanisms, similar to those for active smoking and congestive heart disease (CHD). Glantz and Parmley (1995) reviewed these data, which suggest that ETS causes greater platelet aggregation, increased risk of thrombosis, lower oxygen supply, and greater oxygen demand. A rat model of ischemia and reperfusion suggests that ETS increases myocardial infarct size (Zhu et al., 1994). Many of these effects are believed to be caused by nicotine and carbon monoxide in ETS, but other unidentified agents may also play a role. Analogous to the evidence for mainstream smoking (for which risk drops about 50% within one year of quitting; see Surgeon General, 1990), much of the experimental data that suggest an ETS–heart disease association also support an acute effect of ETS on the heart. In addition, there are also plausible mechanisms of chronic effects, such as accelerated plaque formation due to endothelial cell damage by ETS (Zhu et al., 1993; Penn et al., 1994). Nonsmoking adolescents exposed to ETS measured by urinary cotinine had significantly lower HDL and lower high density/low density lipoprotein (HDL/LDL) ratios than nonsmokers without such exposure (Feldman et al., 1991). Both cross-sectional and longitudinal observational studies have shown that carotid artery intimal-medial thickness is significantly increased in ETS-exposed subjects, although not as much as in active smokers (Howard et al., 1994; Diez-Roux et al., 1995). Taken together, these studies suggest a biologically plausible role for ETS in causing heart disease.

Despite the epidemiologic and mechanistic evidence accumulated to date, the ETS–heart disease association is not as well supported as the ETS–lung cancer association. There are fewer epidemiologic studies, there are more potential confounders that must be controlled in studies of heart disease, and the increase in heart disease risk seen in epidemiologic studies due to active smoking is smaller than is the increase in lung cancer risk due to active smoking.

This last point would seem to make an ETS/heart disease association less plausible than an ETS/lung cancer association. However, caution must be exercised here for several reasons. First, the constituents of ETS are not the same in sidestream and mainstream smoke; for example, ETS is produced at a lower temperature and the relative concentration of CO is higher in ETS than in mainstream smoke. This means that arguments about "cigarette equivalents" based on some specific biomarker may not hold. For example, reliance on urinary cotinine, a metabolite of nicotine, would suggest that those exposed to ETS are absorbing the equivalent of less than what would be absorbed by smoking one cigarette a day—but urinary cotinine may not be the best indicator of absorbed dose. Second, regardless of any argument about the relative dose of ETS versus mainstream smoke and the relative effects expected from the epidemiology of active smoking, experimental data have shown appreciable effects on the heart due to sidestream smoke, as outlined above. Third, the referent group in studies of active smoking generally includes never-smokers exposed to ETS, whereas the referent group in ETS studies is composed of never-smokers not exposed to ETS, so the two types of studies are not strictly comparable. Finally, Glantz and Parmley (1995) have argued that at least some of the effects of both sidestream and mainstream smoke on the heart may involve a saturation mechanism (e.g., platelet activation), whereby exposure beyond a certain point may not substantially increase risk. This argument would imply that dose-response data for active smoking as well as for ETS exposure might not be monotonic for heart disease, and there is some support in the literature for this.

Example—the American Cancer Society Cohort Study

By way of example of ETS/heart disease studies, I describe in more detail here a recent study of heart disease mortality among never-smokers in a large cohort assembled by the American Cancer Society (Steenland et al., 1996).

The cohort consisted of 353,180 never-smoking women and 126,500 never-smoking men enrolled in the American Cancer Society's Cancer Prevention Study–II (CPS-II). These men and women were aged 30 or above at baseline (median 56) and tended to be somewhat more highly educated than the general U.S. population. Three sub-cohorts were built from the overall cohort, based on the type of ETS-exposure data available: (1) a *spousal* cohort based on married pairs in which both spouses were in CPS-II and in which ETS-exposure status of the never-smoking subject was determined by the spouse's smoking status, (2) a *self-report* cohort based on self-reported current exposure to ETS at home, work, and elsewhere, which suffered from approximately 40% missing data, and (3) a *concordant* cohort in which both self-report and the spouse's report were concordant for current exposure at home. The last sub-cohort, although the smallest, would be expected to suffer the least degree of misclassification. For example, in the spousal cohort those allegedly exposed because the spouse reported smoking might actually be nonexposed because the smoking spouse did not smoke at home.

Follow-up occurred from 1982 to 1989. Ischemic heart disease deaths (ICD9 410–414) in the three sub-cohorts listed above numbered 3819, 4154, and 1606. The sum total of heart disease deaths in all prior ETS/heart disease studies numbered slightly over 3000.

Information was collected at baseline by a four-page questionnaire filled out by study subjects. Preliminary data analysis identified variables on the questionnaire that were predictors of heart disease ($P < .10$), and these were included in a model with exposure variables on the grounds that they were potential confounders. Variables in the model included age, history of heart disease or taking of heart disease medication, history of hypertension or hypertension medication, history of diabetes. history of arthritis, body mass index (BMI), educational level, aspirin use, diuretic use, alcohol consumption, employment status (currently employed outside the home or not), and exercise. Less than 10% of study subjects reported a history of heart disease or the taking of heart medication; the data were analyzed both with and without these subjects. Separate analyses were also conducted for those under age 65 at baseline, based on the hypothesis that rate ratios might be elevated primarily in younger subjects, which is the case in studies of mainstream smoking (Thun et al., 1995). The background risk of heart disease from causes other than smoking is rather low before age 65, making the effect of active smoking (or possibly passive smoking) more easily detected in this group. Finally, in the spousal cohort separate analyses were also conducted for those exposed currently at baseline and for those who had been exposed in the past (this was not possible in the self-reported or concordant cohorts because analyses there were limited to current ETS exposure because of the nature of the ETS question on the questionnaire). Based on known relations between active smoking and heart disease (Surgeon General, 1989) we hypothesized that current ETS exposure would have more of an effect than past ETS exposure; this is the opposite of what one would expect for lung cancer.

Approximately 10% of never-smoking men had wives who were currently smoking at baseline, and about 28% of never-smoking women were married to husbands who were currently smoking at baseline. The respective percentages for former spousal smoking were 10% and 32%. Results for the spousal cohort are shown in Table 11-1. Both men and women exposed to cigarette smoke from currently smoking spouses had small increases in risk of death from heart disease compared to those not so exposed (relative risks 1.22 and 1.10, respectively). Because the sample size was so large, the small excess risks could be estimated with some precision; confidence intervals for the observed relative risks excluded the null value of 1.00 for men and were borderline for women. Excess risks were slightly higher for analyses restricted to subjects aged less than 65. When results were analyzed by amount of current smoking exposure, categorical analysis did not show increasing trends in risk with increasing amount smoked by the spouse, for either men or women. Exposure to former smokers did not entail any excess risk for either men or women.

Table 11-2 provides results for self-reported exposure to ETS. Both men and women showed slightly increased risks for current home exposure (rate ratios 1.15 and 1.07, respectively. These findings parallel the findings for spousal exposure. These risks for home exposure were increased in subjects aged less than 65 at baseline (1.34 for men, 1.18 for women). Self-reported exposure at work or in other settings did not show significant consistent increases in risk. Separation of subjects by blue vs. white collar jobs revealed that male blue collar workers had a risk ratio

262   **Topics in Environmental Epidemiology**

Table 11-1. Results for American Cancer Society spousal cohort[a]

Exposure	Rate Ratio (95% CI)
Men (n = 101,227, 2494 deaths)	
Exposed to current smoker	1.22 (1.07–1.40)
<20 cigarettes/day[b]	1.33 (1.09–1.61)
20 cigarettes/day	1.17 (0.92–1.48)
>20 cigarettes/day	1.09 (0.77–1.53)
Exposed to former smoker	0.96 (0.83–1.11)
Men—age <65 at baseline	
Exposed to current smoker	1.33 (1.09–1.63)
Exposed to former smoker	0.95 (0.74–1.20)
Women (n = 208,372, 1325 deaths)[c]	
Exposed to current smoker	1.10 (0.96–1.27)
<20 cigarettes/day[b]	1.15 (0.90–1.48)
20 cigarettes/day	1.07 (0.83–1.40)
21–39 cigarettes/day	0.99 (0.67–1.47)
40+ cigarettes/day	1.04 (0.67–1.61)
Exposed to former smoker	1.00 (0.88–1.13)
Women—age <65 at baseline	
Exposed to current smoker	1.16 (0.92–1.47)
Exposed to former smoker	1.13 (0.90–1.42)

[a]Analyses controlled for age, self-reported history of heart disease, self-reported history of hypertension, self-reported history of diabetes, self-reported history of arthritis, body mass index, educational level, aspirin use, diuretic use, liquor consumption (men), wine consumption (women), employment status (men), estrogen use (women). Deaths refers to heart disease deaths.

[b]Excludes those exposed to cigarette smokers with amount smoked unknown.

[c]For women, exposure includes pipes/cigars as well as cigarettes. However, analyses by amount smoked includes only cigarettes and excludes those amount unknown. Four levels of spousal exposure were used for women (three for men) because of the increased prevalence of heavy smoking among husbands.

of 1.36 (1.01 to 1.83) for self-reported ETS exposure at work, male white collar workers had no excess (risk ratio 0.95). For women, neither blue nor white collar employees showed much increased risk with ETS exposure at work (risk ratios 1.02 and 1.11, respectively). Self-reported exposure outside the home (e.g., work and other settings) may involve greater misclassification than spousal or domestic exposure, given the wide variety of workplace and other social settings and the lack of information from the questionnaire regarding intensity of exposure. If ETS exposure at home were a risk factor for heart disease, one would expect ETS exposure at work or other settings also to be a risk factor, although perhaps not measurable by our crude definitions of exposure.

Table 11-3 presents the analysis for subjects concordant between self-report and spousal report for exposure or for nonexposure to current cigarette smoke at home. These data probably involve the least amount

Table 11-2. Results for self-reported exposure to Environmental Tobacco Smoke from cigarettes in American Cancer Society cohort[a]

Exposure	Rate Ratio (95% CI)
Men	
Currently exposed at home	1.15 (1.01–1.32)
Currently exposed at work	1.03 (0.89–1.19)
Currently exposed elsewhere	1.03 (0.93–1.13)
Men aged <65	
Currently exposed at home	1.34 (1.09–1.65)
Currently exposed at work	1.10 (0.92–1.31)
Currently exposed elsewhere	1.07 (0.90–1.27)
Women	
Currently exposed at home	1.07 (0.98–1.17)
Currently exposed at work	1.06 (0.84–1.34)
Currently exposed elsewhere	0.91 (0.83–1.00)
Women aged <65	
Currently exposed at home	1.18 (0.96–1.45)
Currently exposed at work	1.09 (0.78–1.52)
Currently exposed elsewhere	1.13 (0.90–1.42)

[a]Subjects with missing data on exposure were deleted from analysis. Analysis for exposure at work restricted to those currently employed outside the home. Cohorts for men numbered 78,710 (1751 deaths) for home analysis, 75,237 (768 deaths) for at-work analysis, 72,827 (1770 deaths) for exposure elsewhere analysis. Corresponding numbers for women were 196,358 (2403 deaths), 108,302 (319 deaths), and 146,474 (1880 deaths). Analyses controlled for variables listed in footnote to Table 11–1. Deaths refers to heart disease deaths.

of misclassification of any of the analyses presented. Men show a 23% excess risk and women a 19% excess risk for heart disease death for the currently exposed versus the nonexposed. For women there are some indications of increased risk for those with increased hours of exposure based on self-report, or with the highest reported amount smoked by the spouse, but trends were not consistent. Inverse trends by intensity were observed for men. For men, the overall rate ratio of 1.23 increased to 1.42 for those under 65 at baseline; for women, there was only a slight corresponding increase.

Overall, these results are consistent with previous literature in finding a small increase in risk (approximately 20%), for never-smokers currently exposed to ETS at home, based on the concordant cohort. The analysis of the sub-cohort in which two sources of exposure data were concordant was the least likely to suffer from misclassification of exposure. Such misclassification would likely be nondifferential (the same for those with and without heart disease), and would be expected to bias results toward the null, which might obscure a small excess in heart disease risk.

Findings were slightly stronger for persons under age 65 at baseline

Table 11-3. Analyses for subjects concordant for both self-reported current exposure to cigarettes and exposure to cigarettes based on spouse report in the American Cancer Society[a]

Exposure	Rate Ratio (95% CI)
Men (n=54,668, 1,180 deaths)	
Exposed currently	1.23 (1.03–1.47)
Self-report	
1–2 hours a day	1.23 (0.91–1.67)
3–4 hours a day	1.35 (0.96–1.90)
>4 hours a day	1.13 (0.84–1.51)
Smoking reported by spouse	
<20 cigarettes/day	1.37 (1.04–1.79)
20 cigarettes/day	1.15 (0.86–1.53)
>20 cigarettes/day	1.12 (0.77–1.63)
Men—age <65 at baseline	
Exposed currently	1.42 (1.10–1.83)
Women (n=80,549, 426 deaths)	
Exposed currently	1.19 (0.97–1.45)
Self-report	
1–2 hours/day	0.70 (0.45–1.10)
3–4 hours/day	1.21 (0.85–1.74)
>4 hours/day	1.28 (1.01–1.62)
Smoking reported by spouse	
<20 cigarettes/day	1.22 (0.86–1.72)
20 cigarettes/day	1.14 (0.83–1.57)
21–39 cigarettes/day	1.02 (0.66–1.60)
40+ cigarettes/day	1.28 (0.81–2.01)
Women—age <65 at baseline	
Exposed currently	1.24 (0.89–1.71)

[a]Analyses controlled for variables listed in footnote to Table 11-1. Deaths refers to heart disease deaths. Four categories of current smoking were used for females (three for males) because of the higher prevalence of heavy smoking among husbands.

and the excess was primarily for those currently exposed, consistent with known patterns for active smoking. There were no marked differences in findings when those with heart disease at baseline were excluded, indicating that the effect was not limited to those with prior heart disease.

The lack of positive dose-response trends in many of the results would tend to not support a causal association. However, there are several reasons why a consistent trend of increased risk with more exposure might not be observed. People who are more highly exposed and ill may selectively remove themselves from exposure. In analyses based on married pairs and spousal reports it is possible that the heaviest smokers have died, so that their surviving never-smoking spouse (potentially at higher risk) was not included in the study. Potential misclassification of exposure limits our ability to define quantitative exposure levels for examining dose-response trends. Although this study is large, the number of heart disease deaths in exposed subgroups used for dose-response analyses was often small, exacerbating the problem of misclassification. Finally, Glantz and Parmley (1995) have postulated that some of the effects of cigarette smoke on the heart may reach a saturation point, so that a monotonic dose-response effect may not exist. There is some suggestion of this in recent studies of mainstream smoking (Thun et al., 1995).

Conclusion

Confounding is likely to be more important for studies of ETS and heart disease than for studies of ETS and lung cancer, because of the many known risk factors and the relatively small putative effect being studied. The potential for confounding was reduced in many of the ETS/heart disease studies, however, by controlling for important heart disease risk factors. Residual confounding due to unmeasured or uncontrolled risk factors is not likely to explain the small but measurable increase in CHD risk that is associated with ETS in many different studies of different design and in different countries, many of which also were able to control for the main cardiovascular risk factors.

ETS exposure is inherently difficult to measure accurately, be it retrospectively in case-control studies or prospectively in cohort studies. In this sense it is typical of most exposures in environmental epidemiology, which are generally low and ubiquitous. Misclassification of ETS exposure is likely to be nondifferential, especially in cohort studies not affected by recall bias, so that observed rate ratios are likely to be biased toward the null.

Another issue of misclassification that arises in the epidemiology of never-smokers exposed to ETS is the possible misclassification of former or current smokers as never-smokers. In studies of ETS and lung cancer, the rate of misclassification is thought to be as high as 5% to 10%, primarily former smokers misclassified as never-smokers. This has been of concern in ETS/lung cancer case-control studies because of the potential for upward bias introduced in observed odds ratios. The argument is that cases are more likely than controls to suffer this type of misclassification, because of the association between active smoking and lung cancer. Furthermore, because smokers (or former smokers) are more likely to live with smokers (or former smokers), there is the potential that misclassified case subjects will be more likely to report exposure to ETS, biasing odds ratios upward. The predicted amount of such bias can be estimated based on the degree of misclassification among cases and controls, and the increased likelihood that smokers live with smokers (similar adjustments can be made for cohort studies). Quantitative downward adjustments of odds ratios have been made in the ETS/lung cancer literature for the likely effect of this bias. This problem is much less significant for heart disease, because active smoking is much more weakly associated with heart disease than it is with lung cancer. Therefore the differential nature of such misclassification (higher for cases in case-control studies, higher among the diseased in cohort studies) is much less pronounced in ETS/heart disease studies, and adjustments made to offset upward bias due to this misclassification are negligible.

To summarize, epidemiologic findings to date point to a modestly elevated risk for heart disease due to ETS exposure among never-smokers. Arguments in favor of this association being causal are that it (1) is generally consistent across studies, (2) is controlled for a number of known cardiovascular risk factors in many studies, and (3) parallels findings for active smoking in showing higher risks for younger individuals and those with current (rather than former) ETS exposure. Arguments against a causal interpretation include the fact that (1) the observed relative risks are small and inherently difficult to detect epidemiologically and could be due to confounding by unmeasured risk factors and (2) positive dose-responses are not consistent across studies (however, caveats regarding inconsistent dose-response trends have been outlined above).

Further advances in the epidemiology of ETS and heart disease will require better assessment of exposure in large prospective studies. Personal monitoring for ambient nicotine in some portion of the cohort to validate self-reported ETS exposure would be useful, as would repeated interviews regarding exposure status throughout the follow-up period. Both of these would be expensive and difficult. On the other hand, there exist a number of large cohorts of never-smokers that are being followed prospectively in the United States and elsewhere and in which these approaches are feasible. An alternative to studies of heart disease itself is carefully designed prospective clinical studies of intermediate end points (e.g., platelet aggregation, carotid artery thickness), accompanied by repeated serial objective measurements of exposure on all study subjects, integrated across all sources of exposure.

References

Butler T. 1988. The relationship of passive smoking to various health outcomes among Seventh Day Adventists in California (dissertation). University of California, Los Angeles.

Diez-Roux A, Nieto F, Comstock G, et al. 1995. The relationship of active and passive smoking to carotid atherosclerosis 12–14 years later. Prev Med 24: 48–55.

Dobson AJ, Alexander HM, Heller RF, Lloyd DM. 1991. Passive smoking and the risk of heart attack or coronary death. Med J Aust 154:793–797.

Feldman J, Shenker I, Etzel R, et al. 1991. Passive smoking alters lipid profiles in adolescents. Pediatrics 2:259–264.

Garland C, Barrett-Connor E, Suarez L, Criqui HM, Wingard DL. 1985. Effects of passive smoking on ischemic heart disease mortality of nonsmokers. Am J Epidemiol 121:645–650.

Glantz SA, Parmley WW. 1995. Passive smoking and heart disease; mechanisms and risk. JAMA 273: 1047–1053.

He Y, Li L-S, Wan Z, et al. 1989. Women's passive smoking and coronary heart disease. Chin J Prev Med 23; 19–22.

He Y, Lam TH, Li LS, Li LS, Du RY, Jia GL, Huang JY, Zheng JS. 1994. Passive smoking at work as a risk factor for coronary heart disease in Chinese women who have never smoked. BMJ 308:380–384.

Hirayama T. 1990. Passive smoking (letter). N Z Med J 103:54.

Hole DJ, Gillis CR, Chopra C, Hawthorne VM. 1989. Passive smoking and cardio-respiratory health in a general population in the west of Scotland. BMJ 299: 423–427.

Howard G, Burke G, Szklo M, et al. 1994. Active and passive smoking are associated with increased carotid wall thickness. Arch Intern Med 154:1277–1282.

Humble C, Croft J, Gerber A, Casper M, Hames CG, Tyroler HA. 1990. Passive smoking and 20-year cardiovascular disease mortality among nonsmoking wives, Evans County, Georgia. Am J Public Health 80:599–601.

Jackson RT. 1989. The Auckland Heart Study (dissertation). University of Auckland, New Zealand.

La Vecchia C, D'Avanzo B, Franzosi MG, Tognoni G. 1993. Passive smoking and the risk of acute myocardial infarction (letter). Lancet 341:505–506.

Lee PN, Chamberlain J, Alderson MR. 1986. Relationship of passive smoking to risk of lung cancer and other smoking related diseases. Br J Cancer 54:97–105.

Muscat J, Wynder E. 1995. Exposure to environmental tobacco smoke and risk of heart attack. Int J Epidemiol 24:715–719.

Penn A, Chen L, Snyder C. 1994. Inhalation of steady-state sidestream smoke from 1 cigarette promotes atherosclerotic plaque development. Circulation 90: 1363–1367.

Sandler DP, Comstock GW, Helsing JH, Shore DL. 1989. Deaths from all causes in nonsmokers who lived with smokers, Am J Public Health 79:163–167.

Steenland K, Thun M, Lally C, et al. (1996) Environmental tobacco smoke and coronary heart disease, Circulation 94:622–628.

Surgeon General. 1990. The Health Benefits of Smoking Cessation. US Dept Health and Human Services, Rockville, Maryland.

Surgeon General. 1989. Reducing the Health Consequences of Smoking: 25 years of Progress. US Dept Health and Human Services, Rockville, Maryland.

Svendsen KH, Kuller LH, Martin MJ, Ockene JK. 1987. Effects of passive smoking in the Multiple Risk Factor Intervention Trial. Am J Epidemiol 126:783–795.

Taylor AE, Johnson DC, Kazemia H. 1992. Environmental tobacco smoke and cardiovascular disease. Circulation 86:1–4.

Thun M, Myers D, Day-Lally C, et al. 1996. Age and the exposure-response relations between cigarette smoking and premature death in Cancer Prevention Study II. In: Smoking and Tobacco Control, National Cancer Institute Monograph 6: Changes in Cigarette-Related Disease Risks and Their Implication for Prevention and Control, Washington, DC, National Institutes of Health.

Wells AJ. 1994. Passive smoking as a cause of heart disease. J Am Coll Cardiol 24:546–554.

Zhu B, Sun Y, Sievers R, et al. 1994. Exposure to environmental tobacco smoke increases myocardial infarct size in rats. Circulation 89: 1282–1290.

Zhu B, Sun Y, Sievers R, et al. 1993. Passive smoking increases experimental atherosclerosis in cholesterol-fed rabbits, J Am Coll Cardiol 21:225–232.

Radiation I: 12

Radon

ROSS C. BROWNSON

MICHAEL C. R. ALAVANJA

RADON is a gas that is often attached to particles. Inhaled radon emits ionizing radiation to the lung. Radon's effects have been studied extensively among miners, who were historically exposed to high levels. Although this might generate optimism that the health effects of indoor radon, which involves much lower exposures, would be readily understood as well, this has not been the case.

Radon is a complicated source of radiation exposure because the complexities of both a gaseous agent and small particles must be considered. Exposure assessment must account for home ventilation. Because human exposure is from radon decay products that attach to dust particles, the assessment of dose to the lungs is a complex function of pulmonary physiology and the physical and chemical properties of the air constituents. As with chemical agents, exposure assessment and quantification are inherently challenging.

A second feature is the need to assess literally decades of exposure history. Recent exposure is clearly irrelevant because lung cancer occurs only after a long latency following radiation exposure. Exposures must be estimated as far back as 40 or 50 years. Identifying residences and characterizing exposure in those residences despite modifications to them (or even their destruction) pose difficult challenges. Prospective studies with concurrent monitoring of exposure over periods of decades are unlikely to be conducted, so epidemiologists must seek methods of mitigating the absence of historical records of exposure.

The study of radon and lung cancer has an unusual benefit of clear results from both experimental studies and occupational epidemiology studies. That is, the phenomenon of lung cancer causation due to radon exposure is well-established and relatively well understood based on this research. The studies of miners provide a segment of the dose-response function for lung cancer in humans, a rare achievement in the study of environmental agents. With those data, the question is narrowed to the shape of the dose-response function in the low-dose region of interest for home exposure.

Statistical tools are available to make an extrapolation from miners to home residents with low exposures, with consideration of the biological phenomena of interest. By the time the chain of assumptions is completed, however, the uncertainty in those estimates is far greater than desired for regulatory purposes. Thus, we want direct information on residential radon and lung cancer.

Such direct studies are not needed to determine whether radon causes lung cancer in humans, but rather to quantify the dose-response relationship. In particular, the goal is to quantify that association in a low-dose range which would be predicted to result in relative risks on the order of 1.2 between exposed and unexposed persons. The study size would be so large and the required precision in exposure estimation so high that this goal may ultimately be unattainable.

Nonetheless, the strategies and achievements in this research area are impressive. The search for markers of historical exposure has generated inexpensive dosimeters that can unobtrusively collect exposure information for periods of a year or more, and has led to the evaluation of window glass as an archaeological relic that can reveal the history of radon in the home. On a broader scale, the methods of epidemiology have been advanced through the efforts to standardize protocols, pool studies, quantify the results of exposure misclassification, and select subjects in a manner that is optimal for isolating a presumably modest risk factor, radon, from an extremely powerful one, tobacco. Given the magnitude of lung cancer and the prevalence of radon exposure, we have good reason to continue grappling with subtleties in the dose-response function and each step toward narrowing the bounds of uncertainty has important consequences for risk assessment and regulation.

Radon is a naturally occurring environmental contaminant that is ubiquitous, and its health effects have been the subject of considerable debate in the scientific and public health communities. Although potential radon-related health effects have included nonmalignant lung disease, adverse reproductive outcomes, and leukemia (Committee on the Biological Effects of Ionizing Radiation [BEIR] IV; Henshaw et al., 1990), the only proven effect is lung cancer (Lubin, 1994a). Radon has been well documented as a cause of lung cancer by extensive epidemiologic studies of miners (Lubin et al., 1994b). In addition, animal studies have supported the carcinogenicity of radon (NRC, 1988; Cross, 1992; Cross, 1994).

Although the occupational health risk of radon due to mining exposure has long been known to the scientific community, radon did not receive much public attention until the early 1980s when, during routine monitoring, a radiation worker at a Pennsylvania nuclear power plant was found to be contaminated with radioactivity on his way into the plant when he reported to work (Logue, 1985). This contamination was subsequently traced to elevated radon in the worker's home.

In attempting to assess the risk of lung cancer due to low-level, residential exposure, researchers have commonly extrapolated risk from the studies of miners to the general population. Based on these extrapolations, the excess relative risk is likely to be less than 1.2 for a 25-year exposure at 4 picocuries per liter (pCi/L) (Lubin, 1994a), which represents a high home exposure. The vast majority of U.S. homes are below this level. Among the limitations in extrapolating from studies of miners are uncertainties in miner-based models, dosimetric differences between mines and homes, and the uncertain application of miner-based models derived from adult males to women and children. The joint analysis of data from the 11 underground miner studies suggests that for a fixed cumulative dose there may be greater risk per unit of radon exposure at lower rather than higher exposure rates (Lubin et al., 1994b). If this proves true domestic radon may be more dangerous than would be suspected based on extrapolations from miner data. Yet there is considerable uncertainty as to whether this inverse dose rate effect applies to low-level exposures (Brenner, 1994) like those found in most North American and European homes.

This chapter reviews the evidence on radon as a cause of lung cancer. It covers studies of occupational exposures among miners, experimental animals, and residential exposures. Methodological issues that may affect epidemiologic findings, including potential biases in modeling based on miners' data and potential sources of error in case-control studies of residential radon and lung cancer, are also discussed.

Radon and Its Properties

Radon-222 (hereafter referred to as radon) is an inert gas under usual environmental conditions. It is the naturally occurring decay product of radium-226, the fifth daughter of uranium-238, which is common in the biosphere (National Council on Radiation Protection and Measurement [NCRP], 1987). The decay of radon leads to a series of short-lived, radioactive progeny—polonium-214, polonium-218, bismuth-214, and lead-214. Radon decays with a half-life of 3.82 days. The short-lived isotopes of radon have half-lives from less than a millisecond to 27 minutes (Samet, 1989). Radon is present in most soils and rocks and is therefore common in indoor and outdoor air. It may accumulate at extremely high levels in underground passages and mines (e.g., uranium mines) (Lubin, 1994a).

Two of the decay products of radon, polonium-214 and polonium-218, emit α-particles. Because decay products are electrically charged when created, most of them attach to surfaces and dust particles in the air. A portion of the decay products remains unattached and is referred to as the unattached fraction (Samet, 1989). The unattached decay products can form ultrafine aggregates and appear to be the major source of α-radiation to the lungs (Samet, 1989; Axelson, 1991). In addition to the fraction of unattached radon progeny, several other factors determine the dose of α-radiation to the lungs in humans, including the total volume of air inhaled each minute, the proportion of oral *versus* nasal breathing, and the size distribution of particles in the inhaled air (Samet, 1989; Axelson, 1991; Darby, 1994). These factors are discussed in more detail in a later section.

Units and Methods of Measurement

Radon concentrations in homes are usually measured in terms of the number of disintegrations of radon gas in a fixed time period and a given volume of air. In the International System, concentrations are expressed in terms of becquerels per cubic meter (Bq/m^3), where 1 Bq/m^3 corresponds to one disintegration per second per cubic meter. Concentrations of radon gas also are expressed in terms of picocuries per liter, where 1 $pCi/L = 37 \ Bq/m^3$. The relationship between the concentration of radon progeny and the concentration of radon gas is determined by the equilibrium between the two.

For exposure in miners, the working level (WL) was established as a measure of exposure in the 1950s (Axelson, 1991). One WL is any combination of short-lived radon progeny in 1 liter of air that will ultimately release 1.3×10^5 million electron volts (MeV) of α-energy by decay. The accumulated occupational exposure to radon is expressed in terms of working level months (WLMs), with one WLM equivalent to one WL exposure for 170 hours. One pCi/L is equivalent to about 0.005 WL. The

Table 12-1. Comonly used terms for meauring radon concentration, exposure, and dose

Term	Definition
Bq/m³	Becquerels per cubic meter. A becquerel is one radioactive transformation per second, an SI unit.
pCi/L	10^{-12} curies per liter. A curie is 37×10^9 transformations per second.
WL	A working level is defined as the activity concentration in air that corresponds to 1.3×10^5 MeV of alpha radiation per liter from the ultimate decay of any mix of the radon daughters. It is a level of activity equivalent to that obtained when the daughters are in an equilibrium with a radon concentration of 100 pCi/L.
WLM	One working level month is the esposure to one WL for 170 hours.
Rad	A unit of absorbed dose of radiation equal to 0.01 J/kg or 100 ergs/g.

rad measures the biologically absorbed dose of radiation per unit of tissue. Commonly used terms are summarized in Table 12-1.

Several devices are commonly used to measure radon (Environmental Protection Agency [EPA], 1990). Charcoal cannisters are passive devices that allow continuous adsorption and desorption of radon. These cannisters measure short-term exposure to radon (usually 2 to 7 days). An α-track detector contains a small piece of plastic or film enclosed in a container with a filter-covered opening. Radon diffuses through the filter and α-particles emitted by radon decay products strike the detector and produce submicroscopic damage tracks. The number of tracks produced per unit time is proportional to the radon concentration. The α-track detector can measure an average concentration over a longer period of time (up to one year) and is commonly used in epidemiologic studies. Other types of radon measurement devices include electret-passive environmental radon monitors (E-PERMS), which measures radon with an electrostatically charged disk of Teflon, and continuous radon monitors, which measures radon in a scintillation cell (EPA, 1990).

Distribution of Radon Concentrations and Public Health Recommendations

Radon concentrations in the general U.S. population have been measured widely by the U.S. EPA. The indoor radon concentrations in U.S. homes is approximately log normal, with a small proportion of homes having extremely high levels. The mean concentration of radon in U.S. homes is approximately 1.25 pCi/L (Marcinowski, 1994). In the most recent surveys of the EPA, approximately 6% of the general population has radon concentrations above 4 pCi/L (Marcinowski, 1994). Persons residing in a home at the EPA action level of 4 pCi/L accumulate 40 to 80 WLM (Lubin, 1995).

The EPA (Page, 1993) now estimates that residential radon accounts for 7,000 to 30,000 lung cancer deaths per year in the United States. Similarly, Lubin and Boice estimated that radon may account for approximately 14,000 annual lung cancer deaths, or an attributable risk of about 10% of lung cancer deaths (Lubin et al., 1995). The EPA has established an "action level" of 4 pCi/L (EPA 1990). Because most excess cases of lung cancer would occur at levels less than 4 pCi/L, the "effective" attributable risk of mitigation of levels above 4 pCi/L is 2% to 4% of lung cancer deaths (Lubin et al., 1995).

When initial radon testing shows residential radon at the 4 pCi/L level, EPA recommends additional testing; and if elevated levels are confirmed, various methods of remediation of the housing structure are recommended, depending on the type of housing and level of radon (EPA, 1989). Because of the potential health burden of residential radon exposure, most state public health agencies have set up programs in radon information, testing, or remediation. Other countries have different recommendations. For example, the action level is 5 pCi/L in the United Kingdom and 10 pCi/L in Canada.

Some scientists have criticized the program of the EPA, arguing that no persuasive scientific evidence exists to prove that residential exposure at 4 pCi/L is a health hazard; that humans have repair mechanisms for low-level exposure (Abelson, 1991); that cost-effectiveness of radon remediation has not been demonstrated; or that EPA moved against radon for political reasons—namely, that abatement becomes the home owners' responsibility and does not cost the government (Cole, 1993). Conversely, defenders of the EPA program contend that miner data have clearly established radon as a carcinogen; no evidence for a threshold exposure level exists; and a combined view of human, animal, and molecular studies must be taken (Page, 1993); Alderson, 1994). The cost of remediating U.S. homes for radon has been estimated at $20 billion (Neuberger, 1992).

Review of Literature on the Health Effects of Radon
Miner studies

Underground miners, particularly uranium and tin miners, are potentially exposed to high levels of radon and its progeny. A causal relationship has been clearly demonstrated between underground miners' exposure to radon and lung cancer occurrence (NRC, 1988). Radon in underground mines can reach high levels, with some cohorts receiving as much as 8,000 to 10,000 WLMs (Lubin, 1994b). For comparison, lifetime exposure in a typical U.S. home results in 10 to 20 WLMs.

The risk of lung cancer due to occupational radon exposure has now been convincingly demonstrated based on studies of 20 different populations in Czechoslovakia, the United States, Canada, Sweden, France, Britain, Norway, China, and Australia (Darby et al., 1994). Most of these studies are cohort studies that involve tracking lung cancer deaths among males over time.

Recently, Lubin et al. (1994b) conducted a pooled analysis of 11 cohort studies of underground miners. This review included all studies with at least 40 lung cancer deaths and estimates of individual exposures to radon. Cohorts included miners of iron, fluorspar, tin, and uranium, with over 2,700 lung cancer deaths among 68,000 miners accumulating 1.2 million person-years of exposure to radon. Six studies had information on smoking history and a few had data on other occupational exposures (e.g., arsenic exposure data was available for two cohorts).

Lubin et al. (1994b) utilized a linear excess relative risk (ERR) model:

$$RR = 1 + \beta w$$

where RR is relative risk, w is cumulative exposure to radon progeny in WLM, and β is a parameter representing the unit increase in ERR per unit increase in w. The ERR was linearly related to cumulative exposure to radon (Lubin et al., 1994b). ERR also decreased significantly with attained age, time since exposure, and time after exposure. A clear pattern of risk for the joint association between radon exposure and cigarette smoking was not apparent, although the data were consistent with a pattern of risk intermediate between additive and multiplicative. Among miners, an estimated 39% of the lung cancer deaths in smokers and 73% of the lung cancer deaths in nonsmokers may be due to radon exposure (Lubin et al., 1994b). In addition, this analysis suggested that previous estimates of radon progeny risk for miners may have been overestimated, and radon progeny exposures more than 25 years ago are less hazardous than more recent exposures. Interestingly, adjustment for arsenic exposure in the mine reduced the estimates of radon progeny effects.

Miner studies have also been analyzed to determine the non-lung cancer effects of radon exposure. In a recent analysis of 11 cohorts of underground miners, Darby et al. (1995) found no excess radon-related risk for all non-lung cancers combined (observed-to-expected ratio 1.01). Among individual cancers, slight elevations in risk were noted for leukemia and cancers of the stomach and liver. However, these sites were unrelated to cumulative exposure and are therefore unlikely to be caused by radon exposure in this population.

Animal studies

For over 50 years, animal studies have been conducted to supplement the information on the health effects of radon exposure among underground miners (BEIR IV) (National Research Council 1988). These studies have been carried out primarily in the United States and France. early studies focused on the acute effect of radon exposure; more recent investigations have involved the induction of lung cancer in experimental rats and dogs. In rats, lung cancer has been induced at relatively low exposures (approximately 20 WLM) (BEIR IV) (National Research Council, 1988). To date, no apparent threshold has been observed in rat experiments at occupational and higher exposure levels (Cross, 1994). Although lung cancer induction among dogs does not yet extend to this low-dose range, tumors have been induced at approximately 600 WLM in dogs.

Residential studies

Because of the clear causal relationship between radon exposure and lung cancer risk in miners, considerable interest has developed in determining whether residential exposure to radon results in measurable lung cancer risk.

Ecologic studies

To date, 15 ecologic studies of radon and lung cancer have been reported (Stidley, 1993). In eight of the 15 studies, there was a significant correlation between radon concentration and lung cancer occurrence. In two ecologic studies, an indication of increased risk was suggested, without reaching statistical significance. No suggestion of a relationship was shown in two studies and three studies showed an inverse relationship. Numerous difficulties exist in the interpretation of the ecologic studies of radon and lung cancer (Darby et al., 1994; Stidley and Samet, 1993). Foremost among these are the varying technologies used to measure radon, the inability to account for confounding factors such as cigarette smoking, limited statistical power, and potential bias in the diagnosis of lung cancer. In a comprehensive review of ecologic studies of residential radon and lung cancer, Stidley and Samet (1993) concluded that limitations are so severe that these studies are essentially uninformative. For a relationship like residential radon and lung cancer, ecologic studies may be particularly ineffective in discriminating between a relatively weak effect and no effect.

Case-control studies

The case-control study is the most appropriate and cost effective method for determining the risk of lung cancer in relation to residential radon exposure. Approximately 14 case-control studies of residential radon and lung cancer have been conducted to date. Earlier studies tended to rely on surrogate measures of radon exposure such as housing construction of stone or wood, or whether residents lived on the basement, ground, or upper floors (Darby et al., 1994). More recent studies tend to have larger sample sizes and more accurate and comprehensive exposure assessments.

The seven major studies that have investigated the relationship between residential radon exposure and lung cancer are presented in Table 12-2. Studies are shown that contained 200 or more cases and conducted long-term radon dosimetry. Other case-control studies (Axelson et al., 1988; Edling et al., 1986; Biberman et al., 1993; Lees et al., 1987; Svensson et al., 1989; Lanctot, 1985; Lanes, 1982) are not shown because they contained small sample sizes, conducted short-term radon measurements, or measured radon for only a fraction of the study subjects. An additional case-control study not shown (Lubin et al., 1994c) was a pooled analysis of three earlier case-control studies (Blot et al., 1990; Pershagen et al., 1992; Schoenberg et al., 1990).

In the seven studies in Table 12-2, a fairly wide range of radon concentration was observed, with the lowest readings in New Jersey (median = 0.6 pCi/L) and the highest readings in Stockholm (mean = 3.5 pCi/L) and Finland (mean = 5.7 pCi/L). However, comparisons in readings are problematic because the Swedish and Finnish studies used winter dosimetry, and all other studies used year-long readings.

Studies reported to date are inconsistent in determining whether residential radon exposure results in a statistically significant increase in lung cancer risk. Two studies are presented from the United States. In a case-control study among New Jersey women (Schoenberg, 1990), elevated risk was observed for exposure to radon concentrations of 4 pCi/L or greater. Only 1% of study subjects were exposed to radon concentrations ≥4 pCi/L. No clear pattern of risk by histologic subtype was observed. Limitations included the relatively few subjects with high radon measurements, the reduction of the original, population-based sample of 1306 cases and 1449 controls to 433 cases and 402 controls with long-term radon data available, and the small number of lifetime nonsmoking cases (n = 61), which

Table 12-2. Summary of case-control studies of residential radon exposure and lung cancer with long-term α-Track Dosimetry

Location	Study Period	Study Population	Radon Dosimetry	Confounders Examined	Findings
New Jersey (Schoenberg et al., 1990)	August 1982–September 1983	Females; smokers & nonsmokers; 433 cases, 402 controls	1-year α-track; median of 21 years covered; 1% > 4 pCi/L	Age, respondent type, race, education, smoking, county of residence, vegetable intake, occupation	RR = 4.2 at ≥4 pCi/L; $P = .04$ for trend; no trend for nonsmokers
Shenyang, China (Blot et al., 1990)	September 1985–September 1987	Females; smokers & nonsmokers; 308 cases, 356 controls	1-year α-track; median of 24 years in last home; 20% >4 pCi/L	Age, education, smoking, indoor air pollution	RR = 0.7 at ≥8 pCi/L; no significant trends in smokers or nonsmokers
Finland, 19 southern municipalities (Ruosteenja, 1991)	1980–1985	Males; smokers & nonsmokers; 238 cases, 434 controls	2-month α-track during winter; median of 15 years covered; 40% >4.7 pCi/L	Age, education, smoking, occupation	RR = 1.1 at >5.3 pCi/L; no significant trend
Stockholm, Sweden (Pershagen et al., 1992)	September 1983–December 1985	Females; smokers & nonsmokers; 210 cases, 191 hospital and 209 population controls	1-year α-track; mean of 26 years covered; 28% >4.1 pCi/L	Age, municipality of residence, smoking, passive smoking, diet, occupation	RR = 1.7 at ≥4 pCi/L; $P = .05$ for trend; significant trend in nonsmokers

Study (location)	Dates	Subjects	Exposure assessment	Adjustments	Results
Missouri (Alavanja et al., 1994)	June 1986–June 1991	Females; nonsmokers; 538 cases, 1183 controls	1-year α-track; median of 20 years covered; 7% >4 pCi/L	Age, passive smoking, lung disease, diet, occupation	RR = 1.2 at ≥2.5 pCi/L; no significant trend overall; slight trend for adenocarcinomas
Sweden (Pershagen et al., 1994)	January 1980–December 1984	Both sexes; smokers & nonsmokers; 1360 cases, 2847 controls	3-month α-track during heating season; mean of 23 years covered; 20% >3.8 pCi/L	Age, urbanization, smoking, occupation	RR = 1.8 at >10.8 pCi/L; $P = .05$ for overall trend; no significant trend in nonsmokers
Winnipeg, Canada (Létourneau et al., 1994)	1983–1990	Both sexes; smokers & nonsmokers; 738 cases, 738 controls	6-month α-track; 25% >4 pCi/L	Country of birth, education, smoking, occupation	RR = 1.0 at ≥7.9 pCi/L (bedroom); RR = 0.6 at ≥7.9 pCi/L (basement); no significant trends

makes risk estimates unstable for this subgroup. The other large U.S. study (Alavanja et al., 1994) is discussed in more detail in the next section.

In a study of 308 cases and 356 controls from Shenyang, China, 20% of the homes measured had radon concentrations greater than 4 pCi/L (Blot et al., 1990). Blot et al. (1990) observed no association between radon and lung cancer, regardless of smoking status. However, nonsignificant excess risk was noted among heavy smokers and among cases with the small cell histologic type.

In the Finnish study (Ruosteenja, 1991), odds ratios were elevated between 1.0 and 2.0 in each of the quintiles of radon exposure above baseline, although none achieved statistical significance. The odds ratio at the highest level of radon exposure was 1.13 (95% confidence interval [CI] = 0.57–2.22). No increasing trend in risk with increasing exposure was noted.

Two case-control studies of residential radon and lung cancer have been reported from Sweden (Pershagen, 1992; Pershagen, 1994). In a study from Stockholm (Pershagen, 1992), lung cancer risk tended to increase with increasing radon exposure. A relative risk estimate of 1.7 was observed for radon concentrations above 4 pCi/L. Increasing trends in risk were noted for both never-smokers and current smokers. In a second Swedish study (Pershagen, 1994), a significant positive trend in risk was observed, with a risk estimate of 1.8 at an average radon concentration of over 10.8 pCi/L. The interaction between radon and smoking appeared to be additive, rather than multiplicative.

A recent case-control study from Winnipeg, Canada, included both women and men (738 cases and 738 controls). Despite the fact that Winnipeg homes had some of the highest radon levels in Canada, no association between residential radon levels and lung cancer was observed after adjusting for smoking and occupation (Létourneau et al., 1994).

DETAILED EXAMPLE OF A RECENT CASE-CONTROL STUDY.

A more detailed review of a recently published case-control study from Missouri (Alavanja et al., 1994) illustrates several issues encountered when designing an investigation of residential radon exposure and lung cancer.

OVERALL DESCRIPTION

The Missouri study included white, female patients who were diagnosed with lung cancer between June 1986 and June 1991 through the Missouri Cancer Registry. In addition to the registry-reported diagnosis of lung cancer, tissue slides were simultaneously reviewed by three pathologists for histologic verification (Brownson et al., 1995). Control subjects were a population-based sample of white females selected randomly through driver's license files (aged 64 years and younger) and through Medicare records (aged 65 years and older). Study subjects included both lifetime nonsmokers and former smokers who had stopped smoking 15 years or more before the study interview.

Subjects were interviewed via a comprehensive telephone interview. Surrogate interviews were conducted for 63% of case subjects. Year-long, α-track measurements were made in the homes of 538 case subjects and 1183 controls subjects in which they had lived for at least a year over the past 30 years. One detector was placed in the bedroom and one in the kitchen. Year-long measurements were completed for 78.4% of the period of risk (defined as the period 5–30 years prior to case diagnosis or prior to study enrollment for controls). Multivariate logistic regression was used to calculate odds ratios while adjusting for potential confounders.

RATIONALE FOR SELECTION OF STUDY POPULATION

A nonsmoking female population was selected for study for several reasons:

- Analyses of miners' radon data suggest that the interaction between radon exposure and cigarette smoking is likely to be intermediate between additive and multiplicative; therefore, relative risks for radon exposure would be expected to be larger among nonsmokers than among smokers (Lubin, 1994c), and the proportion of nonsmoking lung cancer cases is more common among women than among men.
- Studying nonsmoking women allowed examination of radon-related risk in the absence of known potential confounders such as cigarette smoking and occupation.
- The Missouri Cancer Registry contains reasonably accurate information on patient smoking history (Brownson, 1989), therefore, selection of nonsmoking cases could be made efficiently.
- Women in the study (average age 71 years) tended to work outside the home infrequently, thereby having longer periods within the home with measurable exposure to radon.

QUALITY CONTROL MEASURES

Because accurate radon measurement is such a key aspect in evaluating the effects of radon (Lubin et al., 1990), the Missouri study conducted three different quality control procedures:

1. A blank, unexposed dosimeter was shipped together with each batch of 20 dosimeters gathered from households in the study. This procedure determined radon exposure incurred during shipping

and also validated the laboratory's ability to accurately assess detectors exposed to low-level radon.

2. A third detector was placed in every 20th household. This detector was placed next to one of the other detectors in the household. If the two side-by-side detectors did not agree within 20%, additional monitoring of that particular household was conducted.

3. A sample of detectors was periodically exposed to known levels of α-radiation in radon chambers at the Geotech Corporation. These detectors were exposed to radon levels of 1.5, 2.5, 5.0, and 7.5 pCi/L.

KEY FINDINGS

The radon levels in the 2664 measured dwellings in the Missouri study had overall arithmetic and geometric means of 1.6 pCi/L and 1.2 pCi/L, respectively. Approximately 7% of study subjects were estimated to be exposed to time-weighted average radon concentrations of >4 pCi/L.

The age-adjusted odds ratios for five time-weighted average levels of radon concentration were 1.00, 1.0 (95% confidence intervals [CI] = 0.7 to 1.4), 0.8 (95% CI = 0.6 to 1.2), 0.9 (95% CI = 0.6 to 1.3), and 1.2 (95% CI = 0.9 to 1.7), indicating no positive trend in risk. Similar patterns in risk were observed when a cumulative measure of dose was used. Additional adjustment for potential confounders such as education, active smoking, passive smoking, previous lung disease, and saturated fat consumption had little effect on risk estimates. Among histologic types of lung cancer, a suggestive positive effect was observed for adenocarcinomas, with an odds ratio of 1.7 at the highest quintile of radon exposure. When analyses were limited to case subjects directly interviewed, a positive linear trend was observed ($P = .06$), suggesting the possibility of residental history misclassification among surrogate respondents.

IMPLICATIONS

The Missouri study was among the first of specifically designed studies to evaluate the effects of residential radon on lung cancer risk. The study included only nonsmokers, obtained long-term radon measurements for the majority of subjects, and conducted several quality control measures. In the Missouri study, an association between low-level radon exposure and lung cancer risk was not clearly demonstrated.

Additional Methodologic Issues

Several additional methodologic issues are important to consider when evaluating the risk of lung cancer due to low-level radon exposure. Much

Table 12-3. Factors potentially influencing the extrapolation between radon exposure and the risk of lung cancer from residential radon exposure

Considered by Dosimetric Modeling	Not Considered by Dosimetric Modeling
Mucus thickness	Inflammation of airways
Clearance rates	Other carcinogens (e.g., arsenic, silica)
Deposition patterns	Smoking
Bronchial morphometry	Sex
Ventilation patterns	Age at risk
Aerosal size distribution	Age at exposure
Exposure rate	

Adapted from National Research Council: Comparative Dosimetry of Radon in Mines and Homes, Washington, DC: National Academy Press, 1991, p. 13.

of the literature about home exposure is based on extrapolations from miners' data, but there are important questions about the certainty of these extrapolations to low exposures in homes given the differences in exposure between miners and the general population.

Validity of extrapolations from miners' data

Because the dose of α-energy delivered to target cells in the lungs cannot be measured directly, modeling approaches are sometimes used to simulate the sequence of events from inhalation of radon progeny to cellular injury by α-particles. By modeling this system in terms of measurable biologic and physical parameters, it is hoped that the health effect measurements and radon exposure measurements from a well-studied miner population can be accurately converted to estimates of health risk in the general population (National Research Council, 1991). However, the accuracy of extrapolation of lung cancer risks from miners to the general population is dependent on the efficacy of modeling physical and biological factors that influence exposure and also on the validity of the unverified assumption that factors not addressed in the models are unimportant. Both modeled and unmodeled factors are enumerated in Table 12-3. Although a more complete discussion of the methods available for quantifying factors that determine the relationship between exposure to radon and the dose of α-particles delivered to target cells in the respiratory tract are described elsewhere (Lippman et al., 1980; Agnew, 1984; Stuart, 1984; NRC, 1991), we will highlight some of the more important aspects of this process.

In general, the absorbed dose is proportional to the amount of activity (i.e., radioactivity) present, usually expressed in becquerels or picocuries, the spatial distribution of the activity in relation to the target cell, and finally to the length of time the activity is present at the target site.

The amount of activity present at a target cell, in turn, depends on the concentration of activity in the ambient air and the breathing rate of the exposed (see list of definitions in Table 12-1). The concentration of radon and its progeny in the air depends on both the degree to which equilibrium has been achieved and on the fraction of the progeny aerosol that has settled or "plated out" on surrounding surfaces. Breathing rate is a function of age and level of physical activity.

Deposition in the respiratory tract depends on breathing rate, the size distribution of the aerosol particle, airway morphometry, and the fraction of the time the individual breathes through his or her mouth. The deposition of radon progeny is non-uniform in the respiratory tract. Heavy breathing results in preferential deposition of large particles higher up in the respiratory system, where it is more easily cleared. The smaller the airway, the smaller the deposition rate for a given volumetric flow rate. Mouth breathing permits larger particles to penetrate to the upper airways of the lung than does nose breathing.

Particle size distribution also is important in any discussion of aerosol deposition in the respiratory tract (Lippman et al., 1980; Agnew, 1984; Stuart, 1984; National Research Council, 1991). As discussed earlier, a distinction often is made in the state of the airborne radon progeny based on apparent attachment to aerosol particles. The unattached fraction (ultrafine mode, 0.5 to 5 nm) refers to those progeny existing as ions, molecules, or small clusters. The attached fraction (accumulation mode, 0.1 to 0.4 μm) is regarded as those radionuclides attached to ambient particles. Per unit ambient air concentration, the unattached fraction is associated with a higher dose to target cells in the lung than is the attached fraction (i.e., 0.2 to 1.3 rad/WLM for attached fraction verses 10 to 20 rad/WLM for unattached fraction (BEIR IV) National Research Council, 1988).

Unfortunately, because the empirical data needed for these analyses are limited, controversy remains concerning the extrapolation of findings from male miners to the general population. Differences in dosimetry in the two settings have been summarized by the "K" factor, which compares the dose of α-energy (in rads) per WLM delivered to target cells in the respiratory tract for the general population with the exposure-dose ratio for miners. At the present time there is no general agreement on how to convert cumulative air measurements of radon daughters (WLM) to measures of dose to target cells (rads) (Natonal Research Council, 1991). For example, the National Council on Radiation Protection and Measurements (NCRP) model increases the risk estimates based on miner studies by 20% for adults in the general population, assuming 0.5 rad/WLM for the mining environment and 0.7 rad/WLM for the indoor environment.

The BEIR IV model (National Research Council, 1988) makes no adjustment, whereas the model of the International Commission on Radiologic Protection (ICRP) reduces the risk by 20% for adults in the general population. In the recent comprehensive analysis of 11 studies of male underground miners (Lubin, 1994b), the assumed "K" factor was 0.7 for adults and 0.8 for children under 10 years.

Attempts are being made to characterize the shape of the dose-response curve at low dose levels by direct observation through large case-control studies. However, these investigations encounter numerous methodologic difficulties, some of which are discussed in the next section.

Challenges to measuring the effects of residential radon exposure

The power of any study to detect and quantify an association between disease and environmental exposures depends critically on the portion of the population with biologically significant exposures and on the quantity, completeness, and reliability of the exposure data. Quantifying the association between lung cancer and residential radon is especially challenging because few homes have been measured for radon historically and current radon measurement may not accurately reflect historic levels. In recent years, although more homes have radon measurements, most measurements are short term (i.e., usually 2 days to 2 weeks). Such readings are of limited value for assessing typical year-round exposures necessary for etiologic analysis because indoor radon concentrations fluctuate substantially by season. In addition, modifications made to a home in the form of adding storm windows and storm doors, adding ceiling and wall insulation, and adding weather stripping are associated with significant differences in indoor radon as illustrated in previously unpublished data from Missouri (Table 12-4). Studies that ignore the effects of these home modifications made during the biologically significant exposure period (presumably 5 to 30 years prior to disease onset) will tend to overestimate earlier exposures to some degree because all forms of home insulation tend to increase indoor radon levels.

Estimating radon in homes previously occupied by study subjects is also complicated by changes that may have been made in locations of bedrooms or other rooms that are important for radon dosimetry (i.e., rooms with relatively long occupancy times). For example, in Missouri, erroneous assessment of the floor on which the bedroom was located could result in rather substantial errors in estimating radon exposure (see Table 12-5). These data show a marked decline in radon levels found in

Table 12-4. Radon concentration (pCi/L) for dwellings classified by insulation type

Type	n	Arithmetic Mean
Wall insulation	2010	1.9
No wall insulation	652	1.5
Attic/ceiling insulation	2451	1.9
No attic/ceiling insulation	319	1.5
Storm doors	2595	1.8
No storn doors	344	1.4
Storm windows	2674	1.8
No storm windows	269	1.4
Weather stripping/caulking	2187	1.8
No weather stripping/caulking	571	1.6

bedrooms located in the basement (2.8 pCi/L) to those on the fourth or higher floors (0.9 pCi/L).

Early surveys of radon concentrations in U.S. homes used screening measurement techniques and strategies first recommended in EPA's "Interim Radon and Radon Decay Product Measurement Protocol" (EPA, 1986). Use of this protocol tended to overestimate the distribution of radon concentrations (Alter and Oswald, 1987). This bias was the result of measurements being made under "closed house" conditions to produce a "worst case scenario"; the measurements were made in a self-selected sample of homes, presumably where a radon problem was suspected; or measurements were made in basements where radon concentrations are often more than twice as high as in other areas of the home. The actual statistical power of epidemiologic studies that were based on these data tended to be lower than expected because they underestimated the sample size actually necessary for etiologic studies.

High residential mobility tends to exacerbate the problem of finding highly exposed study subjects because high residential mobility tends to increase the exposure variability in the population and therefore reduce the number of study subjects with relatively high (i.e., over 4 pCi/L) long-term (e.g., 30-year) time-weighted average radon exposures (Lubin et al., 1990). This point is illustrated in previously unpublished data (Table 12-6). As shown, the proportion of study subjects with mean 25-year time-weighted average above 4 pCi/L decrease monotonically with increasing number of dwellings occupied during this period.

Another important consideration is that radon concentrations in the home reflect radon exposure only if the individual spent time in those

Table 12-5. Radon concentration (pCi/L) in bedrooms classified by location

Location	No. of bedrooms—Missouri	Arithmetic Mean Missouri	Arithmetic Mean U.S.[a]
Basement	186	2.8	3.3
1st floor	1743	1.9	1.3
2nd floor	741	1.5	1.2
3rd floor	67	1.3	1.0
4th floor and above	25	0.9	

[a]From Marcinowski (1994).

homes. Typical residential occupancy factors (i.e., the proportion of time spent at home) vary, depending on the number of vocational and avocational activities taking place outside the home. Because non-residential exposures to radon at schools, workplaces, shopping malls, and so on are more difficult to integrate into a total exposure estimate, they are often ignored in etiologic studies, resulting in additional exposure error.

Errors associated with estimating any of the above-mentioned determinants of exposure further reduces statistical power to detect an effect. Some of this error is associated with missing data. Missing radon data has resulted when the current occupant or landlord refuses measurements, when the dwelling has been torn down, or when structural changes are so severe that a current measurement has little relevance to past radon concentration. Additional error is possible if unreliable measurement techniques are used to assess exposure.

According to Lubin et al. (1990) mobility and errors associated with missing or erroneous exposure data likely to be encountered in case-control studies may make it necessary to increase the number of cases five- to 15-fold to achieve the required study power compared with exposure measured without error for subjects living in a single residence only.

At least one investigator (Lynch, 1994) has chosen to mitigate the effect of residential mobility in reducing statistical power and increasing radon measurement errors by restricting the study subjects to those who occupied only one home during the past 30 years. Although this methodology has appeal by directly obviating the effect of residential mobility in the study design, it will result in an older population sample that will limit generalizability (see Table 12-7).

An additional challenge to radon and lung cancer epidemiology is the precise measurement of the potential confounding and interaction with smoking. As stated earlier, miners' data suggest that radon and cigarette

Table 12-6. Distribution of dwellings with 25-year time-weighted average radon exposure >4 pC/L, by number of dwellings occupied

No. of Dwellings Occupied	>4 pCi/L	
	No.	Percent
1	41	8.3
2	39	7.4
3	15	5.0
±4	15	3.7
All data combined	110	6.4

smoking interact in an additive, but less than multiplicative manner. Larger and more carefully designed residential studies are needed to measure potential interaction in the home environment.

Emerging technologies for exposure assessment

The enumerated difficulties associated with accurately estimating past radon exposure levels may be circumvented with the application of a method for measuring cumulative levels of radon daughter that become firmly attached to glass surfaces in the home. This technique was first reported by Samuelsson (1988) and others (Lively and Ney, 1987; Lively and Steek, 1991). Mahaffey et al. (1993) adapted the technique for epidemiologic applications.

This technique measures cumulative radon levels by taking advantage of the plating out of radon daughter on macroscopic surfaces such as glass in the home. Subsequent α-decay recoils the nucleus of the radon daughter into the superficial layers of glass to a depth of approximately 0.1 mm, which is a depth that normal cleaning does not affect. Because the first long-lived radon daughter (lead-210; half life, 22 years) becomes firmly attached to the glass in this fashion, the glass "memorizes" the airborne radon activity over several decades. Subsequent α-decay by polonium-210 occurs in a stochiometic relationship to cumulative airborne radon exposure of the glass. Samuelsson measured this decay with a pulse ionization chamber as detector (1988). Mahaffey et al. (1993) counted α-tracks left on CR-39 plastic that was affixed to selected glass objects that were continuously exposed to room air for a period of 30 years prior to the glass radon measurement. Mahaffey et al. (1993) demonstrated that glass suitable for radon dosimetry was found in relative abundance in most Missouri homes. Although this technique holds great promise for more accurately estimating retrospective radon exposure and is currently being evaluated in at least two epidemiologic studies (i.e., Missouri and Iowa),

Table 12-7. Distribution of subjects by age and number of dwellings occupied in past 25 years

No. of Dwellings in Past 25 years	Mean Age (n)
1	73.1 (347)
2	71.8 (353)
3	69.7 (195)
4	65.2 (115)
5	62.7 (69)
6	59.0 (104)

the usefulness of this technique has yet to be demonstrated in any large-scale epidemiologic application (Weinberg, 1995).

Biomarkers of exposure may also be used in conjunction with epidemiologic analyses to refine exposure. Taylor and colleagues (1994) have identified an AGC to ATG transversion at codon 249 of the p53 gene in a high proportion of lung cancers from uranium miners with high radon exposure and have suggested that this mutation may be a marker of radiation-induced lung cancer. This or other biomarkers of exposure would help refine the etiologic analysis, but results thus far have been mixed. Väkäkangus et al. (1992) did not find the codon 249 mutations in their studies of underground miners. Lo and colleagues (1995), in their study of domestic radon exposure in the Cornwall and Devon districts of England purported to have high ambient levels of radon, also did not find the codon 249 mutation. The evidence collected to date would suggest a dose-response relationship for the codon 249 mutation. This would not bode well for using the technique to help assess exposure to domestic radon where the radon doses are usually low, but more studies are necessary to confirm this early study.

Conclusion

The relationship between radon exposure and lung cancer initially may appear paradoxical—miner data clearly demonstrate that radon is a cause of lung cancer, yet the growing body of methodologically sophisticated residential studies have not clearly shown an elevation in lung cancer risk due to low-level, long-term radon exposure. As with many other weak associations, it is difficult to demonstrate a clear increase in risk caused by low-level radon exposure in part because of the methodologic difficulties discussed in this chapter. Studies published since 1990 have begun to address many of these issues. These studies, coupled with several currently in the field (Neuberger, 1992), have considered critical aspects including

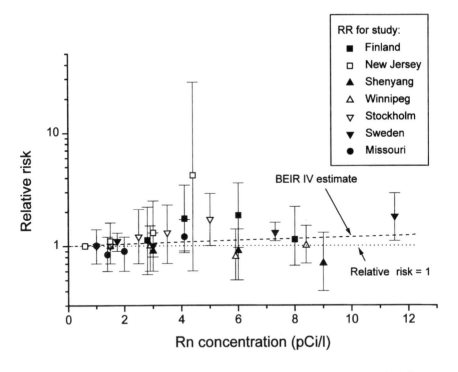

Figure 12-1. Relative risks for lung cancer for the major case-control studies shown in Table 12-2. Also shown are a plot of predicted relative risk for residential exposure from the model of the Committee on the Biological Effects of Ionizing Radiations (BEIR IV) and a plot of a relative risk of 1.0 (reprinted with permission from Am J Epidemiol 1994; 140: 323–332).

better standardization of study protocols and instruments, improved methods of exposure assessment, and clarification of the interaction between smoking and radon exposure. The summary findings of seven recent studies are shown in Figure 12-1. The figure shows multiple risk estimates from each study based on different average dose levels. Also shown is the BEIR IV estimate (National Research Council, 1988), based on a time-dependent model from four studies of miners. The data shown are consistent with either the null hypothesis or the BEIR IV modeling.

As the body of scientific information grow, there also is more opportunity for careful pooling of well-designed epidemiologic studies. Until additional studies of residential radon and lung cancer are completed, particularly in the light of the current social and political environment of scarce public resources, legitimate policy questions will continue to be raised about the expediency of widespread radon testing and remediation of homes with elevated levels.

References

Abelson PH. 1991. Mineral dusts and radon in uranium miners [editorial]. Science 254:774.

Agnew JE. 1984. Physical properties and mechanisms of deposition of aerosols. In: Clarke, SW Pavia D, eds. Aerosols and the Lung: Clinical and Experimental Aspects. Butterworths, Boston.

Alavanja MCR, Brownson RC, Lubin JH, Berger E, Chang J, Boice JD Jr. 1994. Residential radon and lung cancer among nonsmoking women. J Natl Cancer Inst 86:1829–1837.

Alderson L. 1994. A creeping suspicion about radon. Environ Health Perspect 102: 826–830.

Alter HW, Oswald RA. 1987. Nationwide distribution of indoor radon measurements: a preliminary data base. J Air Pollut Control Assoc 37:227–231.

Axelson O, Andersson K, Desai G, et al. 1988. Indoor radon exposure and active and passive smoking in relation to the occurrence of lung cancer. Scand J Work Environ Health 14:286–292.

Axelson O. 1991. Occupational and environmental exposures to radon: cancer risks. Ann Rev Public Health 12:235–255.

Biberman R, Schlesinger T, Margaloit M, et al. 1993. Increased risk for small cell lung cancer following residential exposure to low-dose radon: a pilot study. Arch Environ Health 48:209–212.

Blot WJ, Xu Z-Y, Boice JD Jr, Zhao D-Z, Stone BJ, Sun J, et al. 1990. Indoor radon and lung cancer in China. J Natl Cancer Inst 82:1025–1030.

Brenner DJ. 1994. The significance of dose rate in assessing the hazards of domestic radon exposure. Health Phys 67:76–79.

Brownson RC, Davis JR, Chang JC, et al. 1989. A study of the accuracy of cancer risk factor information reported to a central cancer registry compared with that obtained by interview. Am J Epidemiol 129:616–624.

Brownson RC, Loy TS, Ingram E, Myers JL, Alavanja MCR, Sharp DJ, Chang JC. 1995. Lung cancer in nonsmoking women: histology and survival patterns. Cancer 1995; 75:29–33.

Cole LA. 1993. Elements of Risk: The Politics of Radon. AAAS Press, Washington, DC.

Cross FT. 1992. A review of experimental animal radon health effects data. In: Dewey WC, Edington M, Fry RJM, et al., eds. Radiation Research; A Twentieth Century Perspective. Academic Press, San Diego: 476–481.

Cross FT. 1994. Invited commentary: residential radon risks from the perspective of experimental animal studies. Am J Epidemiol 140:333–339.

Darby SC, Samet JM. 1994. Radon. In: Samet JM, ed. Epidemiology of Lung Cancer. Lung Biology in Health and Disease, Vol. 74. New Marcel Dekker, Inc, New York: 219–243.

Darby SC, Whitley E, Howe GR, Hutchings SJ, Kusiak RA, Lubin JH, et al. 1995. Radon and cancers other than lung cancer in underground miners: a collaborative analysis of 11 studies. J Natl Cancer Inst 87:378–384.

Edling C, Wingren G, Axelson O. 1986. Quantification of the lung cancer risk from radon daughter exposure in dwellings—an epidemiological approach. Environ Int 12:55–60.

Environmental Protection Agency. 1986. Interim indoor radon and radon decay product measurement protocols. National Technical Information Service, Springfield, VA. EPA 520/1:86–104.

Environmental Protection Agency. 1987. Radon Reference Manual. Office of Radiation Programs, Washington, DC. EPA 520/87–20.

Environmental Protection Agency. 1989. Radon Reduction Methods. A Homeowner's Guide, 3rd ed. Office of Radiation Programs, Washington, DC.

Environmental Protection Agency. 1990. Technical Support Document for the 1990 Citizen's Guide to Radon. Office of Radiation Programs, Washington, DC.

Henshaw DL, Eatough JP, Richardson RB. 1990. Radon as a causative factor in induction of myeloid leukemia and other cancers. Lancet 335: 1008–1012.

Hornung RW, Meinhardt TJ. 1987. Quantitative risk assessment of lung cancer in U.S. uranium miners. Health Phys 52:417–430.

Lanctot EM. 1985. Radon in the domestic environment and its relationship to cancer: an epidemiological study. Maine Geological Survey, Department of Conservation, Open File No. 85–88.

Lanes SF. 1982. Lung cancer and environmental radon exposure: a case-control study [dissertation]. University of Pennsylvania, Pittsburgh, PA.

Lapp RE. 1990. Radon health effects? Health Physics Society's Newsletter 18:1,3–5.

Lees REM, Steele R, Roberts JH. 1987. A case-control study of lung cancer relative to domestic radon exposure. Int J Epidemiol 16:7–12.

Létourneau EG, Krewski D, Choi NW, Goddard MJ, McGregor RG, Zielinski JM Du J. 1994. Case-control study of residential radon and lung cancer in Winnipeg, Manitoba, Canada. Am J Epidemiol 140:310–322.

Lippmann M, Yeates DB, Albert RE. 1980. Deposition retention and clearance of inhaled particles. Br J Ind Med 1980; 37:337.

Lively RS, Ney SP. 1987. Surface radioactivity resulting from the deposition of 222 Rn daughter products. Health Phys 52:411–415.

Lively RS, Steek D. 1991. Current status of glass as a retrospective radon monitor. Proceedings of the 1991 International Symposium on Radon and Radon Reduction Technology, Session III: Measurement Methods. Philadelphia, PA.

Lo YM, Darby S, Noakes L, Whitley E, Silcocks RBS, Fleming KA, Bell JI. 1995. Screening for radon 249 p53 mutation in lung cancer associated with domestic radon exposure. Lancet 345:60.

Logue J, Fox J. 1985. Health hazards associated with elevated levels of indoor radon—Pennsylvania. MMWR 34:657–658.

Lubin JH. 1994a. Invited commentary: lung cancer and exposure to residential radon. Am J Epidemiol 140:323–332.

Lubin JH, Boice JD Jr, Edling C, et al. 1994b. Radon and Lung Cancer Risk: A

Joint Analysis of 11 Underground Miners Studies. Rockville, MD: National Institutes of Health, NIH publication 94–3644.

Lubin JH, Liang Z, Hrubec Z, Pershagen G, Schoenberg JB, Blot WJ, et al. 1994c. Radon exposure in residences and lung cancer among women: combined analysis of three studies. Cancer Causes Control 5:114–128.

Lubin JH, Samet JM, Weinberg C. 1990. Design issues in epidemiologic studies of indoor exposure to Rn and risk of lung cancer. Health Phys 59:807–817.

Lubin JH, Boice JD Jr. 1989. Estimating Rn-induced lung cancer in the United States. Health Phys 57:417–427.

Lubin JH, Boice JD Jr, Edling C, et al. 1995. Lung cancer in radon-exposed miners and estimation of risk from indoor exposure. J Natl Cancer Inst 1995;87: 817–827.

Lynch C. 1994. Personal communication. University of Iowa.

Mahaffey JA, Parkhurst MA, James AC, Cross FT, Alavanja MCR, Boice JD, Ezrine S, Henderson P, Brownson RC. 1993. Estimating past exposure to indoor radon from household glass. Health Phys 64:381–391.

Marcinowski F, Lucas RM, Yeager WM. 1994. National and regional distributions of airborne radon concentrations in U.S. homes. Health Phys 66:699–706.

National Council on Radiation Protection and Measurements. 1987. Ionizing Radiation Exposure on the Population of the United States. NCRP Report No. 93. Bethesda, MD.

National Research Council, Committee on the Biological Effects of Ionizing Radiations. 1988. Health Risks of Radon and Other Internally Deposited Alpha-Emitters: BEIR IV/Committee on the Biological Effects of Ionizing Radiations, Board of Radiation Effects Research Effects, Committee on Life Sciences, National Research Council. National Academy Press, Washington, DC.

National Research Council, Panel on Dosimetric Assumptions Affecting the Application of Radon Risk Estimates. 1991. Comparative Dosimetry of Radon in Mines and Homes. Panel on Dosimetric Assumptions Affecting the Application of Radon Risk Estimates, Board of Radiation Effects Research Effects, Committee on Life Sciences, National Research Council. National Academy Press, Washington, DC.

Nero AV, Schwehr MB, Nazaroff WW, Revzan KL. 1986. Distribution of airborne radon-222 concentrations in U.S. homes. Science 23:992–997.

Neuberger JS. 1992. Residential radon exposure and lung cancer: an overview of ongoing studies. Health Phys 63:503–509.

Neuberger JS. 1991. Residential radon exposure and lung cancer: an overview of published studies. Cancer Detect Prev 15:435–443.

Page SD. 1993. The science and policy of EPA's radon program. Health Physics Society's Newsletter. 1993;11: 1,3–4.

Pershagen G, Åkerblom G, Axelson O, Clavensjö B, Damber L, Desai G, et al. 1994. Residential radon exposure and lung cancer in Sweden. Engl J Med 330:159–164.

Pershagen G, Liang Z-H, Hrubec Z, Svensson C, Boice JD Jr. 1992. Residential radon exposure and lung cancer in Swedish women. Health Phys 63:179–186.

Puskin JS, Nelson CB. 1989. EPA's perspective on risks from residential radon exposure. JAPCA 39:915–920.

Ruosteenoja E. 1991. Indoor radon and risk of lung cancer: an epidemiological study in Finland. Finnish Centre for Radiation and Nuclear Safety, Helsinki.

Samet JM. 1989. Radon and lung cancer. J Natl Cancer Inst 81:745–757.

Samet JM. 1992. Indoor radon and lung cancer. Estimating the risks. West J Med 156:25–29.

Samuelsson C. 1988. Retrospective determination of radon in houses. Nature 334:338–340.

Schoenberg JB, Klotz JB, Wilcox HB, Nicholls GP, Gil-del-Real MT, Stemhagen A, Mason TJ. 1990. Case-control study of residential radon and lung cancer among New Jersey women. Cancer Res 50:6520–6524.

Stidley CA, Samet JM. 1993. A review of ecologic studies of lung cancer and indoor radon. Health Phys 65:234–251.

Stuart BO. 1984. Deposition and clearance of inhaled particles. Environ Health Perspect 55:369.

Svensson C, Pershagen G, Klominck J. 1989. Lung cancer in women and type of dwelling in relation to radon exposure. Cancer Res 49:1861–1865.

Swedjemark GA. 1985. Radon and its decay products in housing. PhD thesis. University of Stockholm, Sweden.

Taylor JA, Watson MA, Devereux TR, Michels RY, Saccomanno G, Anderson M. 1994. Mutation hotspot in radon-associated lung cancer. Lancet 343:86–87.

Vähäkangas KH, Samet JM, Metcalf RA, et al. 1992. Mutations of p53 and ras genes in radon-associated lung cancer from uranium miners. Lancet 339:576–580.

Weinberg CR. 1995. Potential for bias in epidemiologic studies that rely on glass-based retrospective assessment of radon. Environ Health Perspect 103:1042–1046.

Radiation II: 13

Electromagnetic Fields

DAVID A. SAVITZ

TOPICS in environmental epidemiology often engender controversy, but few have done so to the degree that the issue of magnetic fields and cancer has. The issue arose recently, in the 1980s, and may seem unique, but the concerns are largely the traditional ones for environmental epidemiology.

Public perception and concern are heightened by a number of characteristics of this agent and its potential health effects. Magnetic field exposure is undetectable and involuntary, and it occurs in homes. To many people it is a mystery. The primary health effect of concern, childhood cancer, is a rare, life-threatening disease, that does not have a close temporal link to exposure and has few established risk factors, making it rather mysterious as well. Public concern and the closely associated media attention have fostered studies in this area. Some have argued that setting priorities in this manner instead of focusing on purely objective criteria is undesirable, but responding to public concerns is one of the legitimate goals for environmental epidemiology, along with identifying preventable causes of human disease and advancing understanding of human biology. A controversy that has resulted in litigation and debate over regulation would surely benefit from more refined epidemiologic understanding.

Several other features of the exposure raise scientific questions that apply to other environmental exposures to varying degrees. In modern society, exposure to electric and magnetic fields is ubiquitous, and the challenge is to identify clear gradients of exposure to see whether those differences are associated with varying disease rates. These same concerns apply to persistent organochlorides (e.g., polychlorinated biphenyls), indoor radon, and pesticide residues in food. In each instance, the agent is clearly present and detectable, but for a number of logistical reasons, it is difficult to cleanly separate persons with higher and lower levels of exposure. Because the exposure is ubiquitous, however, if health risks result from variation in the "normal" range of exposure, the magnitude of the public health effects could be substantial.

Another important methodologic feature of studying magnetic fields is the multiplicity of exposure sources. Like lead or ultraviolet radiation, or some forms of air pollution such as benzene, many environmental settings contribute small amounts of exposure. Thus, the importance of the various sources depends on both the concentration and the amount of time spent in a particular microenvironment. Unless there is an integrative biological marker, such as for lead, we are forced to confront the added dimension of complexity in allocating our environmental sampling and interview time across several sources rather than a single exposure source. In the case of magnetic fields, the level associated with a single source, for example, electric blanket use, is further complicated by variability within the single category, for example, different brands of electric blanket and different modes of use. The barriers to retrospective construction of an accurate, time-integrated measure are daunting, yet because the concern is with rare diseases, true prospective studies are even more difficult.

Finally, in the study of magnetic fields our ignorance of the biologically important exposure measure has been especially problematic. Choice of a measure is made difficult by the absence of much biological theory or experimental work to narrow the possibilities and provide a logical basis. Tradition makes us comfortable with accepting measures of concentration times time as valid markers of chemical exposure, yet more detailed consideration of human physiology and assessment of target organ dose would rarely provide a firm basis for that assumption. Investigators of magnetic fields and cancer have often used the default measure of average exposure, but with more self-consciousness regarding the relevant measure and time period than is typical. Many of the same questions are as applicable to more extensively studied phenomena such as ozone and respiratory disease or lead exposure and neurobehavioral effects.

The epidemiologic evidence on the health effects of electric and magnetic fields lends itself to varying interpretations, with recurrent observations of modest associations between such exposures and cancers in children and leukemia and brain cancers in adults. However, the associations are typically small enough to raise the question of whether they are truly present at all, and studies of similar quality sometimes do not find such associations.

Superimposed on this suggestive but inconclusive epidemiologic literature is an equally controversial literature in biophysics and other laboratory disciplines. On theoretical grounds, some physicists and biophysicists have forcefully argued that biological effects of these very low energy fields cannot occur (Foster, 1993), and have taken on the mission of explaining how epidemiologists must have gone astray. Despite this debate regarding biophysical mechanisms as the basis for assessing the plausibility of the epidemiologic evidence (Carpenter and Arpetyan, 1994), erroneous epidemiologic findings could only be the product of methodologic flaws within the studies themselves (Savitz, 1994).

Experimental studies of electric and magnetic fields have so far yielded little evidence of biological changes that would be expected to result in cancer, but a range of biological consequences have been reported (Carpenter and Arpetyan, 1994). One pathway in particular, involving effects on the pineal gland and alterations in melatonin production (Stevens et al., 1992), has attracted interest and led to epidemiologic inquiry. The observation of biologic changes, but none clearly linked to cancer, further fuels the controversy over the interpretation of the ambiguous epidemiologic findings. Limited understanding of mechanisms tends to enhance the burden on epidemiology to somehow resolve the controversy.

Exposures of Interest

The type of exposures that environmental epidemiologists have studied needs to be carefully circumscribed. The electromagnetic spectrum includes x-rays, visible light, radar, and microwaves, as well as power-frequency (50 or 60 Hertz) electric and magnetic fields (Carpenter and Arpetyan, 1994). Even the rubric "non-ionizing radiation" covers the portion of the spectrum of frequencies with a wide range of biological responses. With only a few exceptions (e.g., Robinette et al., 1980), the entire epidemiologic literature addresses fields in the extremely low frequency range (less than 300 Hertz), specifically the fields resulting from generation, distribution, and use of electric power. Such fields are 60 Hertz in North America and 50 Hertz in Europe and many other parts of the world. Although there may be some commonalities in biological effects across field frequencies, the most reasonable assumption would be that studies of power-frequency fields have little or no relevance to other types of electromagnetic fields. Current controversies regarding siting of broadcast towers, microwave relays, and use of cellular telephones concern much higher frequencies and vastly different exposure circumstances than the focus of this chapter. In addition, the sizable literature on occupational exposure to electric and magnetic fields will not be addressed here, with reviews available elsewhere (Savitz and Ahlbom, 1994; Theriault, 1991).

Even given the restriction to power-frequency electric and magnetic fields, there is substantial uncertainty about what field characteristics should be the focus of attention. There is some agreement that magnetic fields are of greater concern than electric fields, at least in residential settings. At the frequencies of interest, electric fields are readily shielded by building materials so that fields from power lines near a home do not influence electric field exposures in the home. Even the surface of the human body shields the interior of the body, such that electric fields produce only a surface charge (Tenforde and Kaune, 1987). In contrast, magnetic fields pass through essentially all common materials with no attenuation, so that outside power lines influence fields in the home; the field just beyond the outer wall is quite similar to that just inside the wall. Analogously, the field at the surface of the body is similar to the internal field (e.g., in the marrow or brain tissue).

Although the absence of a known mechanism by which magnetic fields would be expected to influence cancer should not inhibit epidemiologic research that tries to determine whether it does, this lack of understanding poses particular challenges for the epidemiologist. Primary among them is the uncertainty over the form of exposure that should be evaluated, with such obvious options as time-weighted averages, peaks, time above threshold, and variability. Each makes implicit assumptions about the type of exposure that is biologically relevant with the truth at present unknown. By default, and in parallel with chemical agents, we have focused mostly on the time-weighted average. This is consistent with the research interest in sources of prolonged elevated exposures that will substantially influence the time-weighted average such as the typical field level in homes (determined, in part, from outside power lines near the home) and electric blankets (which are used for prolonged periods of time) and far less attention on very high-field, short-use appliances such as electric hair dryers or electric power tools.

Health Outcomes of Concern

Various health concerns have been raised in relation to residential magnetic field exposure, including cancers in adults (Wertheimer and Leeper, 1982; Severson et al., 1988), depression and suicide (Poole et al., 1993;

McMahan et al., 1994;, Perry et al., 1981), and adverse reproductive outcomes (Juutilainen et al., 1993; Wertheimer and Leeper, 1989). However, the primary focus for the public, the research community, and this review is on childhood cancer. The methodological issues in exposure assessment are quite similar independent of the health outcome. Because all are relatively rare events (with the exception, perhaps, of depression), retrospective exposure assessment is typically required. That is, because of the disease rarity, true prospective studies are infeasible, and therefore prospective exposure monitoring cannot be incorporated into the studies.

In addition, for childhood cancer, the period between exposure and disease is potentially on the order of several years, further diminishing the prospects for direct measurement of the etiologically relevant exposure. Although the presumed etiologic period for childhood cancer is shorter than that for adults, essentially the entire period from pregnancy to shortly before diagnosis may be relevant to etiology, an interval lasting up to 15 years. In designing and evaluating epidemiologic studies, the time to which the exposure is applicable and the underlying assumptions about the etiologic period deserve careful evaluation.

To address childhood cancer, we must therefore reconstruct exposure retrospectively, using any available tools. That is, we use historical records, people's memory, and environmental markers that are still available to estimate the exposures that existed in the past. Even ostensibly direct measures like in-home magnetic field measurements or personal monitors have been used so far only as candidate markers for past exposure, competitors with self-reported history or inferred exposure from power lines near the home. Much of the controversy has focused on whether "indirect" markers of exposure such as power lines are valid relative to "direct" markers such as measured fields in the home. Relative to the time periods of concern, both are indirect markers and it is an empirical question (that has not been fully resolved) which is the better indirect marker.

Overview of the Epidemiologic Literature
Childhood cancer

A rather sizable literature has developed over the years since Wertheimer and Leeper (1979) initially published the results of their study of wiring configurations near residences and childhood cancer. In addition to the substantive results of their case-control study, some of the ideas that they introduced remain key, controversial issues. Case-control studies have evolved over a long period of time (Schlesselman, 1982; Rothman, 1986), and the basic strategy of comparing exposure histories of properly selected cases and controls is rather well understood. However, the exposure assessment methods proposed by Wertheimer and Leeper (1979) were novel.

The assessment of the magnetic field exposure history of the cases and controls in their study was based solely on the configuration of the electric power lines near the subjects' homes. Several assumptions were made, which are discussed in more detail below. They argued that external characteristics of the power lines could be used to infer the approximate current flow along those lines; that current flow along the lines is roughly proportional to the levels of magnetic fields produced by the line; that residential magnetic field exposure levels are largely determined by those fields from outside power lines; and that typical residential magnetic fields are a dominant contributor to total exposure. Virtually every one of those points has been challenged, with some resolved and some remaining important points of disagreement.

Among the many criticisms directed at Wertheimer and Leeper's (1979) study, most were actually suggestions of nondifferential exposure misclassification caused by the inherent limitations in using a wiring configuration code as a marker of magnetic field exposure. Such deficiencies, inherent in the code as applied to cases and controls, would be suggestive of stronger actual associations than those that were observed. Only the unblinded coding of residences by the study authors was a plausible source of differential misclassification that could have given rise to a spurious positive association. The investigators did code a subset of residences using an independent, blinded coder, with corroboration of their results, but the criticism was not fully countered.

Detailed reviews of the subsequent studies are available elsewhere (Savitz and Ahlbom, 1994; Bates, 1991; Washburn et al., 1994) and will not be repeated here, with the exception of the Swedish study that serves as the primary case example in this chapter (Feychting and Ahlbom, 1993). Instead, the general methods and patterns in the literature will be summarized.

The studies have used a variety of exposure measures, each with methodological strengths and weaknesses, and, not surprisingly, some disparities in the results. Wiring configuration codes, identical to or closely related to those developed by Wertheimer and Leeper (1979), have provided the most consistent evidence of an association with childhood cancer (Savitz et al., 1988) or childhood leukemia alone (London et al., 1991). All three studies (Wertheimer and Leeper, 1979; Savitz et al., 1988; London et al., 1991) report odds ratios in the range of 1.5 to 3.0, somewhat higher in Wertheimer and Leeper's (1979) study than in the others. Variants of wiring configuration were not found to be associated with childhood leukemia in a study in Rhode Island (Fulton et al., 1980), but disparities in the calendar time period of occupancy of cases and controls is likely to have produced a bias (Wertheimer and Leeper, 1980). Because of a general migration out of the central city to the suburbs, with larger yards and lower prevalence of high wire codes, the earlier average occupancy dates of controls appears to have reduced the observed odds ratios. Although the earlier studies found associations of equal or greater magnitude with childhood brain tumors compared to those for childhood leukemia (Wertheimer and Leeper, 1979; Savitz et al., 1988), two recent, well-designed studies did not identify such associations (Preston-Martin et al., 1996; Gurney et al., 1996), though these studies also suffered from many of the limitations common to earlier ones (Poole, 1996).

Several investigators have considered a range of electrical facilities in proximity to homes (Tomenius, 1986; McDowall, 1986; Myers et al., 1990), but these are only remotely related to wiring configuration codes and most would be not be expected to capture relatively subtle distinctions in exposure. For example, using overly generous cutpoints of distance from above-ground power lines would mean that most persons classified as "exposed" would not have had truly elevated exposures.

Several studies of childhood cancer have also included measurements of magnetic fields in the home, typically collected in conjunction with the interview. These protocols range from an instantaneous "spot" measurement of electric or magnetic fields (Savitz et al., 1988) to a 24-hour measurement (London et al., 1991). In contrast to the array of assumptions underlying a wire code, only one assumption is made in the use of magnetic field measurements: the levels seen at the time of measurement are reflective of the levels that were present over the historical period of etiologic inference. This ostensibly straightforward question actually turns out to be as complex as the question about the validity of wire codes as a marker of historical exposure.

The conventional interpretation that analyses using magnetic field measurements have produced weaker links with childhood cancer than those using wire codes is only partially correct. The key limitation in the analyses of measured fields and childhood cancer in studies from both Denver (Savitz et al., 1988) and Los Angeles (London et al., 1991) is incomplete coverage. Due to residential mobility and respondent refusal, the Denver study had only 35% of case homes measured, and the Los Angeles study achieved around 50% coverage. Any results, positive or negative, from such analyses should be interpreted cautiously. Within the constraint of those limited samples, both studies produced a similar pattern: weak associations were found between measured magnetic fields and childhood cancer, weaker than those seen for wiring configuration codes.

Thus, while the positive associations observed for wire codes motivate continued research, it would be erroneous to interpret the literature as providing strong evidence against an association of present-day measurements and childhood cancer.

Case study: Swedish study of residential magnetic fields and childhood cancer

The Swedish study of childhood cancer and exposure to magnetic fields from power lines (Feychting and Ahlbom, 1993) provides a useful illustration of the issues in residential exposure assessment. Relative to the studies that preceded it in the United States, the investigators sought to identify an exposure source and setting that was particularly amenable to historical reconstruction and to address the concerns with potential selection bias from the manner in which controls had been identified and recruited in previous studies.

Only long-distance transmission lines are aboveground in Sweden, with distribution lines buried, thus the exposure source of interest was restricted to overhead transmission lines. Corridors of 300 meters around such lines were defined, chosen to be wide enough to include both exposed and unexposed residences but having an elevated prevalence of higher exposure homes. (European studies that are not restricted in some such manner tend to have such low exposure prevalence as to be uninformative, e.g., Coleman et al., 1989; Myers et al., 1990). All persons who lived on property within those corridors between 1960 and 1985 constituted the study base, with cases of childhood cancer among such residents identified through the cancer registry and controls selected from the population registry.

Eligible subjects were identified primarily from a computerized listing of the coordinates of all properties in Sweden. All persons who lived in this corridor were followed from birth or from movement into the corridor through 1985. This roster of persons was matched against records of the cancer registry to identify cases, with medical records then sought from the treating hospital. Controls were selected from the population register in a 4:1 ratio to cases, matched on year of birth, sex, parish, and living in the same power line corridor as the case.

Two main approaches were taken to assess magnetic field exposure:

1. Spot measurements of magnetic fields were taken in homes where cases and controls lived around the time of diagnosis. A protocol involving several locations was taken under low power use condi-

tions in the home, similar to those used in previous studies (Savitz et al., 1988; London et al., 1991).

2. Calculated magnetic fields were estimated using information on the spatial arrangement of the lines relative to the home (e.g., height of towers, distance between phases of the power line). In order to develop a predictive model linking the power line characteristics to historical magnetic field exposure levels, information on line load at the time of measurement was assessed so that a statistical relationship between line characteristics, load, and present fields could be established. Then, information on the average line load during the periods of interest (1958–1985) was obtained from records maintained by the electric utility company. This allowed historical loads to be used to calculate historical exposures.

In addition to the direct value of the information produced by this study, the insights regarding exposure assessment are of great importance. Note that in choosing to focus on overhead transmission lines, the investigators were able to define a field source that was amenable to simple engineering-based predictive models. This is in contrast to the complexity of fields determined by overhead distribution lines in the United States, which are not readily modeled with accuracy because of multiple lines in proximity to one another and variable current flows. The wire configuration codes are a simplified, categorical approach to a much more complex relationship between wiring and magnetic fields.

Second, record-keeping practices allowed them to use information on the historical loads to estimate historical exposure. Their historical magnetic field estimates, based on modeling, are a sophisticated variant of a wiring configuration code with refinements possible because of restriction to transmission lines and the opportunity to explicitly account for historical changes in the load on the line. A fairly strong correlation was found between spot measurements of magnetic fields and calculated contemporary fields (r=0.70) which was attenuated somewhat in comparing spot measurements to calculated historical fields (r=0.52). Predictions were notably less accurate for apartments than for single-family dwellings.

In comparing subjects with calculated historical exposures for the period 1960 to 1985 of 0.1 to 0.19 µT, and 0.2 µT or higher to those with calculated exposures of 0.09 µT or less, odds ratios of 1.5 and 1.1 were found for total cancers and 2.1 and 2.7 for leukemia. Using a higher cutpoint of 0.3 µT or higher, the odds ratios were 1.3 for total cancer and 3.8 for leukemia. The imprecision in these estimates should be noted; only 24 cancer cases had exposures of 0.1 µT or higher and 11 leukemia cases were in that range. There were only four brain tumor cases above

0.09 μT, with no increase in risk with higher exposure. The increased risk with increasing exposure for leukemia was limited to residents of single-family homes, for whom the odds ratios were 4.5 (four cases) and 5.6 (five cases) for calculated exposures of 0.1 to 0.19 μT, and 0.2 μT or higher, respectively. Using distance from the line as the exposure marker generated a similar pattern of results, with an increased risk for leukemia among residents within 50 meters of the line. Of great interest for comparison to U.S. studies, spot measurements of magnetic fields (ignoring distance or historical changes in loads) were not associated with an increased risk of leukemia, with odds ratios of 0.2 (1 case) and 0.6 (4 cases) for measured exposures of 0.1 to 0.19 μT, and 0.2 μT or higher.

The primary limitation of the Swedish study, well-recognized by the authors, is imprecision. In contrast to the U.S. studies that preceded it, this study had a nearly perfect method of control selection. The population register allows direct sampling from the study base in contrast to the indirect approaches used in the United States, such as random-digit dialing. The exposure assessment methods, as discussed above, allowed for incorporation of historical changes in line load. The contrast between the results for spot measurements and calculated historical fields would suggest that a true association may be present which is diluted by misclassification when using spot measurements. Similarly, the stronger association for single-family dwellings can be interpreted to suggest that an association is present but blurred when evaluating apartments where the exposures are not determined simply by the outside power lines. Unfortunately, the unique resources that made this study feasible, including a population register, computerized property listings, a national cancer registry, and historical records of line loads do not exist in many other settings. Thus, direct replication of this study is not feasible outside of Scandinavia.

Exposure Assessment Issues
Theoretical concerns

Because of the rarity of the health end points of concern, exposure assessment for individuals has been and is likely to continue to be retrospective. Even when cases can be identified prospectively as they occur, the relevant exposures for etiology will still be in the past. Monitoring magnetic field exposure concurrently for hundreds of thousands of people over periods of several years while cancers occur is not likely to ever be done. Ecologic studies in which cancer rates in communities or perhaps countries that do or do not use electricity are compared would be informative if it were possible to identify such contrasts not accompanied by a wide array of other disparate conditions.

Given this situation, the practical challenge researchers face is to use information currently available to assess exposures in the past. Some past exposures have little promise of accurate reconstruction—for example, driving near power lines, exposures outside the home, school, or workplace. Even within locations of sufficient importance to warrant an attempt at reconstruction, there are only a few options for assessing the exposures likely to have been present in the past and no opportunity to validate those assessments in the absence of historical records of field levels.

Two broad strategies can be applied: reports of contributors to past exposure, such as use of electrical appliances or residential proximity to power lines; and measurements of current field levels as proxies for past field levels. Underlying both of these methods is the notion that some field sources are predictable and are readily identifiable in the past, such as outside power lines near homes that change little over extended periods of time. The former approach is explicit in inquiring about those presumably stable sources, but even present-day measurements as a surrogate for the past rely on an assumption of stability over time. Measurements should reflect a mixture of stable, historically relevant field determinants as well as temporally unstable influences, which would add noise to the estimation of exposures in the past.

The question that guides exposure assessment efforts is a purely empirical one: What measures best approximate historical individual magnetic field levels? Because of the interest in prolonged as opposed to transient exposure, this may be interpreted as a question of what best approximates time-weighted average exposure as opposed to peaks or other parameters of the distribution.

Wiring characteristics in relation to measured fields in homes

A fairly extensive literature addresses the relationship between nearby power line characteristics and measured magnetic fields, beginning with Wertheimer and Leeper's (1979) original report. Studies have evaluated that association in Denver (Savitz et al., 1988), Seattle (Kaune et al., 1987), Los Angeles (London et al., 1991), and more recently in a national sample (EPRI, 1993a). Using the Wertheimer-Leeper code, which divides homes into underground, very low, ordinary low, ordinary high, and very high current configurations (Wertheimer and Leeper, 1982), there is rather consistent evidence of the highest average fields in very high current configuration homes, above-average fields in ordinary high current configuration homes, and little distinction in fields among the lowest three wire configurations. In the largest survey, the 1000-home survey conducted by EPRI (1993a), the median magnetic field measurements were 0.5, 0.4, 0.6, 0.8, and 1.2 across the five levels. Thus, based simply on average fields, there is some discriminatory power but the association is not terribly strong.

In an analysis of variance framework, wire codes are often found to be rather poor predictors of measured magnetic fields, accounting for only 15% to 20% of the total variance (Kaune et al., 1987; Kaune and Savitz, 1994; EPRI, 1993b). Either this reflects a coding system that inadequately captures aspects of the outside power line that have major influences on fields, or else the wire codes accurately reflect the true magnitude of the contribution of wiring to residential field levels, and there are substantial field determinants other than outside power lines.

On the other hand, perhaps efforts to explain total variance in measured fields based on wire codes is inappropriate. In relatively low field, low wire code homes, there is likely to be a major contribution from other sources such as in-home wiring and currents on water pipes, sources that reduce the explanatory power of outside power lines. Measured magnetic fields in homes tend to follow a log-normal distribution, with most values in the low end (0.05 to 0.15 μT) and a tail to the upper end that diminishes rapidly above 0.2 μT. Discriminations among measurements in the low end based on outside power lines are likely to be poor, given that variation is thought to result from many transient or otherwise unidentifiable sources, including meter inaccuracy, interference from in-home wiring or nearby appliances, and the electrical load in the home or neighborhood at the time of measurements. However, discriminating between homes in the low end (dominant part of the distribution) and the tail may be much more feasible because placement in the upper tail is more likely to involve a particular field source, such as a high current configuration of power lines.

A different approach to examining the relationship between outside power lines and magnetic fields examines the accuracy of classification of fields into categories of high and low (rather than absolute value) based on knowledge of outside power line configurations. Using wire codes as a predictor of residential magnetic fields above or below 0.2 μT, for example, Kaune and Zaffanella (1994) found 80% sensitivity (for detecting homes above 0.2 μT using wire codes) and 76% specificity (for detecting homes below 0.2 μT using wire codes). Sensitivity and specificity were in the same range (around 77%) in another similarly designed study (EPRI, 1992).

Thus, the question of how strongly predictive wire codes are for residential magnetic fields does not have a simple answer. There is clearly an association present in the direction predicted by Wertheimer and Leeper (1979, 1982), yet there is substantial variability in measured fields within wire code levels. In the lower end of the distribution, wire codes are poorly predictive; but for discriminating between homes in the lower end and the upper tail of the distribution, wire codes are reasonably effective (sensitivity and specificity in the range of 0.75 to 0.80).

Wire codes, residential magnetic fields, and personal magnetic field exposure

Obviously, the goal in epidemiologic studies is not to find a useful historical marker of homes (which do not get cancer) but a marker of the exposures of the occupants of those homes (who do get cancer). Therefore, the exposure of individuals can be viewed as the ultimate predictive goal to which both wire codes and residential magnetic fields must be compared.

The question of what proportion of total exposure or what proportion of the variability in exposure is accounted for by residences is critical to evaluating the adequacy of the exposure proxies. In other words, we need to examine whether the focus on residential magnetic field exposures as opposed to other sources is justified. Instrumentation now available readily allows for monitoring personal exposure over extended periods of time, but few studies have obtained the necessary information to examine the contribution of different environments (including the home) to total personal exposure. The one study that directly addressed this question found that children's total exposure is strongly associated with their residential exposure, with a correlation coefficient of 0.97 (Kaune et al., 1994). Although there are other sources of magnetic fields encountered in schools and other locations in the community, the large number of hours spent in the home appear to make it the dominant contributor to time-weighted average exposure.

Some of the exposure surveys cited above have also looked directly at the relation of wire codes to personal exposure. A report by Rankin et al. (1992) indicated higher personal exposures for persons living in very high current configuration homes (0.30 μT) and ordinary high current configuration homes (0.25 μT) compared to persons living in other homes (0.11 to 0.20 μT). Children's exposures were predicted reasonably accurately by the wire codes of their homes (30% to 60% of total variance) in two small studies (EPRI, 1992; Kaune and Zaffanella, 1994).

Other Health End Points

There have been a wide variety of other health end points evaluated in relation to residential magnetic fields. In the area of adult cancer (reviewed elsewhere [Savitz and Ahlbom, 1994; Coleman and Beral, 1988]), Wertheimer and Leeper (1982) found associations between wiring codes and a number of cancer types, but the limited subsequent research has provided ambiguous results (Severson et al., 1988; Feychting and Ahlbom, 1994). A topic of some interest at present is a potential link between magnetic fields and female breast cancer, as postulated by Stevens et al. (1992). Studies to address that hypothesis are in progress.

The limited literature on neurobehavioral effects of residential exposure (broadly defined) includes studies of limited quality suggestive of an association with suicide (Perry et al., 1981) and studies of higher quality providing mixed evidence regarding depression (Poole et al., 1993; McMahan et al., 1994). Given the hypothesized biological pathways involving melatonin (Stevens et al., 1992), such end points are worthy of attention.

Reproductive health has been considered in relation to electric and magnetic fields primarily from appliances used in workplaces (video display terminals) (Delpizzo, 1994) and residential settings (electric blankets) (Wertheimer and Leeper, 1989). Ambient magnetic fields have received more limited attention, with one report suggestive of an increased risk of early pregnancy loss in homes with elevated magnetic fields (Juutilainen et al., 1993).

Future Directions for Epidemiologic Research
Enhancements to Magnetic Field Assessment

Besides confirming the patterns suggested above for wire codes, residential measurements, and personal exposure, what can be done to enhance the quality of retrospective exposure assessment of residential magnetic fields? Three avenues are suggested, corresponding to engineering refinements, behavioral refinements, and a purely empirical effort to identify predictors of exposure.

Engineering refinements refer to better methods of interpreting wiring configurations (e.g., Kaune & Savitz, 1994), as well as methods of incorporating additional attributes of the home into the exposure classification protocol. Part of the goal is to do a better job estimating the time-weighted average exposures of interest in the past; an additional goal is to develop methods for estimating other attributes of exposure (peaks, pattern of temporal variability, etc.). For example, to evaluate the contribution of in-home wiring, electrical loads of known magnitude can be placed at selected locations in the home. There is no reason to believe that Wertheimer and Leeper (1979, 1982) found at the outset the best possible method of interpreting wiring attributes as markers of residential magnetic field exposure.

Behavioral refinements refer to time-activity profiles, addressing time spent in the home, location within the home, and time spent in other locations. In addition, use and placement of electrical appliances in the home is generally a function of voluntary behavior and can be a substantial source of magnetic field exposure.

Empirical evaluation of exposure determinants would incorporate both of the above realms as well as any others that might be proposed. Given available instrumentation, it is relatively easy to acquire exposure profiles of large numbers of people over extended periods of time. Administering detailed diaries in conjunction with those measurements would allow for development of predictive models based on location and activities. Many of these determinants would undoubtedly not be amenable to historical reconstruction (e.g., use of a particular electrical appliance that was not available in the past), whereas other sources of exposure would be amenable to historical reconstruction (e.g., time spent commuting on electric railways). Quantifying the predictable and unpredictable components of exposure would be of value in its own right, but an empirical prediction equation that would have as inputs historically ascertainable sources of fields should improve on the current situation in which the "model" consists only of power lines near the home.

Extension to other health outcomes

The initial focus on cancer as a possible consequence of elevated exposure to electric and magnetic fields was rather arbitrary. Once this link was pursued, positive findings led to additional research, which has continued to the present. However, there have also been other clinically important outcomes suggested as potential consequences of exposure, including miscarriage (Wertheimer and Leeper, 1989; Lindbohm et al., 1992) and depression (Poole et al., 1993).

A greater understanding of the biological consequences of exposure could obviously help to focus the research, but even the current theories would encourage a wider range of exploration. The postulated mediation by pineal melatonin production (Stevens et al., 1992) would not point exclusively toward cancer but rather to disturbances in circadian rhythms and a well-established link between such disturbances and depression (Beck-Friis et al., 1985).

Biological research that leads to the identification of more common, short-latency outcomes (biomarkers of effect) would facilitate a range of study opportunities. True prospective studies with real-time exposure monitoring over days or weeks could be undertaken, with examination of the exposure circumstances that lead to greater or lesser responses.

Conclusions

It is likely that this research avenue will persist for some time, regardless of the results of ongoing epidemiologic studies. Although advocates on both sides of the issue argue that our understanding is sufficient to know what to do (nothing or something, depending on their point of view), most who evaluate this body of research find it perplexing. As the literature grows in size and quality, the marginal contribution of each study tends to diminish. More focused efforts are needed to address key individual issues: Is selection bias likely to account for associations between wiring configuration codes and childhood cancer? Are wire codes or in-home measurements better predictors of individual exposure over extended periods of time? These may be embedded in new studies of exposures and health outcomes or they may be free-standing methodological evaluations. Regardless, the clarification of the methodological issues and resolution of them is more efficient and intellectually satisfying than just accruing new studies hoping that the issue will be resolved when weight of evidence leans sufficiently far in one direction or another.

References

Adey WR. 1988, Cell membranes: the electromagnetic environment and cancer promotion. Neurochem Res 13: 671–677.

Bates MN. 1991. Extremely low frequency electromagnetic fields and cancer: the epidemiologic evidence. Environ Health Perspect 95: 147–156.

Beck-Friis J, Kjellman BF, Aperia B, Unden F, Von Rosen D, Ljunggren J-G, Wetterberg L. 1985. Serum melatonin in relation to clinical variables in patients with major depressive disorder and a hypothesis of a low melatonin syndrome. Acta Psychiatr Scand 71: 319–330.

Blanchard JP, Blackman CF. Clarification and amplification of an ion parametric resonance model for magnetic field interactions with biological systems. Bioelectromagnetics 1994; 15:217–238.

Carpenter DO, Ayrapetyan S, Eds. 1994. Biological effects of electric and magnetic fields. Vol. I, Sources and Mechanisms; Vol. 2, Clinical Applications and Therapeutic Effects. Academic Press, San Diego, CA.

Coleman MP, Bell CM, Taylor HL, Primic-Zakelj M. 1989. Leukaemia and residence near electricity transmission equipment: a case-control study. Br J Cancer 60: 793–798.

Coleman M, Beral V. 1988. A review of epidemiological studies of the health effects of living near or working with electricity generation and transmission equipment. Int J Epidemiol 17: 1–13.

Delpizzo V. 1994. Epidemiological studies of work with video display terminals and adverse pregnancy outcomes (1984–1992). Am J Ind Med 26: 465–480.

EPRI. 1992. Assessment of Children's Long-Term Exposure to Magnetic Fields (The Geomet Study). Contract TR-101406, Research Project 2966-04, Electric Power Research Institute, Palo Altro, Calif.

EPRI. 1993a. Survey of Residential Magnetic Field Sources: Volumes 1 and 2, Goals, Results, and Conclusions. EPRI TR-102759-V1/V2; Project 3335-02. Prepared by High Voltage Transmission Center, Electric Power Research Institute, Palo Alto, Calif.

EPRI. 1993b. The EMDEX Project Residential Study Interim Report. EPRI TR-102011; Project 2966-01. Prepared by T. Dan Bracken, Inc. Electric Power Research Institute, Palo Alto, Calif.

Feychting M, Ahlbom A. 1993. Magnetic fields and cancer in children residing near Swedish high-voltage power lines. Am J Epidemiol 138; 467–81.

Feychting M, Ahlbom A. Magnetic fields, leukemia, and central nervous system tumors in Swedish adults residing near high-voltage power lines. Epidemiology 1994;5:501–509.

Foster KR. Weak magnetic fields: a cancer connection? In: Foster KR, Bernstein DE, eds. Phantom Risks: Scientific Inference and the Law. MIT Press, Cambridge, MA: 47–85.

Fulton JP, Cobb S, Preble L, Leone L, Forman E. 1980. Electrical wiring configurations and childhood leukemia in Rhode Island. Am J Epidemiol 111: 292–296.

Gurney JG, Mueller BA, Davis S, Schwartz SM, Stevens RG, Kopecky KJ. 1996. Childhood brain tumor occurrence in relation to residential power line configurations, electric heating sources, and electric appliance use. Am J Epidemiol 143:120–128.

Juutilainen J, Matilainen P, Saarikoski S, Laara E, Suonio S. 1993. Early pregnancy loss and exposure to 50-Hz magnetic fields. Bioelectromagnetics 14: 229–36.

Kaune WT, Darby SD, Gardner SN, Hrubec Z, Iriye RH, Linet MS. 1994. Development of a protocol for assessing time-weighted average exposures of young children to power-frequency magnetic fields. Bioelectromagnetics 15: 33–51.

Kaune WT, Savitz DA. 1994. Simplification of the Wertheimer-Leeper wire code. Bioelectromagnetics 15:275–282.

Kaune WT, Stevens RG, Callahan NJ, Severson RK, Thomas DB. 1987. Residential magnetic and electric fields. Bioelectromagnetics 8: 315–335.

Kaune WT, Zaffanella LE. 1994. Assessing historical exposures of children to power-frequency magnetic fields. J Exp Anal Environ Epidemiol 4: 149–170.

Koontz MD, Mehegan LL, Dietrich FM, Nagda NL. 1992. Assessment of Children's Long-Term Exposure to Magnetic Fields (The Geomet Study). Electric Power Research Institute Report No. TR-101406. Electric Power Research Institute, Palo Alto, Calif.

Lindbohm M-L, Hietanen M, Kyyronen P, Sallmen M, von Nandelstadh P, Taskinen H, Pekkarinen M, Yikoski M, Hemminki K. 1992. Magnetic fields of video display terminals and spontaneous abortion. Am J Epidemiol 136: 1041–1051.

London SJ, Thomas DC, Bowman JD, Sobel E, Cheng T-C, Peters JM. 1991. Exposure to residential electric and magnetic fields and risk of childhood leukemia. Am J Epidemiol 134: 923–937.

McDowall ME. 1986. Mortality of persons resident in the vicinity of electricity transmission facilities. Br J Cancer 53: 271–279.

McMahan S, Ericson J, Meyer J. 1994. Depressive symptomatology in women and residential proximity to high-voltage power lines. Am J Epidemiol 139: 58–63.

Myers A, Clayden AD, Cartwright RA, Cartwright SC. 1990. Childhood cancer and overhead powerlines. A case/control study. Br J Cancer 62: 1008–1014.

Perry FS, Reichmanis M, Marino AA, Becker RO. 1981. Environmental power-frequency magnetic fields and suicide. Health Phys 41: 267–277.

Poole C. 1996. Invited commentary: evolution of epidemiologic evidence on magnetic fields and childhood cancer. Am J Epidemiol 143:129–132.

Poole C, Kavet R, Funch DP, Donelan K, Charry JM, Dreyer NA. 1993. Depressive symptoms and headaches in relation to proximity of residence to an alternating-current transmission line right-of-way. Am J Epidemiol 137: 318–330.

Preston-Martin S, Navidi W, Thomas D, Lee P-J, Bowman J, Pogoda J. 1996. Los Angeles study of residential magnetic fields and childhood brain tumors. Am J Epidemiol 143: 105–119.

Rankin RF, Bracken TD, Senior RS. 1992. Comparison of Measured Magnetic Fields and Wire Code Schemes—EMDEX Project: Residential Study. First World Congress for Elect. & Magnetism in Biology and Medicine; Lake Buena Vista, Florida.

Robinette CD, Silverman C, Jablon S. 1980. Effects upon health of occupational exposure to microwave radiation (radar). Am J Epidemiol 112: 39–53.

Rothman KJ. 1996. Modern Epidemiology. Little, Brown and Company, Boston.

Savitz DA. 1994. In defense of black box epidemiology. Epidemiology 5: 550–552.

Savitz DA, Ahlbom A. 1994. Epidemiologic evidence on cancer in relation to residential and occupational exposures. In: Carpenter DO, Ayrapetyan S eds. Biological Effects of Electric and Magnetic Fields, Vol. 2. San Diego, CA: Academic Press: 233–261.

Savitz DA, Wachtel H, Barnes FA, John EM, Tvrdik JG. 1988. Case-control study of childhood cancer and exposure to 60-Hz magnetic fields. Am J Epidemiol 128:21–38.

Schlesselman J. 1982. Case-Control Studies. Design, Conduct, Analysis. Oxford University Press, New York.

Severson RK, Stevens RG, Kaune WT. 1988. Acute non-lymphocytic and residential exposure to power frequency magnetic fields. Am J Epidemiol 128:10–20.

Stevens RG, Davis S, Thomas DB, Anderson LE, Wilson BW. 1992. Electric power, pineal function, and the risk of breast cancer. FASEB J 6:853–860.

Tenforde TS, Kaune WT. 1987. Interaction of extremely low frequency electric and magnetic fields with humans. Health Phys 53:585–606.

Theriault GP. 1991. Health effects of electromagnetic radiation on workers: epidemiologic studies. In: Bierbaum PE, Peters JM, eds. Proceedings of the Scientific workshop on the Health Effects of Electric and Magnetic Fields on Workers. US DHHS, National Institute for Occupational Safety and Health, Cincinnati, Ohio.

Tomenius L. 1986. 50-Hz electromagnetic environment and the incidence of childhood tumors in Stockholm county. Bioelectromagnetics 7:191–207.

Washburn EP, Orza MJ, Berlin JA, Nicholson WJ, Todd AC, Frumkin H, Chalmers TC. 1994. Residential proximity to electricity transmission and distribution equipment and risk of childhood leukemia, childhood lymphoma, and childhood nervous system tumors: systematic review, evaluation, and meta-analysis. Cancer Causes Control 5:299–309.

Wertheimer N, Leeper E. 1979. Electrical wiring configurations and childhood cancer. Am J Epidemiol 109:273–284.

Wertheimer N, Leeper E. 1980. Re: Electrical wiring configurations and childhood leukemia in Rhode Island (Letter). Am J Epidemiol 111:461–462.

Wertheimer N, Leeper E. 1982. Adult cancer related to electrical wires near the home. Int J Epidemiol 11:345–55.

Wertheimer N, Leeper E. 1989. Fetal loss associated with two seasonal sources of electromagnetic field exposure. Am J Epidemiol 129:220–224.

Wilson BW, Wright CW, Morris JE, Buschbom RL, Brown DP, Miller DL, Somers-Flannigan R, Anderson LE. 1990. Evidence for an effect of ELF electromagnetic fields on human pineal gland function. J Pineal Res 9:259–69.

Effects of Lead in Children and Adults

14

DAVID BELLINGER

JOEL SCHWARTZ

FEW environmental agents have such diverse uses and such a long history of suspected and recognized toxicity as lead. The circumstances in which lead is encountered are varied; regardless of the original source, lead is persistent so that exposure can occur via community air pollution, soil contamination, and water pollution. There are also many relatively isolated sources, such as the workplace environment (e.g., smelters), lead water pipes in homes, lead-contaminated paint, lead-soldered cans, and lead-glazed pottery.

Fortunately, biological markers that integrate across exposure sources have been developed and evaluated, with blood lead being one of the most readily available measures. The "right" biological marker depends, of course, on the health event of interest. As we focus on increasingly subtle consequences of lead, the demand for precise assessment of the relevant exposure has grown. Lead poisoning is easily linked to lead but detection of a decrement of one or two points on a test of intelligence or a rise of two or three millimeters mercury in blood pressure is far more dependent on the accuracy of the exposure indicator. Blood lead reflects recent exposure; interest in the possible influence of historical lead exposures on increased blood pressure in adults and on the decline in neurobehavioral function in the elderly has directed researchers to examine bone lead as a marker of long-term stores.

Another key feature of lead is the diversity of consequences and differing dose-response functions across different end points. In some instances, the effects differ only by severity, lower levels of lead being associated with increasingly subtle damage to cognitive development while the thresholds for overt encephalopathy are far higher than the levels normally encountered. A consequence of these differing dose-response functions is that regulation to protect health depends greatly on the health end point of interest. Philosophically, the most sensitive end point should be protected, but in the case of lead, we are not entirely sure which it is.

Many environmental agents are associated with social class, most exposing poorer segments of the population to a greater extent than wealthier people. Lead, however, is a more extreme case in which disentangling general effects of poverty from specific effects of lead is quite difficult. First, lead exposure is probably more closely linked to lower socioeconomic status than many agents. Second, neurobehavioral development in children is probably more strongly affected by a variety of social class–related factors than many other health measures. Diet, intellectual stimulation at home and school, and even the very ability to perform well on standardized tests may be adversely affected by poverty, and hence may mix with the influence of lead.

A final point that lead illustrates very nicely is the importance of considering not just the tail of the distribution of health outcomes (i.e., the most seriously affected) but rather the entire spectrum. While the consequences of a small decrement in intellectual function or small rise in blood pressure are of little clinical significance, and may well be below any appreciable adverse effect on an individual, shifting the population's IQ distribution may be of large consequence. If we were unable to measure neurobehavioral function or blood pressure accurately on a continuous scale, and instead could only observe profound mental retardation or malignant hypertension, the influence of lead might well be indiscernible.

Lead is unique among chemical pollutants in terms of the large number of potential pathways and sources of exposure as well as the amount of data available on human exposures and their health effects. As a result, risk assessments for lead rest on an empirical foundation that is unusually broad and detailed, requiring little extrapolation from high doses to low doses or from animal models to humans. This wealth of data can be traced, at least in part, to lead's economic value in modern industrialized society and to the long period of time that humans have exploited lead's useful properties.

Widespread dispersion of lead into the environment began over 5,000 years ago. Approximately half of the 300 million metric tons of lead produced throughout history persists in the form of environmental contamination (National Research Council [NRC], 1993), with the current yearly "anthropogenic" mobilization of lead into the biosphere estimated to be approximately 1,160,000 tons (Nriagu and Pacyna, 1988). Lead concentrations in isolated, undisturbed media such as Greenland ice cores, marine sediments, and tree rings provide a chronological record of deposition rates and long-distance transport. They reveal concentrations that may exceed "natural" concentrations by more than two orders of magnitude, at least in the Northern Hemisphere. Two particularly sharp increases in deposition occurred in the 18th and early 20th centuries, due most likely to production changes associated with the Industrial Revolution and to the introduction of tetraethyl lead as an octane-boosting gasoline additive, respectively. If one were to set about to design a strategy for dispersing lead in ways that maximize the likelihood of human exposures, one could hardly do better than to arrange to have it emitted as submicron-sized particles from the exhaust of the ubiquitous automobile and to be incorporated into the paint applied to the interior and exterior surfaces of homes.

Current Blood Lead Levels in the U.S. Population

The Third National Health and Nutrition Examination Survey (NHANES III, 1988 to 1991, phase 1) provides the most recent nationally representative data on blood lead levels (Brody et al., 1994). The geometric mean blood level in the U.S. population was 2.8 μg/dL. Children aged 1 to 2 years had the highest geometric mean level, 4.1 μg/dL, and the highest prevalence of levels greater than 10 μg/dL (11.5% vs. 4.5% in the entire population). As in NHANES II (1976–1980), young (1-to 5-year-old) low-income black children living in large urban areas had the highest mean level (9.7 μg/dL).

Secular Changes in the Blood Lead Levels of the U.S. Population

Population blood lead levels declined by 78% over the decade between NHANES II and NHANES III, from 12.8 μg/dL to 2.8 μg/dL (Pirkle et al., 1994). Comparable decreases were evident in all sex, race/ethnicity, age, urbanicity, and income level subgroups. In NHANES II, 88.2% of children aged 1 to 5 years had a blood lead level greater than 10 μg/dL and 24.7% a level greater than 20 μg/dL, with a mean blood lead of approximately 15 μg/dL (Mahaffey et al., 1982).

Sources and Pathways of Exposure

The dramatic decline in population exposures is most likely a result of federal regulation of exposure sources with highly centralized distribution systems. The amount of lead added to gasoline declined 99.8% between 1976 and 1990 and the proportion of domestically produced food and soft drink cans containing lead solder declined from 47% (1980) to 0% (1991) (Pirkle et al., 1994). Regression analyses of data collected during the NHANES II survey suggested that eliminating lead from gasoline would reduce mean blood lead levels by approximately 9 μg/dL (Schwartz et al., 1985) and the results of NHANES III are consistent with this.

Less centralized lead sources and pathways of exposure are not as amenable to control and must be addressed on a more local level. These media include lead in paint already in place, lead-contaminated dust and soil, and lead in drinking water. The Agency for Toxic Substances and Disease Registry (1988) estimated that 4.4 million children aged 6 months to 5 years live in pre-1940 housing in metropolitan areas, the housing most likely to harbor leaded paint. The potential hazard associated with living in a home with leaded paint was characterized by Schwartz and Levin (1991) using data from the Chicago lead-screening program (N=200,000, 1976–1980). The relative risk of lead toxicity (defined as a blood lead level >30 μg/dL), given residence in a home with lead paint hazard (versus a home without lead paint hazard), was 15.8 in the summer, 12.8 in the spring, and 5.7 in the fall/winter. In many other studies, residence in homes with a lead paint hazard was associated with higher childhood blood lead levels (Clark et al., 1985; Rabinowitz et al., 1985).

Dust and soil integrate lead from various sources, such as vehicle exhaust, stationary (point) sources (e.g., secondary smelters, battery plants, municipal incinerators), and leaded paint from the exterior surfaces of structures. It does not degrade over time, remaining in place until dispersed by natural (e.g., wind, rain) or anthropogenic processes (e.g., excavation). The natural level in rural soils is typically less than 30 parts per million (ppm) (NRC, 1993), but soil lead concentrations in inner-city neighborhoods or areas proximal to smelters or heavily traveled roadways may exceed 10,000 parts per million (Environmental Protection Agency [EPA], 1986). Cross-sectional studies suggest a positive association between soil lead levels and blood lead levels in children (a 2 to 7 μg/dL increase for each 1000 ppm increase in soil lead, depending on factors such as particle size distribution, lead species, other sources, and extent of hand-to-mouth activities) (EPA, 1986).

Lead in drinking water rarely derives from source water, instead entering at several points near the end of the distribution system: connectors, service line, soldered joints in copper plumbing, drinking fountain, brass fixtures. House-to-house variability is attributable to physical characteristics of the water (e.g., its corrosivity or pH) and characteristics of the delivery system (e.g., the age of lead-soldered joints, the area of leaded surfaces to which water has access, water temperature, and length of time water "stands" in contact with leaded materials) (NRC, 1993). The EPA recently issued standards for lead in drinking water requiring water utilities to reduce water corrosivity.

Exposure Standards

The lead-screening guideline is the basis for classifying a child's risk and candidacy for diagnostic evaluation. In the past 25 years, this guideline has been revised downward several times, from 60 µg/dL in the 1960s, to 40 (1970), 30 (1975), 25 (1985), and 10 (1991). Parental counseling and environmental investigation are currently recommended for children whose blood lead levels are persistently between 15 and 19 µg/dL. Children with levels greater than 20 µg/dL should be referred for medical evaluation. The choice of 10 µg/dL as the definition of "poisoning" was generally health-based, although the Centers for Disease Control and Prevention (CDC) acknowledged that ". . . no threshold has been identified for the harmful effects of lead" (CDC, 1991, p. 2).

No corresponding system exists for classifying adults' risk except among workers, most of whom are covered by the Occupational Safety and Health Administration (OSHA) lead standard (OSHA, 1978). A blood lead level of 50 µg/dL is viewed as cause for "medical removal protection." Unlike most occupational standards, it addresses reproductive toxicity, recommending but not mandating an upper limit of 30 µg/dL for any worker (male or female) who anticipates having a child. Reconsideration of the OSHA standard is indicated given the amount of data accumulated since it was promulgated nearly 20 years ago.

Natural Lead Exposures

Despite recent reductions in population exposures, current bone lead concentrations are 500 to 1000-fold higher than the concentrations measured in skeletons from the preindustrial era (Patterson et al., 1991). Extrapolating bone lead: blood lead ratios from contemporary humans and animals to skeletal remains from the earlier era, Flegal and Smith (1992b) estimated that the natural blood lead level of humans is 0.016 µg/dL, 600-

fold lower than the level currently used to define childhood lead poisoning (i.e., 10 µg/dL).

Pharmacokinetics

Lead is absorbed mainly through the respiratory and gastrointestinal tracts. Up to half of inhaled lead is retained in the lungs and absorbed, although the rate depends on physical characteristics (e.g., particle size distribution), and host characteristics (e.g., smoking status). Absorption in the gut varies with age and time since food consumption. The fractional absorption is 10% to 15% in adults (Heard and Chamberlain, 1982) but may be as high as 50% in infants and children (Ziegler et al., 1978).

Exposure Assessment

Alternative biologic markers: blood, bone, and tooth lead

Many of the complexities of lead exposure assessment stem from the way in which an individual's body burden is distributed among different pools and the dynamic equilibrium among them. The major pools or compartments are blood, soft tissues, and mineralized tissues. Each compartment can itself be subdivided. For instance, 99% of lead in blood is associated with red cells, with the balance in plasma and extracellular fluid. Although small, the latter pool represents a diffusible fraction that is probably the most bioavailable and thus of greatest toxicologic significance. Metabolic balance studies show that whole blood lead has a half-life of 25 to 30 days (Rabinowitz et al., 1976), the basis for the oft-cited statement that a blood lead level reflects primarily recent exposure. The bulk of body lead burden resides in mineralized tissue, although the fraction of total body burden so sequestered is greater for adults than children (90% to 95% versus ~75%) (U.S. EPA, 1986). Bone itself appears to include multiple compartments (Aufderheide and Wittmers, 1992), with lead in spongy trabecular bone (e.g., patella, calcaneus) perhaps being somewhat more exchangeable with the circulation than is lead in more compact cortical bone (e.g., tibia). These differences in the kinetic characteristics of lead in different body pools have important implications for exposure assessment. Because alternative exposure biomarkers sample different pools, they differ as well in their "exposure averaging times"—the periods over which they integrate an individual's exposure (e.g., bone lead > chelatable lead > erythrocyte protoporphyrin > blood lead). The dose-response relationship estimated for a particular health end point will be most meaningful if the exposure index used to characterize dose is relevant to the underlying toxicologic mechanism. For example, in a cohort of carpenters, patella lead concentration was inversely related to hemoglobin and hematocrit, although neither hematologic parameter was associated with current blood lead (Hu et al., 1994). Bone lead, with its longer exposure averaging time, may be a better index than is blood lead of a chronic "subclinical" effect of lead on hematopoiesis.

Until recently, the opportunity to measure lead in mineralized tissues other than teeth was limited to autopsy series. This has changed with the refinement of noninvasive in vivo techniques for measuring bone lead concentration using x-ray fluorescence (XRF). K-line XRF, so named because it induces electrons in the K-shell of a lead atom to fluoresce, is currently the method most widely used although methods that excite electrons in the L-shell are also available (Todd and Chettle, 1994). A critical difference between K-and L-line methods is the volume of bone tissue sampled, with K-XRF measuring whole bone lead to a greater extent than does L-XRF. Some evidence suggests that L-XRF assesses a more bioavailable pool of lead (Rosen et al., 1991). To date, L-XRF methods have more often been used than K-XRF methods to assess bone lead in pediatric populations (e.g., Rosen et al., 1991), although technical considerations, such as radiation dose or measurement precision, do not currently favor the use of either technique in this age group (Todd and Chettle, 1994).

Rather than being metabolically inert, as formerly believed, lead in bone may be mobilized under a variety of physiologic or pathophysiologic conditions associated with increased bone turnover and remodeling, such as pregnancy (Silbergeld, 1991), postmenopausal osteoporosis (Silbergeld et al., 1988), immobilization osteoporosis (Markowitz and Weinberger, 1990), and thyrotoxicosis (Goldman et al., 1994). From the standpoint of exposure assessment, mobilized bone lead is important because it may represent a significant endogenous source of lead exposure, complicating the use of blood lead level as the end point in assessing the impact of contemporaneous exposures or interventions (e.g., the impact of lead paint abatement or soil lead abatement on children's blood lead levels).

The potential mobilization of bone lead during pregnancy is a particular concern. Changes over pregnancy in the ratios of the natural stable isotopes of lead in blood are consistent with the hypothesis that hormonal processes that regulate calcium metabolism may also increase efflux of bone lead stores that reflect remote (i.e., past) exposures (Manton, 1985; Inskip et al., 1992). Case studies (Thompson et al., 1985) and epidemiologic studies (Silbergeld et al., 1988; Muldoon et al., 1994; Symanski and Hertz-Picciotto, 1994; Kosnett et al., 1994; Rothenberg et al., 1994) provide corroborating but not conclusive evidence. The increase in blood lead following menopause is attributed to a physiologic osteoporotic process (Silbergeld et al., 1988). Women who have been pregnant or who have breastfed infants tend to have lower postmenopausal blood lead levels or smaller increases in blood or bone lead following menopause, presumably because of a greater depletion of bone lead stores over the course of prior pregnancies. Stable isotope ratio studies of women who migrated to areas in which environmental lead has "isotopic signatures" distinctly different from those of the environmental lead in the homeland (and thus from lead accumulated in bone) would clarify the extent to which, and the circumstances under which, endogenous lead contributes to a pregnant woman's blood lead and thus to the exposure of her fetus.

The concentration of lead in children's shed deciduous teeth has frequently been used as an accessible surrogate index of bone lead stores and interpreted as a measure of cumulative postnatal deposition of lead (e.g., Needleman et al., 1979, 1990; Smith et al., 1983; Winneke et al., 1983; Hansen et al., 1989; Rabinowitz et al., 1991; Fergusson et al., 1993; Greene and Ernhart, 1993; McMichael et al., 1994). As generally used, such indices do not permit a detailed reconstruction of a child's exposure history. Recent stable isotope studies suggest, however, that the concentration in the incisal end of the crown most likely reflects in utero exposure; the concentration in the cervical portion (i.e., enamel plus coronal dentin) reflects exposure from birth to shedding (Gulson and Wilson, 1994). The epidemiologic utility of tooth lead as an exposure index is reduced by the narrow window of time within which shed teeth are available for collection and by the fact that lead concentration varies according to tooth type, portion of tooth sampled (i.e., whole tooth vs. secondary dentin), and position in the jaw (Grandjean et al., 1986; Purchase and Fergusson, 1986; Paterson et al., 1988).

Assessment of fetal exposure

Because it is not feasible to measure lead in the fetal brain, the critical target organ for developmental neurotoxicity, investigators must depend on the concentration of lead in surrogate tissues. Transplacental passage of lead is efficient, probably via passive diffusion (Goyer, 1990), and the correlation between the concentration of lead in maternal venous blood at term and umbilical cord blood approaches 0.90 (Graziano et al., 1990). The concentrations of lead in umbilical cord tissue or placental body do not correlate highly, however, with indices of maternal or fetal blood lead level (Baghurst et al, 1991). Among the possible reasons: these indices sample different fetal lead pools; individuals vary in the efficiency of transplacental transfer of lead; or fetal status influences the rate of lead accumulation in different tissues. In addition, exposure indices that are highly correlated with one another (e.g., maternal blood lead and cord or neonatal blood lead levels) do not always bear similar relationships to a given health end point (Ernhart et al., 1986; Dietrich et al., 1991). A more detailed understanding of the biokinetics of lead in the maternal-fetal unit is needed to clarify the relationships among alternative biomarkers of exposure and to identify the best biomarkers of delivered dose for different dimensions of fetal growth and maturity.

Health Effects Associated with Lead

In the following section, the associations between lead exposure and two important health end points are briefly examined: development and blood pressure.

Development

TERATOGENICITY

At high doses, lead has devastating impact on fetal growth and development (Cantarow and Trumper, 1944). Although prenatal exposure in animals (hamsters, rats, chicks) may produce a urorectocaudal pattern of anomalies (Winder, 1993), including structural anomalies in the nervous system (Morrissey and Mottet, 1980), epidemiologic evidence that lead is a human teratogen is limited. In a cohort of 4354 infants, the prevalence of minor physical anomalies (e.g., hemangioma, lymphangioma, hydrocele) was increased approximately twofold among infants with cord blood lead levels greater than 15 µg/dL (Needleman et al., 1984), although no specific syndrome was identified. Two studies with much smaller sample sizes failed to replicate this finding (McMichael et al., 1986; Ernhart et al., 1986). Given the unavailability of good information in these studies about critical exposure parameters such as dose and timing, only limited inferences can be drawn about lead's teratogenicity in humans.

INTRAUTERINE GROWTH AND MATURITY

Significant lacunae also exist in our knowledge about lead's impact on intrauterine growth and development. In some cohorts, increased lead was associated with shorter periods of gestation (McMichael et al., 1986; Dietrich et al., 1987; Rothenberg et al., 1989). In others, either no association (Factor-Litvack et al., 1991) or a slight positive association was found (Bellinger et al., 1991a). A similar lack of consistency characterizes the findings on lead and birth weight. Some studies reported an inverse association similar in magnitude to the association between cigarette smoking and birthweight (Bornschein et al., 1989). Others reported an association between lead and fetal growth only when the end point was defined as "intrauterine growth retardation," "small for gestational age," or "low birth weight" (Bellinger et al., 1991a). In one study of a large cohort of women with a wide range of blood lead levels (up to 50 μg/dL), no association was found between birthweight and any of several indices of fetal exposure, including mid-pregnancy, delivery, and umbilical cord blood lead levels (Factor-Litvak et al., 1991). Among the possible explanations for the inconsistencies are differences among studies in the exposure index used (and the biokinetic compartment of the maternal-fetal unit sampled), the level of and variability in prenatal exposures, patterns of confounding and confounder adjustment strategies, and outcome definition and classification (Andrews et al., 1994; Hertz-Picciotto and Neutra, 1994).

FUNCTIONAL DEVELOPMENT

Case studies suggest that in utero exposures sufficient to produce maternal toxicity are associated with poor outcomes in children, including encephalopathy, seizures, developmental delay, and other signs of neurological dysfunction (Bellinger and Needleman, 1985). Lower levels more typical of population exposures appear not to be associated with detectable long-term neurobehavioral effects. In most of the studies reporting early lead-associated developmental impairment (e.g., Bellinger et al., 1987; Dietrich et al., 1987), the associations were either attenuated by the time the children reached preschool age or expressed in a form not detected by the global assessment instruments used (Bellinger et al., 1991b; Dietrich et al., 1991). One exception is a study of relatively heavily exposed children living near a smelter, in which intellectual performance at age 4 years was inversely related to prenatal blood lead levels (integrated average of mid-pregnancy and delivery levels) (Wasserman et al., 1994).

In contrast, elevated postnatal exposures in children are associated with persisting intellectual performance deficits. Several meta-analyses, using somewhat different procedures to combine data from overlapping sets of studies, converge on the conclusion that a 10 μg/dL increase in blood lead is associated with a 1 to 3 point drop in school-age IQ (Needleman and Gatsonis, 1990; Schwartz, 1994a; Pocock et al., 1994). Although the effect estimates from different studies are not heterogeneous in a formal statistical sense, they do vary considerably. This may be attributable to methodological factors such as misclassification (of exposure, outcome, or confounders), cohort differences in exposure profiles (and thus toxicokinetic factors), host characteristics (i.e., pattern and distribution of confounders and effect modifiers such as social class, genotype, other neurotoxic exposures), or other factors (Bellinger, 1995).

Blood pressure

Small reductions in blood pressure have been identified as a major benefit of reducing lead exposure. Although this issue has received less attention than have the cognitive effects of lead exposure, it has been the subject of considerable toxicologic and epidemiologic investigation.

TOXICOLOGIC STUDIES

A substantial number of studies indicate that exposure to moderate levels of lead increases blood pressure in vivo in animals (Perry and Erlanger, 1978; Revis et al., 1981; Boscolo and Carmignani, 1988; Fouts and Page, 1942; Iannaconne et al., 1981; Webb et al., 1981; Bogden et al., 1991; Nakhoul et al., 1992; Lal et al., 1991; Skoczynka et al., 1986). Lead-exposed animals demonstrate an increased responsiveness to alpha-adrenergic stimulation (Boscolo and Carmignani, 1988; Iannaconne et al., 1981; Carmignani et al., 1983; Chai and Webb, 1988; Webb et al., 1981), suggesting an effect of lead on vascular tone via the disturbance of calcium metabolism. Lead is known to increase intracellular calcium stores. Alpha-adrenergic stimulation results in the release of calcium stores from the endoplasmic reticulum. This produces increased vascular contraction through calcium's role as a messenger for smooth muscle contraction. A toxicant that increases both free and stored intracellular calcium concentrations would be expected to increase resting tone and to increase responsiveness to alpha-adrenergic stimulation. This hypothesis is supported by the reduced effectiveness of isoproterenol in lowering blood pressure in lead-exposed animals (Skoczynka et al., 1986) and by the prolonged elevation of blood pressure following administration of norepinephrine in exposed rats (Skoczynka et al., 1986).

In in vitro studies of isolated tail arteries, lead exposure resulted in both increased pressure (Piccinini and Favalli, 1977; Boscolo and Carmignani, 1988; Chai and Webb, 1988) and increased responsiveness to alpha-adrenergic stimulation (Webb et al., 1981). The contractile response to lead was increased in the presence of a protein kinase C stimulant and decreased in the presence of a protein kinase C inhibitor, again suggesting an effect of lead on calcium pathways regulating smooth muscle tone. Lal et al. (1991) reported that elevations in blood pressure were first apparent within 2 weeks of exposure. In summary, the experimental literature indicates that lead increases blood pressure using pathways known to be important in human hypertension.

EPIDEMIOLOGIC STUDIES

A recent meta-analysis examined the results from 15 general population studies of the association between blood lead and blood pressure (Schwartz, 1995). Table 14-1, reproduced from that paper, shows the results of the individual studies. They consistently show positive associations that are roughly similar in magnitude. The meta-analysis indicated that a change in blood lead concentration from 10 µg/dL to 5 µg/dL would be expected to produce a 1.25 mm Hg decrease in systolic blood pressure (95% CI 0.87 to 1.63 mm Hg). The results were not very sensitive to deletion of the study with the most significant results, the study with the largest estimated effect size, or to the hypothetical addition of eight new studies with an estimated effect size of zero and with the average standard error of the existing studies. Given this consistency, it seems unlikely that these results are due to confounding, particularly since the administration of lead to animals under experimental protocols results in elevations of blood pressure.

Methodological Issues

Obtaining precise estimates of the magnitude and nature of the associations between lead exposure and particular health end points has proven difficult. Among the reasons are two problems commonly encountered in epidemiologic investigations: (1) the measurement of critical dose and its appropriate expression for the purpose of estimating dose-effect relationships and (2) the identification and control for factors that may confound the association between exposure and outcome. Each of these issues is discussed with reference to the two end points chosen as examples, development and blood pressure.

Issues in modeling dose-effect relationships

Current data provide little support for the existence of a threshold below which lead has no adverse developmental or neuropsychological impact. One impediment to the search for a threshold is the analytical challenge of measuring both low levels of lead burden and subtle variations in development within the normal range Detecting any association that may exist in the range of 0 to 10 µg/dL may strain the sensitivity of available neurobehavioral measures. In addition, in most of the cohorts assembled

Table 14-1. Effect of reduction in blood lead from 10μg/dL to 5 μg/dL on systolic blood pressure in adult males.

First Author and Year of Study	Effect Size (mm Hg)	Standard Error	Age Range
Orsaud, 1985	1.74	0.73	24–55
Schwartz, 1988	2.24	0.86	20–74
Pocock, 1988	1.45	0.49	40–59
Kromhout, 1988	3.15	1.20	57–76
Elwood (Wales), 1988	0.25	0.49	18–64
Elwood (Caerphilly), 1988	0.39	0.63	49–65
Neri, 1988	1.05	0.70	NA
Moreau, 1988	1.50	0.76	23–57
deKort, 1988	0.90	0.39	25–60
Sharp, 1988	0.80	1.25	28–64
Morris, 1990	3.17	1.59	NA
Egelund, 1992	1.26	0.62	NA
Møller (cross-section), 1992	1.86	0.63	40–51
Møller (longitudinal), 1992	0.90	0.74	40–51
Hense, 1993	1.45	0.51	28–67

in the past, relatively few children had blood lead levels below 10 μg/dL, reducing the precision with which the form of any relationship within that range could be characterized. In one study, however, a significant inverse association was found between blood lead level and IQ in a cohort in which 90% of the children had a blood lead level below 13 μg/dL (Bellinger et al., 1992).

Identifying the age or ages at which children are most vulnerable to lead toxicity would clearly advance efforts to target screening and intervention programs most efficiently. This issue is complicated by the fact that lead exposure is generally chronic, and in most high-risk environments children's blood lead levels display a high degree of intra-individual stability ("blood lead tracking") (Baghurst et al., 1992; Dietrich et al., 1993). In addition, because of the time-course of behaviors such as hand-to-mouth activity, blood lead level tends to be confounded with age and, in most cohorts, peaks at approximately 2 years. Under such circumstances, an investigator is largely limited to assessing the contributions of exposure indices that reflect cumulative lead exposure rather than indices that reflect exposures during well-defined and circumscribed developmental epochs. These caveats notwithstanding, it appears that blood lead levels measured in the 1-to 3-year age range are most strongly associated with school-age IQ. In one study blood lead at age 2 years was a stronger predictor of IQ at age 10 years than was maximum blood lead level measured over the course of the study despite the fact that for many children blood lead level did not peak at age 2 years (Bellinger et al., 1992). In studies of children with heavier exposures, blood lead levels measured between 15 months and 4 years were most predictive of IQ at age 7 years (Baghurst et al., 1992), levels measured between 3 and 6 years of age were most predictive of IQ at age 6.5 years (Dietrich et al., 1993), and levels measured after 2 years of age were most predictive of cognitive performance at age 4 (Wasserman et al., 1994).

In drawing inferences about periods of critical vulnerability, the distinction between age at exposure to lead and age at measurement of lead burden must be respected. As noted, because lead in blood has a relatively short half-life, blood lead tends to be discounted as anything more than a marker of very recent exposure. The half-life may be considerably longer in children, however, especially among those with relatively high exposures (Succop et al., 1987), at least in part because of the active remodelling of bone in early childhood. The level of lead in blood at age 2 years, as at all ages, integrates exogenous and endogenous inputs. Even if age 2 represents the height of nervous system vulnerability to lead, efforts to reduce exposure specifically at this age are unlikely to be sufficient because of the possibility of high endogenous inputs due to remote exposures. This demonstrates why pharmacokinetic factors need to be carefully considered in interpreting epidemiologic associations between a toxicant and a health end point.

In cross-sectional studies, exposure classification is often based on a blood lead concentration measured at school age. This strategy entails a risk that a child's exposure status at a potentially critical prior point in development will be misclassified. Only if exposure remains relatively stable, which is most likely if the major source is airborne or soil/dust lead from a point source such as a smelter, will a blood lead level at school age accurately reflect a child's early exposure. Even then, the school age measurement may convey mainly information about children's rank ordering rather than the absolute magnitude of lead burden. The misclassification risk is likely to be asymmetrical, involving classifying as "unexposed" a child with substantial exposure as a toddler, when blood lead typically peaks. Even if children's rank ordering in terms of blood lead level is preserved, the tendency for blood lead levels to decline during middle childhood increases the risk of error in estimating the dose associated with adverse outcomes. If it were earlier (higher) exposures that were responsible for later neurobehavioral impairment, the most likely error would be to infer that impairment occurs at lower blood lead levels than it actually does.

Use of the major alternative exposure index in epidemiologic studies of children, the concentration of lead in bone (or shed deciduous teeth), does not fully address these misclassification problems. Although a tooth lead level integrates exposure over a longer period of time than does a blood lead level, like blood lead it may poorly characterize a child's exposure in early stages of development. Although progress is being made, the analytical methods generally available do not permit working backwards from the spatial distribution of lead in a tooth to reconstruct specific features of dosing history (specifically temporal variation). Tooth lead is commonly interpreted as an index of cumulative exposure from birth to the time of exfoliation. Although experimental animal studies suggest that lead binds irreversibly in teeth (NRC, 1993), some human data raise the possibility that lead may move in and out of deciduous teeth, at least initially. In a cohort for whom serial blood lead levels were available, dentin lead levels more closely reflected exposure proximate in time to exfoliation than it did remote exposures, such as those occurring in the first few postnatal years (Rabinowitz et al., 1993). Therefore, a low tooth lead level does not necessarily imply that a child's blood lead level was not elevated at some critical early period.

The impossibility of "translating" either a tooth lead level or a bone lead level into a blood lead level limits the public health utility of these exposure indices. Because of practical constraints on sample availability (for shed teeth) and the relative unavailability of the hardware and laboratory resources needed to measure tooth or bone lead levels, it is unlikely that either will ever serve as the basis for exposure standards, although in the future an XRF method could conceivably serve as the basis for lead screening.

In many of the examples presented, lead was treated as a continuous exposure variable. As such, the models used implicitly specify a dose response relationship. Lead was assumed to be *linearly* associated with IQ or blood pressure on either the natural or the logarithmically transformed scale. Such assumptions about dose-response relationships should be examined. First, we need to assess whether any observed significant associations are dominated by a few extreme points, e.g., extreme responses by a few individuals with high exposures. While such an association may reflect a threshold (no effect until a certain dose is reached), it may also reflect the chance occurrence of a few observations. Second, the hypothesis being tested is that a significant *linear* association holds between exposure and outcome. If the true association is nonlinear, a significant association may be missed. Schwartz (1994b) showed how a highly significant *nonlinear* association between serum cholesterol and all-cause mortality appears nonsignificant if a *linear* dependence is specified. Thus, an examination of the shape of the dose-response relationship provides some guidance on how best to specify the continuous exposure variable (e.g., are transformations necessary, is the relationship linear, quadratic, exponential, or some more complex form?). Finally, better knowledge of the dose-response relationship provides some guidance as to the anticipated effect of changes in exposure (if the association is judged to be causal).

This issue has received insufficient attention, primarily because exposure variables used in epidemiology are often binary (yes/no) or categorical (low, medium, high). As exposure assessment improves in quality (and price), continuous exposure measures will more often be available and we must deal with them appropriately. The lead and blood pressure studies illustrate some of the issues. First, most studies used the natural logarithm of blood lead as the index of exposure rather than untransformed blood lead or some other transformation. The justification usually given is that a logarithmic transformation gives a normally distributed exposure variable. But this misses two points. First, it is the residuals of a regression that should be normally distributed, not the exposure variable itself. Second, the regression model selected specifies a dose-response curve. If blood pressure or IQ is regressed against untransformed blood lead values, we specify a linear change with increasing dose. If blood pressure is regressed against the logarithmic transform of blood lead, we specify that each successive 5 μg/dL increment in blood lead has less and less effect on blood pressure (or IQ).

The correct specification for the blood lead variable presumably depends on the mechanism of action, that is, on what happens in cells. The distribution of lead exposure in the population, by contrast, is determined by what happens in tailpipes and breweries. Rather than assuming a linear or linear-logarithmic relationship, the investigator should rely on theoretical models when they exist, or examine the data to identify the shape of the dose-response relationship. Only one of the population studies of blood pressure (Pirkle et al., 1985) examined the linearity of the dose-response relationship, and chose the logarithmic transform because it fit the data better than did linear, quadratic, or square root transforms. Two of the studies (Orssaud et al., 1985; Pocock et al., 1984; 1988) examined plots of adjusted blood pressure by categories of blood lead, and found a curvilinear dose-response curve, similar to a logarithmic curve.

An example of one way to address the problem of specifying the lead exposure variable is to plot the residuals of blood pressure after adjustment for age and body mass index against the residuals of blood lead after similar adjustment. This is called a partial regression plot and shows the relationship between lead and blood pressure adjusted for confounders. Unfortunately for weak associations such as those involving environmental toxicants, the scatter is too great to clearly show the shape of the relationship. One way to explore the shape of the relationship between a continuous exposure variable and an outcome is to use nonparametric smoothing. The role of such smoothing has been discussed both for lead epidemiology (Schwartz, 1993) and for general epidemiology (Schwartz, 1994b). A nonparametric smooth is a weighted moving average (or a generalization of one, see Hastie and Tibshirani, 1990, for details) and as such can easily fit nonlinearities in the data. In a weighted moving average, a window is drawn about each value of adjusted blood lead and a weighted average is taken of all the adjusted blood lead and blood pressure measurements in the window. That is the best prediction of the expected value of adjusted blood pressure at that adjusted blood lead. The weights decline with distance from the middle of the window. As the window moves from left to right, it traces a predicted curve of adjusted blood pressure versus adjusted blood lead. This plot provides our best guess as to what the shape of the relationship is and can serve as a guide in choosing a transformation for the exposure variable. These methods can also be used for hypothesis testing. The generalized additive model (Hastie and Tibshirani, 1990) allows the association between two variables to be tested without having to specify the specific form (e.g. quadratic, linear, etc.) in advance. It also allows testing for whether this smooth plot fits the data better than a simple linear relationship does.

Figure 14-1 shows a nonparametric smooth plot of adjusted blood pressure versus adjusted blood lead, using data for males in NHANES II. The curve suggests some leveling out of the dose-response curve at higher blood lead levels. The curve even turns down at the highest blood lead levels, although the number of points is small. This suggests a nonlinear relationship, perhaps polynomial or logarithmic. Animal studies using experimental protocols have reported the same phenomenon (e.g. Victery et al., 1982).

A recent analysis of lead and IQ using nonparametric smoothing (Schwartz, 1994a) reexamined data from the Boston Prospective Lead Study and found what appears to be a linear relationship, with little evidence that expressing blood lead logarithmically provides a better fit to the data. Investigators risk misspecifying the relationship by basing their modeling on the distribution of blood lead in their sample—that is, choosing a logarithmic transformation for blood lead because it produces a normal distribution. For the blood pressure studies, a logarithmic transformation seems not to have been a bad choice. For studies of cognitive effects, however, this choice seems more problematic.

Issues in modeling confounders

LEAD AND DEVELOPMENT

Concern that lead at subclinical doses may affect children's intellectual function has provided much of the impetus for the tremendous effort

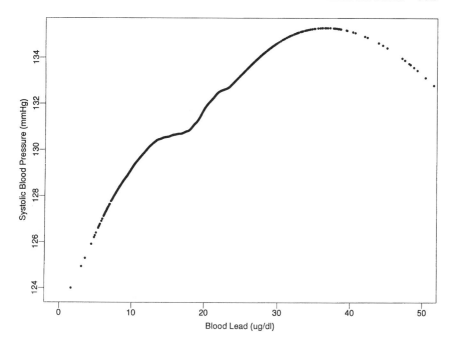

Figure 14-1. A smoothed plot of adjusted systolic blood pressure (after control, by regression, for age, age squared, body mass index, and race) versus the adjusted blood lead level in adult males in the Second National Health and Nutrition Examination Survey (NHANES II).

mounted to characterize the neurotoxicity of lead. Because trials involving random assignment of children to exposure groups are not feasible, investigators are limited to observational studies that capitalize on variability in the amount of lead to which children are exposed. Because of this, as well as of the fact that many factors influence intellectual function, much of the controversy in this literature focuses on how potential confounders are measured and controlled. On a population basis, higher blood lead levels tend to be more prevalent among children whose development is imperiled for many reasons other than lead exposure (e.g., poverty). As usually framed, the issue is: How much of the developmental morbidity in a more highly exposed cohort is attributable solely to elevated lead exposure and how much to competing risk factors? Incorrect inferences may take the form of a type I error (i.e., erroneously attributing to lead developmental variance that actually reflects residual confounding by poor medical care, poor nutrition, etc.) or a type II error (i.e., erroneously concluding that lead exposure is not associated with development because a weak lead "signal" cannot be measured with sufficient precision to achieve statistical significance because of the variability in outcome produced by other risk factors whose occurrence is correlated with higher lead exposure).

Two approaches have traditionally been taken to the problem of confounding in observational lead studies. Most frequently, investigators have attempted to distinguish the developmental variance attributable to lead from the variance attributable to the correlated risk factors by estimating lead's coefficient after adjusting statistically for them. Because inclusion of additional factors in the regression model often produces incremental reductions in the magnitude of the lead coefficient, the possibility that the coefficient would be reduced to zero by adjustment for unmeasured confounders cannot be rejected (Pocock et al., 1994). In addition, heterogeneity in terms of potentially confounding characteristics can decrease power by increasing the standard error of the lead coefficient.

Alternatively, some investigators have attempted to dissociate the contributions of lead exposure and correlated risk factors by their choice of sampling frame. Just as the impact of air pollution on lung function might best be evaluated in a cohort from which smokers are excluded (e.g., Mills et al., 1991), a subtle exposure-related perturbation of performance may be most easily measured in a cohort of children who, apart from lead exposure, are at generally low risk of developmental problems. For instance, in an effort to dissociate elevated lead exposure and other developmental risk factors, one cohort was recruited from a delivery hospital serving a largely middle and upper-middle class population (Bellinger et al., 1989b). Because many of these factors were not correlated with blood lead level in this cohort, they did not confound the association between lead and development as they could have if a higher lead level had been a marker of generally increased risk (Bellinger et al., 1989b). In general, sample restriction to reduce collinearity between lead and other risk factors is preferable to statistical adjustment for such confounders. The efficiency of adjustment depends on the degree of collinearity between the exposure index and potential confounders. In simulation analyses, given a certain "true" correlation between lead and development, the magnitude of the correlation "adjusted" for social class differs depending on the size of the correlation between lead and social class (Bellinger et al., 1989a).

Issues of model specification remain contentious. Adjustment for certain variables, such as social class and maternal IQ, is *de rigueur* in lead studies, yet an argument can be made that including them in a regression model leads to greater bias than does excluding them. In many studies, for instance, the outcome is adjusted for social class before the association between lead and the outcome is estimated because, in many cohorts, lower social class is associated both with higher blood lead level and with poorer development. Thus, the investigator assumes a priori that adjustment is appropriate. This practice requires the assumption that any outcome variance that is shared by social class and blood lead level "belongs," in truth, to social class and should be excluded from the portion of outcome variance considered in estimating lead's contribution. It is plausible, however, to hypothesize that some of the association between social class and development is attributable to the fact that children in the lower classes tend to be exposed to more lead. Moreover, social class may convey information about a child's lead burden that is not conveyed by a marker of short-term exposure such as blood lead. Thus, two components of the association between social class and development can be distinguished, one that is dependent on lead and one that is independent of lead. Simply including social class in a regression model blurs this distinction by ignoring the former component and attributing all the social class–related variation in outcome to the latter component (Bellinger et al., 1989a).

The role of maternal IQ in this nexus of variables is also complex. Maternal IQ tends to be one of the strongest predictors of child IQ. The need to adjust for it seems straightforward, yet it is important to acknowledge the possibility that a woman's past or current lead exposure, which is usually not measured in studies of postnatal lead exposure and child development, has affected her own IQ as well as her ability to provide her child with an optimal rearing environment. Under this scenario, controlling for maternal IQ may bias the estimate of the contribution of lead to her child's development. The validity of adjusting for measures of rearing environment quality can be questioned on the grounds that parental and offspring interaction is a complex system in which components are conditioned by one another. In animal models, lead-induced behavioral perturbations in offspring elicit different patterns of nurturing behaviors from parents (Zenick et al., 1979; Barrett and Livesey, 1983) which, in turn, may affect the subsequent development of offspring. These examples are presented in extreme form to illustrate the point that the issue of which variables to adjust for in studies of lead and development is far from straightforward. They should not be interpreted as a call to abandon efforts to control for non-lead factors statistically, but as indicating a need for thoughtful consideration of the assumptions that underlie regression-based assessment of the relationship between lead and development.

Statistical techniques that address some of these issues have been applied for three decades in the social sciences, although they are rarely used in epidemiology. Often we can hypothesize a complex pathway from exposure to health end point. Some variables may be outcomes in themselves and, at the same time, intermediate steps in the relationship be-

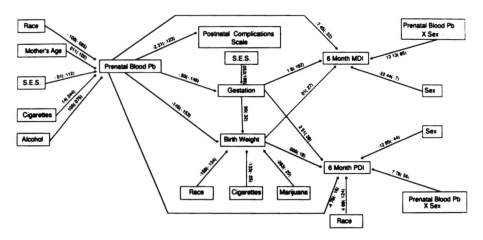

Figure 14-2. A structural equation model of Mental Development Index (MDI) and Psychomotor Development Index (PDI) scores at 6 months of age for infants in the Cincinnati Prospective Lead Study (Buncher et al., 1991). The number on a path represents a regression coefficient (standard error). "S.E.S." is socioeconomic status.

tween exposure and another outcome. Under some circumstances, then, adjustment for them may be inappropriate (Weinberg, 1992). For example, prenatal lead exposure has been associated with reduced birth weight and gestational age in some studies. Gestational age can be treated as an outcome, or as an intermediate step between prenatal lead exposure and lower birthweight. However, prenatal lead exposure may also affect birthweight by mechanisms that are unrelated to gestational age. We might draw diagrams showing these potential pathways, as indicated in Figure 14-2 (from Buncher et al., 1991). The goal is to evaluate the significance of each of these pathways. Prenatal lead exposure has also been associated with Mental Development Index (MDI) scores on the Bayley Scales. Is this merely a consequence of the lower birthweight of more highly exposed children, or are other pathways involved? Again, a path diagram can be constructed. The paths on Figure 14-2 can be described by a collection of regression models. These include models in which birthweight and gestational age are end points, as well as models in which they are also considered independent variables. A technique called structural equation modeling was developed to permit the simultaneous estimation of all of the bivariate regression equations. This approach enables one to prune back paths that make no significant contribution, and hence to form hypotheses about potential mechanisms as well as to identify associations.

One issue that has been the topic of spirited debate is whether birth-weight should be controlled for in the regression of MDI (possibly biasing downward the lead coefficient) or should not be controlled (possibly biasing the lead coefficient upward). Structural equation models avoid this bind because the estimated effect of lead is the sum of its effects via all of its pathways, yielding an unbiased estimate. As in all epidemiology, replication and confirmation are needed before one can have confidence in the inferences drawn from such analyses. However, these models allow us to ask questions that are otherwise difficult to ask.

Another aspect of modeling that warrants comment is the distinction between confounding and effect modification. Confounding refers to the distortion of the true relationship between an exposure and a disease by a third factor. This can be addressed by statistical adjustment. Effect modification refers to differences in the true exposure–disease relationship depending on the level of a third factor. In studies of the relationship between lead and development, confounding tends to receive greater consideration than does effect modification. Although it is known that a chemical's toxicity depends on exposure parameters, intrinsic host characteristics, and environmental factors (Doull, 1980), little credence is given to the possibility that there is not a single "best" estimate of the dose-response relationship between lead and development that each study should arrive at if all confounders are measured and appropriately adjusted for. In other words, differences between studies in cohort characteristics, in patterns of exposure (e.g., timing, duration), and in other key aspects of the developmental environment may contribute to interstudy differences in the effect estimates derived. That the magnitude of the effect estimate is contingent on such factors is implicit in the finding, reported in several studies, of a significant statistical interaction between lead and social class. This implies that two cohorts differing substantially in social class distribution may yield different effect estimates, even if within each study adjustment is made for social class. This has been termed "cross-study effect modification" (Bellinger, 1995). In a meta-analysis, Schwartz (1994a) evaluated possible effect modification by several factors, but the power of these analyses was limited by the small number of studies available.

LEAD AND BLOOD PRESSURE

Many of the issues raised in the discussion of potential confounders of the lead–development relationship apply to the lead–blood pressure relationship as well. Some variables that have been treated as potential confounders in most studies may also be viewed as either sources of lead exposure, modifiers of the effect of lead, or as pathways for the effect of lead. These issues will be dealt with specifically regarding a number of the key confounders, but some general points may be useful here. One is that the selection of a sample can be critical in resolving these issues. Restriction to narrow age ranges or to individuals who never smoked are effective tools for dealing with potential confounding. If alcohol is both an important source of lead exposure and a potential independent predictor of blood pressure, it may be possible to choose a sample in which the independent effects of both exposures are more readily seen. For example, choosing a sample with a narrow range of alcohol consumption and/or a large variability in lead exposure due to other sources will minimize the difficulty.

The following section discusses two variables that may confound the association between lead and blood pressure.

AGE

In Western countries, both blood pressure and blood lead increase with age, creating the potential for confounding. Several approaches can be used to disentangle the effects of age and lead on blood pressure. Restriction is one option, i.e., restricting the sample to individuals within a narrow age range, or to an age range in which the correlation between age and blood lead is small. In the NHANES II survey, the correlation between blood lead and age was an order of magnitude lower in the 40–54 year age group than in the 20–40 year age group. By focusing on the former group, Pirkle et al. (1985) eliminated confounding of the lead and blood pressure relationship by age. They found a higher regression coefficient in that restricted age group than Schwartz (1988) found in the entire sample. This suggests that overadjustment for age may be an issue. However, Hertz-Picciotto and Croft (1993) pointed out that effect modification is an alternative explanation. Lead may have a different effect in different age groups.

Some data in the NHANES II support this view. We split participants into three age groups: 20–44, 45–59, and 60+ years. In regressions controlling for age, age squared, body mass index, and race, the association between systolic blood pressure and the logarithm of blood lead systematically increased across the age groups ($\beta=3.25$ t=2.78; $\beta=4.36$ t=2.00; and $\beta=5.62$ t=2.85 respectively). Nonparametric smoothing revealed some interesting additional aspects. Figure 14-3 shows smoothed plots of the residual of systolic blood pressure versus the residual of blood lead (after controlling for age, race, and body mass index) in the three age groups. Below a residual log blood lead of about 0.4 (corresponding to a blood lead level of 28 μg/dL) the curves for the three age groups have

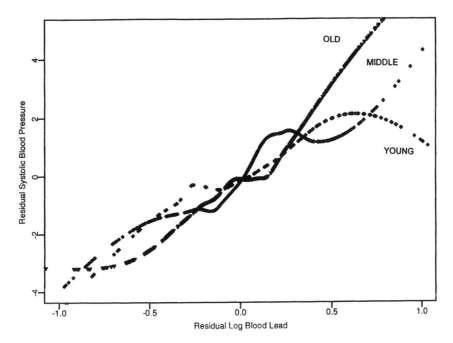

Figure 14-3. Smoothed plots of the residual systolic blood pressure (after control, via regression, for age, age squared, body mass index, and race) in adult males in NHANES II in three age strata: young (20–44 years), middle (45–59 years), and old (60–74 years).

the same slope and appear roughly linear on the log scale. The curves differ above that level, however. Assuming that random error is not responsible for these differences, the data suggest that for younger subjects blood pressure flattens out and actually turns down with increasing blood lead. For middle-aged males, the slope is similar to the slope at lower blood lead levels. For older subjects, the slope actually increases. Whatever accounts for these differences is relevant only at blood lead levels rarely seen today without either some unusual exposure (e.g., occupation) or very heavy drinking. This modification of the interaction with level would be difficult to detect without the use of smoothing Figure 14-4 shows the smoothed plots of residual blood pressure versus residual log blood lead in the three age groups before and after control for age. Controlling for age has little effect. For younger subjects the curves are on top of each other, and for the other two age groups the small shifts are not even consistent as to whether the effect of lead is larger or smaller before control for age. These two figures suggest that age is not a confounder if age

YOUNG

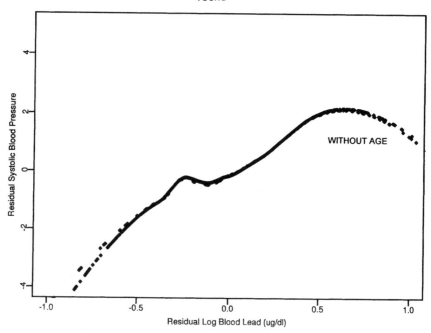

WITHOUT AGE

MIDDLE

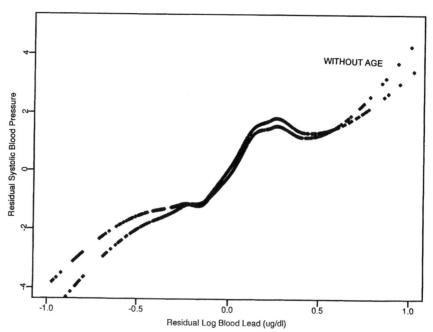

WITHOUT AGE

OLD

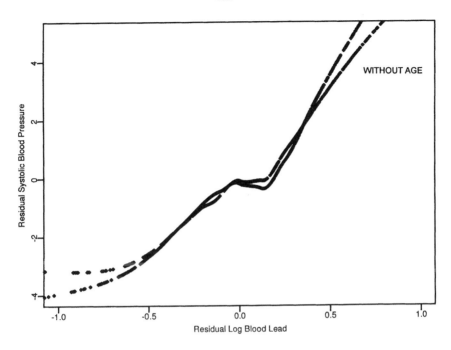

Figure 14-4. (a,b,c) The same smoothed plots as Fig. 14-3 for each age category, with the smoothed plot without adjustment for age superimposed. After stratification, control for age has little impact on the association.

intervals are sufficiently narrow, but that the relationship between lead exposure and blood pressure does differ across age groups. In other words, age is an effect modifier of this relationship.

ALCOHOL

The treatment of alcohol also poses challenges. Alcoholic beverages may contain substantial amounts of lead, particularly in Europe. In addition, alcohol may increase gut absorption of lead from other sources. Either way, alcohol is associated with internal lead dose. A high level of alcohol may also be a risk factor for elevated blood pressure, although the evidence is weaker for more moderate alcohol levels. As with age, control for alcohol may understate the association between lead and blood pressure, but ignoring alcohol may overstate it. One approach is to find a sample where, first, alcohol is a minor source of lead exposure and, second, where lead levels vary widely due to other sources, reducing the collinearity. The NHANES II study has several advantages in this regard.

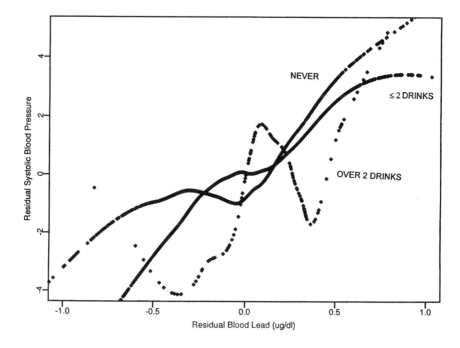

Figure 14-5. The smooth plots of residual systolic blood pressure (after control, via regression, for age, age squared, body mass index, and race) versus residual blood lead for three categories of alcohol consumption: never drinker, less than two drinks per day, and greater than two drinks per day. The relationship is much noisier in the heavy drinkers.

First, the lead content of U.S. wine and beer is considerably lower than was the case at the time in Europe. Second, in contrast to Europe, there was substantial variation over this period in U.S. blood lead levels due to changes in the amount of lead added to gasoline. Finally, per capita alcohol consumption is lower in the United States than in Europe.

The best approach to reducing confounding by alcohol is also restriction. In the NHANES II sample, the number of "never" drinkers and the variation in lead exposure from sources other than alcohol were sufficient to make this feasible. If the regression between systolic blood pressure is restricted to never drinkers, the overall association does not change much ($\beta = 3.76$, $t = 2.01$) although power is obviously reduced. Excluding only "heavy" drinkers (more than two drinks per day) also had little impact (gb = 4.25, $t = 4.22$). However, smoothed partial regression plots of the relationship between systolic blood pressure and blood lead stratified by alcohol consumption reveal an interesting feature (Fig. 14-5). While the associations are similar in never drinkers and light drinkers, the association in heavy drinkers is much noisier, although it does show a general upward trend. Hence, we would expect noisier relationships in samples with heavier drinking. Whether this reflects effect modification, increased noise due to the less healthy state of the subjects, or something else warrants further investigation.

Conclusion

The abundance of research on lead over the past two decades has yielded a wealth of knowledge about exposure pathways, health effects, and mechanisms of toxicity. It has provided the empirical basis for dramatic shifts both in the way the lead problem is perceived in the lay, medical, and public health communities and in the vigor of regulatory activity. As the recent NHANES III survey suggests, the combined effect of these trends has been a sharp reduction in population exposures and, one presumes, in many types of lead-associated morbidity.

At the same time, lead research provides clear illustrations of many of the methodological challenges that attend observational research on topics in environmental epidemiology, including exposure assessment, confounding and model specification for biological phenomena that are multi-determined, and characterization of dose-response and dose-effect relationships. The fact that many of these issues remain contentious despite the tremendous investment of research resources in lead epidemiology and toxicology confirms the conceptual and practical difficulties of addressing them.

References

Agency for Toxic Substances and Disease Registry. 1988, The Nature and Extent of Lead Poisoning in Children in the United States: A report to Congress. U.S. Department of Health and Human Service, Atlanta.

Andrews K, Savitz D, Hertz-Picciotto I. 1994. Prenatal lead exposure in relation to gestational age and birth weight: a review of epidemiologic studies. Am J Ind Med 26: 13–32.

Annest J, Pirkle J, Makuc D, et al. 1983. Chronological trend in blood lead levels between 1976 and 1980. N Engl J Med 308: 1373–1377.

Apostoli P, Maranelli G, Micciolo R. 1992. Is hypertension a confounding factor in the assessment of blood lead reference values? Sci Total Environ 120: 127–134.

Aufderheide A, Wittmers L. 1992. Selected aspects of the spatial distribution of lead in bone. Neurotoxicol 13: 809–820.

Baghurst P, Robertson E, Oldfield R, et al. 1991. Lead in the placenta, membranes, and umbilical cord in relation to pregnancy outcome in a lead-smelter community. Environ Health Perspect 90: 315–320.

Baghurst P, McMichael A, Wigg N, et al. 1992. Environmental exposure to lead and children's intelligence at the age of seven years. The Port Pirie cohort study. N Engl J Med 327: 1279–1284.

Barrett J, Livesey P. 1983. Lead induced alterations in maternal behavior and offspring development in the rat, Neurobehav Toxicol Teratol 1:65–71.

Bellinger D. 1995. Interpreting the literature on lead and child development: the neglected role of the experimental system. Neurotoxicol Teratol 17: 201–212.

Bellinger D, Needleman H. 1985. Prenatal and early postnatal exposure to lead: developmental effects, correlates, and implications. Int J Mental Health 14: 78–111.

Bellinger D, Leviton A, Waternaux C, et al. 1987. Longitudinal analyses of prenatal and postnatal lead exposure and early cognitive development. N Engl J Med 316: 1037–1043.

Bellinger D, Leviton A, Waternaux C. 1989a. Lead, IQ, and social class. Int J Epidemiol 18: 180–185.

Bellinger D, Leviton A, Waternaux C, et al. 1989b. Low-level lead exposure and early development in socioeconomically advantaged urban infants. In: Smith M, Grant L, Sors A, eds. Lead Exposure and Child Development: An International Assessment. Kluwer Academic Publishers, Boston. 345–356.

Bellinger D, Stiles K, Needleman H. 1992. Low-level lead exposure, intelligence and academic achievement: a long-term follow-up study. Pediatrics 90: 855–861.

Bellinger D, Leviton A, Rabinowitz M, et al. 1991a. Weight gain and maturity in fetuses exposed to low levels of lead. Environ Res 54: 151–158.

Bellinger D, Sloman J, Leviton A, et al. 1991b. Low-level lead exposure and children's cognitive function in the preschool years. Pediatrics 87: 219–227.

Bornschein R, Grote J, Mitchell T, et al. 1989. Effects of prenatal lead exposure on infant size at birth. In: Smith M, Grant L, Sors A, eds. Lead Exposure and Child Development: An International Assessment Kluwer Academic Publishers, Boston: 307–319.

Bogden J, Gertner S, Kemp F, et al. 1991. Dietary lead and calcium: effects on blood pressure and renal neoplasia in Wistar rats. J Nutr 121: 718–728.

Boscolo P, Carmignani M. 1988. Neurohumoral blood pressure regulation in lead exposure, Environ Health Perspect 78: 101–106.

Brody D, Pirkle J, Kramer R, et al. 1994. Blood lead levels in the US population. Phase 1 of the Third National Health and Nutrition Examination Survey (NHANES III, 1988 to 1991). JAMA 272: 277–283.

Buncher R, Succop P, Dietrich K. 1991. Structural equation modeling in environmental risk assessment. Environ Health Perspect 90: 209–213.

Cantarow A, Trumper M. 1944. Lead Poisoning. Williams & Wilkins, Baltimore.

Carmignani M, Boscolo P, Ripanti G, Finalli V. 1983. Effects of chronic exposure to lead and/or cadmium on some neurohumoral mechanisms regulating cardiovascular function in the rat. In: Proceedings of the Fourth International Conference on Heavy Metals in the Environment. CEP Consultants, Edinburgh. 557–560.

Centers for Disease Control. 1991. Preventing Lead Poisoning in Young Children. A Statement by the Centers for Disease Control. U.S. Department of Health and Human Services, Atlanta.

Chai S, Webb R. 1988. Effects of lead on vascular reactivity. Environ Health Perspect 78: 85–89.

Clark C, Bornschein R, Succop P, et al. 1985. Condition and type of housing as an indicator of potential environmental lead exposure and pediatric blood lead levels. Environ Res 38: 46–53.

Cory-Slechta D. 1990. Exposure duration modifies the effects of low level lead on fixed-interval performance. Neurotoxicology 11: 427–442.

deKort W, Zwennis W. 1988. Blood lead and blood pressure: some implications for the situation in the Netherlands. Environ Health Perspect 78:67–70.

DerSimonian R, Laird N. 1986. Meta-analysis in clinical trials. Control Clin Trials 7: 177.

Dietrich K, Krafft K, Bornschein R, et al. 1987. Low-level fetal lead exposure effect on neurobehavioral development in early infancy. Pediatrics 80: 721–730.

Dietrich K, Succop P, Berger O, et al. 1991. Lead exposure and the cognitive development of urban preschool children: the Cincinnati Lead Study cohort at age 4 years. Neurotoxicol Teratol 13: 203–211.

Dietrich K, Berger O, Succop P, et al. 1993. The developmental consequences of low to moderate prenatal and postnatal lead exposure: intellectual attainment in the Cincinnati Lead Study cohort following school entry, Neurotoxicol Teratol 15: 37–44.

Doull J. 1980 Factors influencing toxicology, in Casarett and Doull's Toxicology: The Basic Science of Poisons, 2nd. ed., Doull J, Klaassen K, Amdur M (eds), Macmillan Publishing Co., Inc, New York, 70–83.

Egeland G, Burkhart G, Schnorr T, et al. 1992. Effects of exposure to carbon disulfide on low density lipoprotein cholesterol concentration and diastolic blood pressure. Br J Ind Med 49: 287–293.

Elwood P, Davey-Smith G, Oldham P, Toothill C. 1988. Two Welsh surveys of blood lead and blood pressure. Environ Health Perspect 78: 119–121.

Environmental Protection Agency. 1986. Air Quality Criteria for Lead, vol. III. EPA-600/08–83/028aF-Df. Research Triangle Park, NC.

Ernhart C, Wolf A, Kennard M, et al. 1986. Intrauterine exposure to low levels of lead: the status of the neonate. Arch Environ Health 41: 287–291.

Evis M, Dhaliwal K, Kane K, Moore M, Parratt J. 1987. The effects of chronic lead treatment and hypertension on the severity of cardiac arrhythmias inducted by coronary artery occlusion or by noradrenalin in anesthetised rats. Arch Toxicol 59: 336–340.

Factor-Litvak P, Graziano J, Kline J, et al. 1991. A prospective study of birthweight and length of gestation in a population surrounding a lead smelter in Kosovo, Yugoslavia. Int J Epidemiol 20: 722–728.

Fergusson D, Horwood L, Lynskey M. 1993. Early dentine lead levels and subsequent cognitive and behavioural development. J Child Psychol Psychiatry 34: 215–227.

Flegal A, Smith D. 1992a. Current needs for increased accuracy and precision in measurements of low levels of lead in blood. Environ Res 58: 125–133.

Flegal A, Smith D. 1992b. Lead levels in preindustrial humans. N Engl J Med 326: 1292–1294.

Fouts P, Page I. 1942. The effect of chronic lead poisoning on arterial blood pressure in dogs. Am Heart J 24: 329–331.

Goldman R, White R, Kales S, et al. 1994. Lead poisoning from mobilization of bone stores during thyrotoxicosis. Am J Ind Med 25: 417–424.

Goyer R. 1990. Transplacental transport of lead. Environ Health Perspect 89: 101–105.

Grandjean P, Lyngbye T, Hansen O. 1986. Lead concentration in deciduous teeth: variation related to tooth type and analytical technique. J Toxicol Environ Health 19: 437–445.

Grandjean P, Hollnagel H, Hedegaard L, Christensen J, Larsen S. 1989. Blood lead-blood pressure relations: alcohol intake and hemoglobin as confounders. Am J Epidemiol 129: 732–739.

Graziano J, Popovac D, Factor-Litvak P, et al. 1990. Determinants of elevated blood lead during pregnancy in a population surrounding a lead smelter in Kosovo, Yugoslavia. Environ Health Perspect 89: 95–100.

Greene T, Ernhart C. 1993. Dentine lead and intelligence prior to school entry: a statistical sensitivity analysis. J Clin Epidemiol 46: 323–339.

Gulson B, Wilson D. 1994. History of lead exposure in children revealed from isotopic analyses of teeth. Arch Environ Health 49: 279–283.

Hansen O, Trillingsgaard A, Beese I, et al. 1989. A neuropsychological study of children with elevated dentine lead level: assessment of the effect of lead in different socio-economic groups. Neurotoxicol Teratol 11: 205–213.

Hastie T, Tibshirani R. 1990. Generalized Additive Models. Chapman and Hall, London.

Heard M, Chamberlain A. 1982. Effect of minerals and food on uptake of lead from the gastrointestinal tract of humans. Hum Toxicol 1: 411–415.

Hense H, Filipiak B, Keil U. 1993. The association of blood lead and blood pressure in population surveys. Epidemiology 4: 173–179.

Hertz-Picciotto I, Croft J. 1993. Review of the relation between blood lead and blood pressure. Epidemiol Rev 15: 352–373.

Hertz-Picciotto I, Neutra R. 1994. Resolving discrepancies among studies: the influence of dose on effect size, Epidemiology 5: 156–163.

Hill A. 1965. The environment and disease: association or causation? Proc R Soc Med 58: 295–300.

Hu H. 1991. A 50 year follow-up of childhood plumbism: hypertension, renal function, and hemoglobin levels among survivors. Am J Dis Child 145: 681–687.

Hu H, Watanabe H, Payton M, et al. 1994. The relationship between bone lead and hemoglobin. JAMA 272: 1512–1517.

Iannaccone A, Carmignani M, Boscolo P. 1981. Reattivita cardiovascolare nel ratto dopocronica esposizione a cadmio o piombo [Cardiovascular reactivity in the rat following chronic exposure to cadmium and lead]. Ann Ist Super Sanita 17: 655–660.

Inskip M, Franklin C, Subramanian K, et al. 1992. Sampling of cortical and trabecular bone for lead analysis: method development in a study of lead mobilization during pregnancy, Neurotoxicology 13: 825–834.

Khera A, Wibberley D, Edwards K, Waldron H. 1980. Cadmium and lead levels in blood and urine in a series of cardiovascular and normotensive patients. Int J Environ Studies 14: 309–312.

Kirkby H, Gyntelberg F. 1985. Blood pressure and other cardiovascular risk factors of long term exposure to lead. Scand J Work Environ Health 11: 15–19.

Kopp S, Barron J, Tow J. 1988. Cardiovascular actions of lead and relationship to hypertension: a review. Environ Health Perspect 78: 91–99.

Kosnett M, Becker C, Osterloh J, et al. 1994. Factors influencing bone lead concentration in a suburban community assessed by noninvasive K X-ray fluorescence, JAMA 271: 197–203.

Kromhaut D. 1988. Blood lead and coronary heart disease risk among elderly men in Zutphen The Netherlands. Environ Health Perspect 78:43–46.

Lal B, Murthy R, Anand M, et al. 1991. Cardiotoxicity and hypertension in rats after oral lead exposure. Drug Chem Toxicol 14:305–318.

Mahaffey K, Annest J, Roberts J, et al. 1982. National estimates of blood lead levels: United States 1976–1980. N Engl J Med 307:573–579.

Manton W. 1985. Total contribution of airborne lead to blood lead, Br J Ind Med 42:168–172.

Markowitz M, Weinberger H. 1990. Immobilization-related lead toxicity in previously lead poisoned children. Pediatrics 86:455–457.

McMichael A, Vimpani G, Robertson E, et al. 1986. The Port Pirie cohort study: maternal blood lead and pregnancy outcome. J Epidemiol Community Health 40: 18–25.

McMichael A, Baghurst P, Vimpani G, et al. 1994. Tooth lead levels and IQ in school-age children: The Port Pirie Cohort Study. Am J Epidemiol 140:489–499.

Mills P, Abbey D, Beeson W, et al. 1991. Ambient air pollution and cancer in California Seventh-Day Adventists. Arch Environ Health 46:271–280.

Moller L, Kristensen T. 1992. Blood lead as a cardiovascular risk factor. Am J Epidemiol 136:1091–1100.

Moreau T, Orssaud G, Juget B, Busquet G. 1982. Blood lead levels and arterial pressure: initial results of a cross sectional study of 431 male subjects. Rev Epidemiol Sante Publique 30:395–397.

Moreau T, Hannaert G, Orssaud G, et al. 1988. Influence of membrane sodium transport upon the relation between blood lead and blood pressure in a general male population. Environ Health Perspect 78:47–52.

Morris C, McCarron D, Bennett W. 1990. Low-level lead exposure, blood pressure, and calcium metabolism. Am J Kidney Dis 15:568–574.

Morrissey R, Mottet N. 1980. Neural tube defects and brain anomalies: a review of selected teratogens and their possible modes of action. Neurotoxicology 2: 125–162.

Muldoon S, Cauley J, Kuller L, et al. 1994. Lifestyle and sociodemographic factors as determinants of blood lead levels in elderly women. Am J Epidemiol 139: 599–608. 1994

Multiple Risk Factor Intervention Trial Research Group. 1982. Multiple Risk Factor Intervention Trial: Risk factor changes and mortality results. JAMA 248: 1465–1477.

Nakhoul F, Kayne L, Brautbar N, Hu M, McDonough A, Eggena P. 1992. Rapid hypertensinogenic effect of lead: studies in the spontaneously hypertensive rat. Toxicol Ind Health 8:89–102. 1992

National Research Council. 1993. Measuring Lead Exposure in Infants, Children, and Other Sensitive Populations. National Academy Press, Washington, D.C.

Needleman H, Gatsonis C. 1990. Low-level lead exposure and the IQ of children. JAMA 263: 673–678.

Needleman H, Rabinowitz M, Leviton A, et al. 1984. The relationship between prenatal exposure to lead and congenital anomalies, JAMA 251:2956–2959.

Needleman H, Gunnoe C, Leviton A, et al. 1979. Deficits in psychologic and classroom performance of children with elevated dentine lead levels. N Engl J Med 300: 689–695. 1979

Neri L, Hewitt D, Orser B. 1988. Blood lead and blood pressure: analysis of crosssectional and longitudinal data from Canada. Environ Health Perspect 78: 123–126.

Nriagu J, Pacyna J. 1988. Quantitative assessment of worldwide contamination of air, water and soils by trace metals. Nature 333:134–139.

Occupational Safety and Health Administration. 1978. Occupational exposure to lead: final standard Fed Reg 43:52952–52960.

Orssaud G, Claude J, Moreau T, Tellouch J, Juget B, Festy B. 1985. Blood lead concentrations and blood pressure. BMJ 290:244.

Paterson L, Raab G, Hunter R, et al. 1988. Factors influencing lead concentrations in shed deciduous teeth. Sci Total Environ 74: 219–233.

Patterson C, Ericson J, Manea-Krichten M, et al. 1991. Natural skeletal levels of lead in *Homo sapiens* uncontaminated by technological lead. Sci Total Environ 107:205–236.

Perry H, Erlanger M. 1978 Pressor effects of chronically feeding cadmium and lead together. In: Hemphill D, ed. Trace Substances in Environmental Health—XII: Proceedings of the University of Missouri's 12th Annual Conference on Trace Substances in Environmental Health. University of Missouri, Columbia, MO: 268–275.

Piccinini F, Favalli L, Chiari M. 1977. Experimental investigations on the contraction induced by lead in arterial smooth muscle, Toxicology 8:43–51.

Pirkle J, Schwartz J, Landis J, Harlan W. 1985. The relationship between blood lead levels and blood pressure and its cardiovascular risk implications. Am J Epidemiol 121:246–258.

Pirkle J, Brody D, Gunter E, et al. 1994. The decline in blood lead levels in the United States. The National Health and Nutrition Examination Surveys (NHANES). JAMA 272:284–291.

Pocock S, Shaper A, Ashby D, Delves T, Whitehead T. 1984. Blood lead concentrations, blood pressure, and renal function, BMJ 289:872–874.

Pocock S, Shaper A, Ashby D, Delves T, Clayton B. 1988. The relationship between blood lead, blood pressure, stroke, and heart attacks in middle-aged British men. Environ Health Perspect 78:23–30.

Pocock S, Smith M, Baghurst P. 1994. Environmental lead and children's intelligence: review of the epidemiological evidence. BMJ 309:1189–1197.

Purchase N, Fergusson J. 1986. Lead in teeth: the influence of the tooth type and the sample within a tooth on lead levels. Sci Total Environ 52:239–250.

Rabinowitz M, Wetherill G, Kopple J. 1976. Kinetic analysis of lead metabolism in healthy humans. J Clin Invest 58:260–270.

Rabinowitz M, Leviton A, Bellinger D. 1985. Home refinishing, lead paint, and infant blood lead levels. Am J Public Health 75:403–404.

Rabinowitz M, Wang J, Soong W-T. 1991. Dentine lead and child intelligence in Taiwan, Arch Environ Health 1991 46:351–360.

Rabinowitz M, Leviton A, Bellinger D. 1993. Relationships between serial blood lead levels and exfoliated tooth dentin lead levels: models of tooth lead kinetics, Calcif Tissue Int 53:338–341.

Revis N, Zinsmeister A, Bull R. 1981. Atherosclerosis and hypertension induction by lead and cadmium ions: an effect prevented by calcium ion. Proc Natl Acad Sci USA 78:6494–6498.

Rosen J, Markowitz M, Bijur P, et al. 1991. Sequential measurement of bone lead content by L x-ray fluorescence in $CaNa_2EDTA$-treated lead-toxic children. Environ Health Perspect 93:271–277.

Rothenberg S, Schnaas L, Cansino-Ortiz S, et al. 1989. Neurobehavioral deficits after low level lead exposure in neonates: The Mexico City Pilot Study. Neurotoxicol Teratol 11:85–93.

Rothenberg S, Karchmer S, Schnaas L, et al. 1994. Changes in serial blood lead levels during pregnancy. Environ Health Perspect 102:876–880.

Schroeder H, Balassa J. 1965. Influence of chromium, cadmium, and lead on rat aortic lipids and circulation cholesterol. Am J Physiol 209:433–437.

Schwartz J. 1988. The relationship between blood lead and blood pressure in the NHANES II survey. Environ Health Perspect 78:15–22.

Schwartz J. 1991. Lead, blood pressure, and cardiovascular disease in men and women, Environ Health Perspect 91:71–75.

Schwartz J. 1993. Beyond LOEL's, p values, and vote counting: methods for looking at the strengths and shapes of associations. Neurotoxicology 14:237–246.

Schwartz J. 1994a. Low-level lead exposure and children's IQ: a metaanalysis and search for a threshold, Environ Res 66:42–55.

Schwartz J. 1994b. The use of generalized additive models in epidemiology. Invited paper presented at the XVII International Conference, International Biometric Society; 55–80.

Schwartz J. 1995. Lead, blood pressure, and cardiovascular disease in men. Arch Environ Health 50:31–37.

Schwartz J, Pitcher H, Levin R, Ostro B, Nichols A. 1985. Costs and benefits of reducing lead in gasoline: final regulatory impact analysis. (EPA Report no.: 230-05-85-006). U.S. Environmental Protection Agency, Washington, D.C.

Schwartz J, Pitcher H. 1990. The relationship between gasoline lead and blood lead in the United States, J Off Stat 5:421–431.

Schwartz J, Levin R. 1991. The risk of lead toxicity in homes with lead paint hazard. Environ Res 54:1–7.

Sharp D, Osterloh J, Becker C, et al. 1988. Blood pressure and blood lead concentration in bus drivers. Environ Health Perspect 78: 131–137.

Shurtleff D. 1974. Some characteristics related to the incidence of cardiovascular disease and death: Framingham study, 18 year follow up. Section 30, DHEW Publication No. 74–599. Department of Health, Education and Welfare.

Silbergeld E. 1991. Lead in bone: implications for toxicology during pregnancy and lactation, Environ Health Perspect 91: 63–70.

Silbergeld E, Schwartz J, Mahaffey K. 1988. Lead and osteoporosis: mobilization of lead from bone in postmenopausal women. Environ Res 47:79–94.

Skoczynka A, Juzwa W, Smolik R, Szechinski J, Behal F. 1986. Response of the cardiovascular system to catecholamines in rats given small doses of lead. Toxicology 39:275–289.

Smith M. Delves T, Lansdown R, et al. 1983. The effects of lead exposure on urban children: the Institute of Child Health/Southampton study, Dev Med Child Neurol 25: suppl 47.

Staessen J, Sartor F, Roels H, et al. 1991. The association between blood pressure, calcium, and other divalent cations: a population study. J Hum Hypertens 5:485–494.

Succop P, O'Flaherty E, Bornschein R, et al. 1987. A kinetic model for estimating change in the concentration of lead in the blood of young children. In: Lindberg S. Hutchinson T, eds. International Conference. Heavy Metal in the Environment, vol. 2, CEP Consultants, Edinburgh. 289–291.

Symanski E, Hertz-Picciotto I. 1994. Blood lead levels in relation to menopause (abstract 291). Am J Epidemiol 139:S74.

Thompson G, Robertson E, Fitzgerald S. 1985 Lead mobilization during pregnancy, Med J Aust 143:131.

Todd A, Chettle D. 1994. In vivo X-ray fluorescence of lead in bone: review and current issues. Environ Health Perspect 102:172–177.

Victery W, Tyroler H, Volpe R, Grant L, eds. 1988. Summary of discussion sessions:

Symposium on lead-blood pressure relationships. Environ Health Perspect 78:139–155.

Victery W, Vander A, Shulak J, et al. 1982. Lead, hypertension, and the renin-angiotensin system in rats. J Lab Clin Med 99:354–62.

Voors A, Johnson W, Shuman M. 1982. Additive statistical effects of cadmium and lead on heart-related disease in a North Carolina autopsy series. Arch Environ Health 37:98–102, 1982

Wasserman G, Graziano J, Factor-Litvak P, et al. 1994. Consequences of lead exposure and iron supplementation on childhood development at age 4 years, Neurotoxicol Teratol 16:233–240. 1994

Webb R, Winquist R, Victery W, Vander A. 1981. In vivo and in vitro effects of lead on vascular reactivity in rats. Am J Physiol 214:H211–H216.

Weinberg C. 1992. Toward a clearer definition of confounding. Am J Epidemiol 137:1–8.

Weiss S, Munoz A, Stein A, Sparrow D, Speizer F. 1986. The relationship of blood lead to blood pressure in a longitudinal study of working men. Am J Epidemiol 123:800–808.

Winder C. 1993. Lead, reproduction, and development. Neurotoxicology 14:303–318.

Winneke G, Kraemer U, Brockhaus A, et al. 1983. Neuropsychological studies in children with elevated tooth-lead concentrations. II. Extended studies, Int Arch Occup Environ Health 51:231–252.

Zenick H, Pecorraro F, Price D, et al. 1979. Maternal behavior during chronic lead exposure and measures of offspring development. Neurobehav Toxicol 1: 65–71.

Ziegler E, Edwards B, Jensen R, et al. 1978. Absorption and retention of lead by infants. Pediatr Res 12:29–34.

Future Trends in Environmental Epidemiology

15

KYLE STEENLAND

DAVID A. SAVITZ

ALL of the exposures discussed in this book will continue to be the subject of epidemiologic research in the future because they are very common and because their association with health effects in most cases has not been proven or disproven conclusively, at least not at the exposure levels currently encountered in developed countries. The degree to which these associations are accepted as causal and the dose-response relationship will help determine what intervention, if any, should take place to avoid or reduce exposure.

While none of the exposure-disease associations considered in this text is definitely established, the connection between lead and childhood development is probably the most widely accepted. Its acceptance by public health authorities and the American public has led to the elimination of leaded gasoline and leaded paint, which dramatically reduced blood lead levels over the past 30 years (but exposures to lead remain high in much of the underdeveloped world where leaded gasoline is common). Nonetheless, substantial research on lead is likely to continue. There is still debate on whether current low levels of lead contribute to developmental deficits in children, and hence on the exact nature of the dose-response relationship at low levels. The outcome of this debate will affect efforts at further lead abatement. Moreover, the effect of lead on adult blood pressure remains controversial, particularly at the relatively low current levels of exposure in the United States.

Perhaps the next most well-established association discussed in this book is that between environmental tobacco smoke and some childhood disease, and to a lesser extent, between ETS and lung cancer. While these associations remain somewhat unsettled among epidemiologists, they have been rather widely accepted by the general public and have led to intervention by public health authorities, primarily by way of reducing exposure to ETS in public settings such as restaurants and office buildings. Future interventions are contingent on continued studies seeking to solidify or weaken the evidence regarding ETS. The putative association between ETS and heart disease is perhaps the one with the most public health impact, and epidemiologic studies in this area, while substantial, remain the least developed.

The health effects of other exposures covered in earlier chapters are less well established and will continue to be the focus of much research. For some issues there is virtually no epidemiologic evidence at all, despite public concern. For example, the possible health effects of low levels of pesticide residues in food are as yet unproven; of particular concern are children who consume relatively high levels of these residues (National Research Council, 1993).

The health effects of air pollution are a field of study that has been pursued for years but is sure to grow in the future. The past decade has produced a large body of literature indicating that small particulate air pollution at current levels in urban air is correlated with a significant amount of daily morbidity and mortality from cardiorespiratory disease. Some new data also suggest chronic effects on lung cancer (Pope et al., 1995) and acute effects of carbon monoxide on congestive heart failure (Morris et al., 1995). The data on acute or chronic effects of ozone and NO_2 are not as consistent; perhaps the strongest evidence relates to the acute effects of ozone on susceptible populations (Romieu et al., 1995). Methodological challenges include the difficulty of separating the effects of correlated air pollutants from each other and the need for longitudinal designs to study the chronic effects of air pollutants.

Radon in homes is a common exposure but an association with lung cancer has not been established. Public health interventions to decrease exposures have been limited to date. The Environmental Protection Agency has recommended that steps be taken to reduce levels in homes where they are above 4 picocuries, but because the evidence is uncertain this recommendation has not had much impact to date. Detecting a lung cancer effect at the low levels of ambient exposure is difficult for the science of epidemiology, which may have insufficient resolution to confirm or refute such small effects. If a linear dose-response relationship is assumed for low-level exposure, it is clear that a reduction in current exposure would yield a substantial health benefit. Lubin et al. (1995) have conducted a pooled analysis of data from miners exposed to high doses of radon. Based on the dose-response observed for miners, these authors estimate that 10% of lung cancers in the United States may be attributable to low doses of radon in homes. However, the data from direct observational studies of radon in homes have wide confidence levels and are consistent with such a positive effect, but also with no effect. Progress in this area will require better methods of reconstructing exposure levels.

Electromagnetic fields is another area where more studies seem warranted, although the biological plausibility of a carcinogenic effect is questionable. Some studies suggest an association with cancer in children, but the epidemiologic evidence is not consistent. The ubiquitous exposure to EMF, however, drives the research. Again, exposure measurement issues are key; lacking a clear mechanism, the relevant measure of exposure is uncertain.

Water quality, including levels of chlorinated hydrocarbons or infectious agents, will clearly remain an important concern. Water treatment is necessary to prevent infection but introduces chlorinated hydrocarbons in the water that may cause cancer, with large potential public health implications. Again, retrospective exposure assessment is key to learning more about this possible association. Infectious agents in the water at low levels are common, but their possible contribution to endemic disease has been little studied (Payment et al., 1991). Disease outbreaks due to infectious agents continue to occur despite improvements in overall water quality, and new agents such as *Cryptosporidium* appear to be responsible. At a time when there is pressure to reduce public monies for water quality, such outbreaks are likely to continue.

A recurring theme in the above discussion has been the need to improve exposure assessment, a critical issue for all epidemiology but especially for the low-level, ubiquitous exposures considered in environmental epidemiology. The strategies for improvement have both statistical and biological components. As has been recognized for workplace exposures (Rappaport and Smith, 1991), there is a need to systematically evaluate levels of human exposure to environmental agents based on something more than sporadic or convenience samples. Targeted environmental sampling efforts are called for as a major aspect of epidemiologic studies, with clear quantitative goals regarding the accurate measurement of individual exposure, taking into account sources of variability and error.

Biological markers also have potential value as integrative markers of exposure across time (Rothman et al., 1995). This has long been appreciated for such indices as carboxyhemoglobin or blood lead levels that reflect short-term exposures. Indicators of long-term exposure are needed as well to help characterize exposure to such agents as radon, ozone, or magnetic fields, which are quite difficult to reconstruct in studies of chronic health effects. Major advances could occur if suitable biological indicators of long-term exposures became available.

Besides the topics covered in this book, whole new areas of environmental epidemiology are likely to develop in the future because of concerns about global environmental changes. The most obvious are the possible health effects of ozone depletion and of global warming. In both these areas recent data have confirmed suspected relationships between pollution produced by man and atmospheric or climate changes. The accelerated depletion of stratospheric ozone since the 1970s has been confirmed by direct measurement in the stratosphere and has been shown to be highly correlated with man-made halogenated hydrocarbons over the poles (Armstrong, 1994; UN Environmental Programme [UNEP], 1994). Ultraviolet (UV) radiation at ground level is not monitored systematically around the globe. The Antarctic is one region where there have been systematic measurements, and there empirical data show the expected correlation between ozone depletion and surface ultraviolet radiation (UVB) (Fig. 15.1) (UNEP, 1994). International agreements to reduce halocarbons may succeed but compliance is not assured. Assuming full compliance, and assuming a causal relationship between ozone depletion and UV radiation, estimates are that UVB levels will peak from

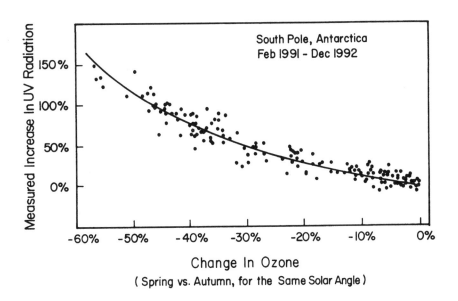

Figure 15-1. Increases in erythemal (sunburning) UV radiation due to ozone reductions (UNEP, 1994).

the year 2000 to 2010 at about 5% to 30% above 1970 levels. Models suggest little change thereafter until 2040, when levels should decline gradually back to baseline by 2080. Natural cloud cover protects against UV radiation; recent analysis have taken cloud cover into account (Lubin and Jensen, 1995). Most of the increased ground level UV radiation will occur in temperate climates above 30° latitude in both hemispheres.

Fluctuations of carbon dioxide (CO_2) and temperature over time can be measured via polar ice cores for a period of more than 200,000 years. Time-series analyses have indicated a high correlation between these two measures that would appear to be causal from theoretical consideration of the ability of CO_2 to trap reflected heat from the earth's surface. There has been a large increase in CO_2 levels over the past 100 years as the result of human activity, and CO_2 levels are expected to double over the next 100 years at present rates. The observed increase of 1° Fahrenheit over the past 100 years appeared to be somewhat less than what would be predicted by models, but recent adjustment of the models to take into account the cooling effect of man-made sulfate aerosols (which deflect incoming solar radiation) has led to conformity of observed warming trends with predicted ones (Charlson and Whigby, 1994). The most recent report of the Intergovernmental Panel on Climate Change (IPCC) indicates a consensus in the field that global warming due to CO_2 and other man-made pollutants is in fact occurring (IPCC, 1995). The best estimate of the IPCC is an increase of 3.5°F (range of estimate 1.5° to 6.0°) by year 2100 if no action is taken to reduce emissions of "greenhouse" gases. By way of reference, the average global temperature is 5 to 9°F warmer now than during the last ice age.

The health effects of these and other man-made trends in the global environment (e.g., soil depletion, decrease in biodiversity) are difficult to predict (see McMicheal, 1993, for an overview). The health effects of ozone depletion are the clearest; an increase in skin cancer, a likely increase in cataracts, and a possible damage to immmune function (Armstrong, 1994).

There is good evidence that UV radiation causes skin cancer; UVB specifically is clearly linked to non-melanoma skin cancer, but it is less clear what type of UV radiation is responsible for melanoma. Dose-response analyses suggest that a 1% increase in UV radiation will result in 0.7% to 0.8% increase in melanoma incidence, and a 1.5% to 2.0% increase in non-melanoma skin cancer, but these estimates are by no means certain. The United Nations Environment Programme (UNEP) has estimated that a 10% loss of ozone over three decades would lead to an additional 300,000 cases of non-melanoma skin cancer and 4500 additional cases of melanoma worldwide (UNEP, 1991). Large well-designed studies across geographical regions of differing UV exposure need to be conducted. Mutations specific to UV radiation in the skin may make it possible to determine much more accurately the dose-response relationship.

Cataracts currently cause visual loss for an estimated 17 million people worldwide, expected to increase to 40 million by 2025. There is a correlation between cataract prevalence and UV radiation geographically, and UVB is known to cause cataracts in animals. It seems likely that UVB causes cataracts, and there is some initial epidemiologic evidence from cross-sectional studies to this effect (see Taylor et al., 1988). Crude estimates suggest that a 1% increase in UVB radiation would be expected to increase the prevalence of cataracts by 1% to 3%. Further epidemiologic studies of the prevalence of specific types of cataracts in relation to UVB need to be conducted.

It is known that UVB can impair cell-mediated immunity in humans, locally and perhaps systemically. The potential effects of this on human health are unknown but conceivably greater than effects on cataracts and skin cancers.

Health effects due to global warming are much more difficult to assess because many are indirect. Direct effects include increased deaths from heat stroke during heat waves such as the one that affected Chicago in 1995. An increase in temperature will cause an increase in sea levels (20 inches by 2010) due to glacial melting and an increase in extreme weather patterns (perhaps already observable; see *NY Times*, May 23, 1995). Less obvious indirect effects on human disease will occur because of change in temperature. The IPCC has estimated that the percentage of the world population in malaria zones will increase from 45% to 60% by the year 2100 if present trends continue, leading to an increase of 50 to 80 million cases annually against a background of 500 million cases (IPCC, 1995). Regions affected by dengue fever will also expand.

The array of environmental health concerns a decade from now will undoubtably include many or perhaps even all of those of present concern. However, the current list is likely to expand in several ways. Human development has a tendency to introduce novel exposure circumstances and novel agents, with questions about the corresponding health effects. In addition, environmental agents that have been present for many years rise to public attention for almost mysterious reasons. Persistent chlorinated hydrocarbons have been present in water for many years, yet the resurgence of interest in their potential health effects is a rather recent phenomenon. Electromagnetic fields have been present since electricity came into use, yet until the early 1980s, health concerns with low-level exposure were absent. Even established hazards such as particulate air pollution have had several stages of interest with dormant periods in between. New technology can increase the level of established toxins; for example, electric vehicles should decrease ozone in urban air but may substantially increase the amount of lead in the air because of their lead batteries (Environmental Health Letter, 1995). Finally, technology can improve the ability to measure established toxins. For example, the ability to measure lead in the bone has opened up new ways to study this exposure with a biological marker that integrates exposure over time. It is impossible to predict the future, yet we can hope that this text has provided an overview of the methods used by environmental epidemiologists, and that these methods and others to be invented can serve us in meeting future challenges.

References

Armstrong B. 1994. Stratospheric ozone and health. Int J Epidemiol 23: 873–885.

Charlson R, Wigley T. 1994. Sulfate aerosol and climatic change. Sci Am 270: 48–57.

Environmental Health Letter. 1995. Lead emissions may increase with popularity of electric vehicles. Environmental Health Letter 34: 97.

IPCC (Intergovernmental Panel on Climate Change), draft of second assessment report, Working Group II, in press, 1995

Lubin J, Boice J, Edling C, et al. 1995. Lung cancer in radon-exposed miners and estimation of risk from indoor exposure. J Natl Cancer Inst 87: 817–827.

Lubin D, Jensen E. 1995. Effects of clouds and stratospheric ozone depletion on ultraviolet radiation trends. Nature 377: 710–713.

McMichael A. 1993. Global environmental change and human population health: a conceptual and scientific challenge to epidemiology, Int J Epidemiol 22: 1–8.

Morris R, Naumova E, Munasinghe R. 1995. Ambient air pollution and hospitalization for congestive heart failure among elderly people in seven large US cities. Am J Public Health 85: 1372–1377.

National Research Council. 1993. Pesticides in the Diets of Infants and Children. National Academy Press, Washington, DC.

Payment P, Richardson L, Siemiatycki J, et al. 1991. A randomized trial to evaluate the risk of gastrointestinal disease due to consumption of drinking water meeting current microbiological standards. Am J Public Health 81: 703–708.

Pope C, Thun M, Namboodiri M. 1995. Particulate air pollution as a predictor of mortality in a prospective study of US adults. Am J Respir Crit Care Med 151: 669–674.

Romieu I, Meneses F, Sierra-Monge J, et al. 1995. Effects of urban air polllutants on emergency visits for childhood asthma in Mexico City. Am J Epidemiol 141: 546–553.

Rappaport S, Smith T, eds. 1991. Exposure Assessment for Epidemiology and Hazard Control. Lewis, Chelsea, Michigan.

Rothman N, Stewart W, Shultte P. 1995. Incorporating biomarkers into cancer epidemiology: a matrix of biomarker and study design categories. Cancer Epidemiol Biomarkers 4: 301–311.

Taylor H, West S, Rosenthal F, et al. 1988. Effect of ultraviolet radiation on cataract formation. N Engl J Med 319: 1429–1433.

UN Environmental Programme (UNEP). 1994. Scientific Assessment of Ozone Depletion: Executive Summary. Nairobi.

Index

Additive risk model, 40
Aflatoxin and cancer, 78
Air pollution, 357
  acute episodes, 119, 127–128
  monitoring, 121, 126, 160–161
  particulates, *see* particulate air
    pollution
Albumin adducts and environmental
    tobacco smoke, 246–247
Alpha particles, 272
American Cancer Society,
    environmental tobacco smoke
    cohort studies, 230–231, 260–
    265
American Heart Association, 257
Aminobiphenyl, *see* hemoglobin
    adducts
Anti-oxidants, and cancer, 80–81
Armitage model, 38
Arsenic, 91
Asthma, pollution and, 149–150, 168,
    169–171, 184–185, 188–189
Attributable deaths, due to ETS,
    257

Beta-carotene and diet, 80–81
Bias
  in ecologic studies, 13
  towards the null, 23–25

Biological markers, 314, 352–353
  and environmental tobacco smoke,
    235, 245–248
Breast cancer and diet, 80

Cadmium in diet, 67–70
Cancer and diet, *see* diet
Carbon dioxide, 353–354
Carbon monoxide and environmental
    tobacco smoke, 209–214, 258
Carboxyhemoglin and environmental
    tobacco smoke, 209
Carcinogenesis, multi-stage model, 38
Carcinogenicity
  correlation between animal and
    human data, 31–32
  in animal studies, 33–34
Causal inference
  and meta-analysis, 47
  in human studies, 35
Causes of epidemics and endemics, 4
Childhood disease and environmental
    tobacco smoke, *see*
    environmental tobacco smoke
Children
  nitrogen dioxide and, 173–175
  particulate effects and, 154–155
Chlorination by-products, 93–100
  bladder cancer, 95–97

Chlorination by-products (*continued*)
  carcinogenicity, 94–97
  ecologic studies, 94
  exposure assessment, 97–100
  Iowa study, 95–97
  production, 93
Cigarette equivalents in measuring
    environmental tobacco smoke,
    246, 259
Clinical studies, 171, 187
Clusters
  boundaries, 18
  causes, 18
  confirmation, 17–18
  definition, 17
  false, 19
  occupational, 18–19
  surveillance for, 19–21
Colon cancer and diet, 80–81
Confounding
  air pollution studies, 132–138
  air pollution studies, weather, 133–136
  air pollution studies, other
    pollutants, 136–138
  in studies of environmental tobacco
    smoke, 240, 265
  lead, social class, 315, 330–335
  radon studies, smoking, 287–288
Controls, live versus dead, *see* surrogate
Cotinine and environmental tobacco
    smoke, 214–219, 227, 235, 245–
    246
Cryptosporidium, 106–110
  Milwaukee outbreak, 107–110
Cuban neuropathy and diet, 76–78

DDT, and cancer, 79
Diet
  cancer and, 78–81
  chemical contamination, 66–67
  endemics and, 78–81
  epidemics and, 67–78
  microbe contamination, 65
  natural toxins in food, 64
Dose-response
  in heart disease and environmental
    tobacco smoke studies, 264–265
  in risk assessment, *see* risk
    assessment

  lead and blood pressure, 325–330
Doses, species-equivalent, 37
Durkheim, and ecologic fallacy, 15

Ecologic fallacy, 13
Ecologic studies
  confounding, 12–14
  cross-level bias, 16
  definition, 11
  degree of bias 16
  inherent 17
  mixed design, 12
  model misspecification, 14
  nondifferential misclassification,
    16
  of water contamination, 94
  temporal sequence, 12
Electromagnetic fields
  adult cancer and, 298–299, 308
  childhood cancer and, 298–304
  exposure assessment, 300–302, 304–
    307, 308–309
  exposure metric, 296
  exposure sources, 296
  field frequency, 297–298
  historical changes, 304–305
  laboratory studies, 297
  measurements, 301–302
  neurobehavioral effects, 298–299,
    308, 309
  personal exposure, 307
  power lines, 299–304
  properties, 298
  reproductive health and, 298–299,
    308, 309
  Swedish study, 302–304
  wire code, 300–301, 305–307
Endemics, 4, 90, 103–104
Environmental Protection Agency
    (EPA) and environmental
    tobacco smoke, 228–230
Environmental tobacco smoke (ETS)
  child health and, 350
  childhood lung disease and, 201–
    202, 208
  childhood ear infection and, 202
  heart disease, plausibility, 259
  heart disease studies, overview, 257–
    258

heart disease, mechanisms, 258–259
heart disease, example, 260–265
lung cancer studies, overview, 228–234
measurement of, 208–218, 240–241, 245–248
methodologic issues in lung cancer studies, 236–245
prevalence of exposure in children, 201
sudden infant death and, 208
workplace studies of lung cancer and, 241–245
Eosinophilia-myalgia syndrome, 76
Epidemics, 3, 90, 105–106
Epidemiology
environmental, definitions, 3, 7
observational, 11
Equivalent, lifetime exposures, 44–45
Ergotism, 66
Estrogen-like chemicals and cancer, 79
Etiology, multifactorial, 5, 18
ETS heart disease studies, design of, 258
Experiments, natural, 5
Exposure
measurement error, Berkson model, 22–24
measurement error, classic model, 21–24
measurement error, violations of classic model, 23
misclassification, 21, 24–25
retrospective assessment, 5
Exposure assessment, methods, 98–100, 113–114, 172, 352
Extrapolation, high to low dose, 269–271

Fat and cancer, see diet and cancer
Fluoride, 91
Fruits and cancer, see diet and cancer

Gas stoves, 167, 172–173
Global warming, 353–355

Harvesting, 120, 141–143
Hazard identification in risk assessment, see risk assessment

HDL and evironmental tobacco smoke, 259
Heart disease, and environmental tobacco smoke, see environmental tobacco smoke
Hemoglobin adducts, of 4–amino–biphenyl, and environmental tobacco smoke, 246–247
Hill, Bradford, 219

Index of precision in risk assessment, 41
Indoor pollution, 168, 172–175, 273–274
Industrial processing, of food, 66
Infectious agents, waterborne, 100–112
exposure routes, 100
monitoring, 100
Itai-itai disease, 67–70

Laboratory studies, 186–187
Lead
biological markers, 314, 319–321
blood lead levels, 316
blood pressure, 324–325
bone, 318–319
confounding by age, 336–339
confounding by alcohol, 340–341
confounding by social class, 315, 330–335
development, 322–324, 350
fetal exposure, 321–322
history, 315–316
modeling confounders, 330–335
modeling dose-response, 325–330
neurological development, 323–324
sources, 317–318
standards, 318 Leukemia, clusters, 20
Linear model in ecologic studies, 14
Linear relative risk model, 39–40
Lung cancer and environmental tobacco smoke, see environmental tobacco smoke

Maximum, tolerated dose in animal carcinogenicity studies, 34
Measurement error, see exposure, measurement error

Meat and cancer, *see* diet and cancer
Meta-analysis
    definition, 46–47
    example, 50–55
    fixed-effect model, 48
    heterogeneity, 49, 56
    particulates, 129–130, 158–159
    publication bias, 48, 56
    random effect model, 49
    water contamination studies, 95
    weighting by precision, 48
Methylmercury, in diet, 70–71
Microbes, in food, *see* diet, microbe
        contamination
Microbial contaminants, *see* infectious
        agents, waterborne
Minimata disease, 71
Misclassification of smokers as never
        smokers, environmental tobacco
        smoke studies, 235, 265
Missing exposure data, 96
Mixtures, pollutant, 92
Model
    biologically-based, 38
    misspecification, *see* ecologic studies
    multi-stage linearized, for
        carcinogenesis, 38
    random effect, *see* meta-analysis
Multiple exposure sources, 296

Neuropathy and diet, *see* Cuban
        neuropathy
Newton, and methyl-mercury
        intoxication, 70
NHANESIII, and environmental
        tobacco smoke, 227
Nickel workers, risk assessment and, 40–
        45
Nicotine and environmental tobacco
        smoke, 214, 258
Nitrates, 92
Nitrogen dioxide
    asthmatics and, 169–171
    children, 173–175
    clinical versus epidemiologic studies,
        169–171
    ecologic studies, 176–178
    exposure measurement, 172
    indoor, 172–175

    infections, 171
    mechanisms, 169
    panel studies, 173–175
    short-term versus chronic effects,
        178
    sources of, 168
NNK and environmental tobacco
        smoke, 248

Ozone
    acute effects, 187–190
    acute versus chronic effects, 184,
        186, 195
    asthmatics, 184–185, 188–189
    chronic effects, 190–191
    clinical studies, 187
    depletion, 353
    infection, 190
    laboratory studies versus
        epidemiology, 186–187
    mortality, 191
    other pollutants and, 194–195
    pulmonary function, 187–188, 191–
        194
    sources, 185—186
    standards, 186
    summer camp study, 191–194
    sunlight, 185–186

PAH adducts and environmental
        tobacco smoke, 246–247
Particulate air pollution, 119–161
    asthma and, 149–150
    characteristics, 122–123
    clearance, 124–125
    confounding, 132–138
    deposition, 123–125
    epidemiologic evidence, 128–155
    exposure assessment, 125–127
    hospitalization and, 144–149
    lung function and, 154–155
    meta-analysis and, 129–130
    mortality and, 128–144
    particle size, 122–123
    respiratory symptoms and, 150–154
    temporal factors, 138–141
Platelet aggregation and
        environmental tobacco smoke,
        258

Polybrominated biphenyls (PBBs), 73
Polychlorinated biphenyls (PCBs), 71–73
Polychlorinated dibenzofuans (PCDFs), 72
Pooled-data, analysis, 47
Public concern, and EMF, 295

Questionnaires versus biomarkers in ETS exposure measurement, 208–209, 241

Radon
   animal studies, 276
   confounding by smoking, 287–288
   ecologic studies, 276–277
   exposure assessment, 269, 270, 285–288
   extrapolation from miners, 269, 270, 271, 283–285
   lung cancer, 274–282, 351
   lung cancer in ecologic studies and, 13, 16
   measurement instruments, 273, 288–289
   miner studies, 274–276
   Missouri study, 280–282
   properties, 271–272
   remediation guidelines, 273–274
   residential changes, 285–286
   residential studies, 276–282
   units, 272–273
Recall bias, in studies of lung cancer and environmental tobacco smoke, 234–235
Renal dysfunction and cadmium in diet, 67
Risk, excess, 44–45
Risk assessment
   animal-based, 31–34
   definition, 30
   dose–response, animal data, 36–38
   dose-response, human data, 38–45
   dose-response, relative risk model, 39–40
   example, 40–45
   hazard identification, 30, 33–35
   human-based, 32–34
   uncertainties, 45–46

Risk, quantification, 30, 43–45
Rothman, K. and clusters, 19

Sellafield, leukemia cluster, 19
Sharpshooter, boundaries in ecologic studies, 18
Silicosis and lung cancer, example of meta-analysis, 50–55
Small area, and clusters, 20
Small effects, 95, 119, 121, 129, 167, 289, 296–297, 314
Standardized mortality ratio (SMR) in dose response models, 39–43
Statistical methods, dose-response modeling, lead and blood pressure, 325–330
Surrogate respondents, in studies of lung cancer and environmental tobacco smoke, 236–240

Temporal course of exposure and disease, 113–114, 138–141, 299, 326–330
Thiocyanate and environmental tobacco smoke, 214
Threshold for carcinogenicity, 36
Time–series studies, 11, 120, 130–144
   methods, 131–136
Tobacco amblyopia, 77
Toxic oil syndrome, 73–76
Trihalomethanes, see chlorination by-products
Trytophan, 76

Ultraviolet radiation, 353–354
Unit risk estimate, 40

Water
   exposure routes, 89–90
   monitoring, 108–111
   treatment, 89
Weighting in meta-analysis, see meta-analysis
Workplace and ETS, see environmental tobacco smoke, workplace

Yu-cheng disease, 72–73
Yusho disease, 71–72